The International Library of Psychology

PSYCHOTHERAPY

Founded by C. K. Ogden

The International Library of Psychology

GENERAL PSYCHOLOGY
In 38 Volumes

I	The Neurosis of Man	*Burrow*
II	Creative Imagination	*Downey*
III	The Caveman Within Us	*Fielding*
IV	Men and their Motives	*Flugel*
V	The Mind in Sleep	*Fortune*
VI	The Mind and its Body	*Fox*
VII	Practical Psychology	*Fox*
VIII	Man for Himself	*Fromm*
IX	The Law Within	*Fuller*
X	The Nature of Laughter	*Gregory*
XI	Readings in General Psychology	*Halmos et al*
XII	The Psychologist at Work	*Harrower*
XIII	The Psychology of Philosophers	*Herzberg*
XIV	Emotion	*Hillman*
XV	The Foundations of Common Sense	*Isaacs*
XVI	The Psychology of Consciousness	*King*
XVII	The Sciences of Man in the Making	*Kirkpatrick*
XVIII	The Person in Psychology	*Lafitte*
XIX	Man's Unconscious Passion	*Lay*
XX	Psychological and Biological Foundations of Dream-Interpretation	*Lowy*
XXI	Nervous Disorders and Character	*Mckenzie*
XXII	An Historical Introduction to Modern Psychology	*Murphy*
XXIII	Modern Theories of the Unconscious	*Northridge*
XXIV	The A B C of Psychology	*Ogden*
XXV	The Psychology of Thought and Feeling	*Platt*
XXVI	Introductory Psychology	*Price-Williams*
XXVII	Empirical Foundations of Psychology	*Pronko et al*
XXVIII	Psychotherapy	*Schilder*
XXIX	The Psychology of Time	*Sturt*
XXX	The Origins of Love and Hate	*Suttie*
XXXI	Art and the Unconscious	*Thorburn*
XXXII	The Elements of Psychology	*Thorndike*
XXXIII	Telepathy and Clairvoyance	*Tischner*
XXXIV	Human Psychology as Seen Through the Dream	*Turner*
XXXV	The Psychology of Self-Conciousness	*Turner*
XXXVI	The Psychology of Economics	*Weisskopf*
XXXVII	The Measurement of Emotion	*Whately Smith*
XXXVIII	How to be Happy Though Human	*Wolfe*

PSYCHOTHERAPY

PAUL SCHILDER

ROUTLEDGE

First published in 1938 by
Routledge and Kegan Paul Ltd

Reprinted in 1999 by
Routledge

2 Park Square, Milton Park, Abingdon, Oxfordshire OX14 4RN
711 Third Avenue, New York, NY 10017

Transferred to Digital Printing 2006

First issued in paperback 2014
Routledge is an imprint of the Taylor and Francis Group, an informa company

British Library Cataloguing in Publication Data
A CIP catalogue record for this book
is available from the British Library

Psychotherapy
ISBN 978-0-415-21040-9 (hbk)
ISBN 978-0-415-75805-5 (pbk)
General Psychology: 38 Volumes
ISBN 978-0-415-21129-1
The International Library of Psychology: 204 Volumes
ISBN 978-0-415-19132-6

CONTENTS

PREFACE TO THE FIRST EDITION

THIS BOOK has developed from a conviction that psychotherapy is not an art but a technical procedure based upon scientific principles. It is a part of the science of psychology and psychopathology. It is the physician who treats the suffering of human beings, and man suffers only as a complete person. Every ailment has its psychological aspect. A human relationship must exist between the physician and his patient, and this should be understood by the physician. This relationship is at the basis of every treatment, even when it seems to pertain to the somatic sphere only. It has often been said that for a psychological approach to the patient the physician needs but two mysterious qualities: a personality and intuition. But these two qualities, without knowledge and training, would hardly suffice for surgery. Neither do they for psychotherapy.

There is much that must be learned about human attitudes and conflicts. Only a psychotherapeutic procedure which is based upon knowledge and serious efforts can be useful. Whatever intuition may be, it only comes to those who have prepared themselves by careful study, diligence and experience. The technique of psychotherapy is no less complicated than that of any other branch of medicine for which years of preparation are deemed necessary. A textbook can but indicate the proper direction and give general principles. It may point to problems and it may help people who are in active practice. You would not expect to become a surgeon by merely reading textbooks. This book is intended for the student, the physician and the psychiatrist in their approach to psychotherapy. A textbook such as this might prove interesting to the psychologist, educator, or sociologist, that he may know about the physician's approach to his patients, but not in order to do psychotherapy. Psychotherapy is the task of the physician, but the methods developed in psychotherapy yield important knowledge of human problems. These methods can be utilized in the entire field of applied psychology. But the psychologist, educator, and sociologist must create their own methods according to their specific problems.

In a book on anatomy most of the facts and data are not controversial. Although the author merely repeats what is generally acknowledged, he may have written a useful book. But if a textbook of psychotherapy were to repeat the opinions of authorities only, it would be useless. Many physicians, eminent as neurologists and psychiatrists, do not want to acknowledge psychological facts and refuse to recognize the problems in this field. They assume a right to pass judgment on problems which they do not understand and have not studied, because of their achievements in psychiatry and neurology prior to modern psychology. A psychotherapy concerned with vital problems reckons with their disapproval and gladly accepts it. Psychotherapy in this sense is a young science. It is obliged to be bold in its experimental approach, and therefore uses psychological facts irrespective of their general acceptance.

Modern psychotherapy has to utilize psychoanalysis. It should be done openly. Many physicians who use psychoanalytic principles and results with a more or less arbitrary selection carefully conceal this fact from others and from themselves. In spite of the work of Charcot and Janet, the new psychotherapy begins with Freud. I have formulated my attitude towards Freud and psychoanalysis as clearly as possible. In many points I deviate from the opinions of Freud and the codifications of the psychoanalytic school. I have approached psychoanalysis with the spirit of complete inner freedom. I believe that the progress of psychotherapy and of psychoanalysis will be in this direction. I have embodied into the systematic arrangement of this book the facts found by psychoanalysis, the psychoanalytic theories, and its technical achievements. This book attempts to survey the field of psychotherapy in general, and is not an introduction to psychoanalysis.

Psychoanalysis should be studied from the books and writings of Freud and from the writings of those who follow him more or less faithfully—men like Abraham, Ferenczi, Nunberg, and Fenichel. The books by Ives Hendrick and Karen Stephen may serve as elementary introductions.

The psychology of Jung and Adler can be studied from their books.

Adolf Meyer's work is to date insufficiently formulated.[1] I may point, however, to the papers and the book of Oskar Diethelm and Leo Kanner's *Child Psychiatry.* The works of Jung, Adler, and Meyer are unquestionably of importance in the development of psychotherapy. I have endeavored to show where they influence therapeutic actions.

Nor is this an attempt to write a textbook of psychiatry or a book on neuroses. The discussions on specific forms of mental suffering are introduced to elucidate the principles of psychotherapeutic procedure. After some hesitation it was decided to omit case histories, not only to save space. Case histories in small print which fill space in many books dealing with psychiatry and psychologic problems are rarely read. In addition, they are usually too sketchy and too incompletely discussed to be of value if they were to be studied.

Finally, this book is not intended as a general textbook of psychology. I have attempted to outline the problems of general psychology in three other volumes—*The Image and Appearance of the Human Body, Mind: Perception and Thought in Their Constructive Aspects,* and *Goals and Desires of Man.*[2] These volumes contain, I hope, the justification of many of the statements made in this book. A system of general psychology is necessarily the background of psychotherapeutic procedure. Systems of this type become dangerous when they become too rigid. I cannot say whether I have escaped this danger.

Man lives in a world full of promises and dangers. He tries to know more about this world and approaches it by action. Through a continuous process of trial and error he increases his knowledge, and reality unfolds before him. His deeper satisfactions lie in this drive towards a fuller reality. Conflicts which originate from dangerous situations which he does not care to face may hamper him. Psychotherapy should be considered as an attempt to help human beings fulfill their destiny in a richer world.

Paul Schilder,
1938

[1] Alfred Lief, in *The Commonsense Psychiatry of Dr. Adolf Meyer* (New York, McGraw-Hill Book Company, Inc., 1948), has brought together and edited fifty-two selected papers of Adolf Meyer.

[2] *Mind: Perception and Thought* and *The Goals and Desires of Man* were published posthumously (New York, Columbia University Press, 1942), and were reprinted in 1949.

PREFACE TO THE REVISED EDITION

PAUL SCHILDER'S *Psychotherapy* appeared in the first edition in 1938 as the earliest critical and integrative analysis and synthesis of the many schools of psychiatric thought and therapeutic practices. In itself it offered the first of the polyphasic and constructive approaches to psychotherapy. The use of the shorter and more active therapies and group therapy in a wide range of conditions was considered heretical at the time he was using them. He modified both psychoanalytic theories and practices in ways which are now widely recognized. Furthermore, most of the present concepts of psychosomatic medicine were presented by him, in the English language, as early as 1929, when his paper on "The Somatic Basis of the Neuroses" appeared in the *Journal of Nervous and Mental Disease.*

It was my happy fortune to have been closely associated with Paul Schilder from the time we met in January, 1930, at the Henry Phipps Psychiatric Clinic of the Johns Hopkins Hospital. Later the same year we were working together in the Psychiatric Division of Bellevue Hospital and the New York University College of Medicine. As his wife in the last four years of his life I shared with him many of the clinical experiences and resulting discussions which went into the making of *Psychotherapy,* which was published in 1938. During that time and before his death in 1940, he wrote some forty scientific papers, many of which were concerned, at least in part, with psychotherapy. This revised edition has been enlarged by adding whole articles or excerpts from these later writings. There have been some minor changes in the organization of the book to allow this new material to be added.

As the editor of the second edition, I have made no contributions to the content of the book other than footnotes, which are clearly indicated and which refer mostly to reviews or significant contributions to the subject under discussion appearing since Paul Schilder wrote *Psychotherapy*.

The bibliography has been enlarged accordingly. A new index has been prepared to include all of the new material.

To Chapter 3, "The Symptomatology of Mental Suffering," there has been added a discussion on failure as a symptom from "Success and Failure," *Psychoanalytic Review*, 1938, and some remarks on the symptomatology of criminal behavior from "The Cure of the Criminal and Prevention of Crime," *Journal of Clinical Psychopathology*, 1940.

There have been added to Chapter 5, "Psychic Health as an Experience," discussions on mental hygiene or psychic health of children, adolescents, medical students, and seniles from "The Constructive Approach to Childhood and Adolescence" (written with Frank J. Curran), *Journal of Clinical Psychopathology*, 1940–1941; "Mental Hygiene of the Medical Student," *Medical Bulletin of the Student Association of the New York University College of Medicine*, 1939; and "Psychiatric Aspects of Old Age and Aging," *American Journal of Orthopsychiatry*, 1940.

To Chapter 6, "Technical Tools of Psychotherapy," additions have been made to the section on dream analysis from "Body Image in Dreams," *Psychoanalytic Review*, 1942, and a section has been added on the use of benzedrine in psychotherapy from "The Psychological Effects of Benzedrine Sulphate," *Journal of Nervous and Mental Disease*, 1938.

Chapter 7, "The Relation between Physician and Patient," has been lengthened by two additions. A considerable discussion on the relation of the physician as leader of the group in group therapy has been taken from "Introductory Remarks on the Group," *Journal of Social Psychology*, 1940. At the end of Chapter 7 has been added a part of "The Death of the Leader in Group Psychotherapy," *American Journal of Orthopsychiatry*, 1947, written by Pauline Rosenthal, who was assisting Paul Schilder with the group therapy just before his death. She has reported and discussed the reactions of some of the patients in the group to his death. This seems to be an appropriate contribution to the subject of this chapter.

To Chapter 10, "The Treatment of Specific Types of Neuroses and Psychopathies," have been added discussions on the treatment of neurosis following head injuries, anxiety neurosis, hysteria, depersonalization, obsessions and compulsion, criminal behavior and alcoholism. These discussions were taken from "Neurosis Following Head and Brain Injuries," Chapter 12 in *Injuries of Skull, Brain, and Spinal Cord,* edited by Samuel Brock, 1941; "Types of Anxiety Neuroses," *International Journal of Psycho-Analysis,* 1941; "The Concept of Hysteria," *American Journal of Psychiatry,* 1939; "The Treatment of Depersonalization," *Bulletin of the New York Academy of Medicine,* 1939; "The Structure of Obsession and Compulsion," *Psychiatry,* 1940; and "The Psychogenesis of Alcoholism," *Quarterly Journal of Studies on Alcohol,* 1941.

The first part of Chapter 11, "Psychoanalysis and Psychotherapy of the Psychoses and the Psychology of Shock Treatment," is a reprint of "Influence of Psychoanalysis on Psychiatry," *Psychoanalytic Quarterly,* 1940. The last part is taken from "The Psychological Considerations of the Insulin Treatment of Schizophrenia" (written with Leo Orenstein) and "Notes on the Psychology of Metrazol Treatment of Schizophrenia," *Journal of Nervous and Mental Disease,* 1938 and 1939; and "The Psychology of Schizophrenia," *Psychoanalytic Review,* 1939.

I am very grateful to all these authors, editors, and publishers for their permission to reprint the material cited above in this book.

Lauretta Bender,
1950

Psychotherapy

Chapter 1

SOME GENERAL PRINCIPLES

Patients come to the physician because they suffer. They may suffer from any type of bodily ailment, such as pain, weakness, tension, or nausea. However, their complaints may not pertain to the body, but to their thinking, their emotions, or their inability to work. The difficulty may be that they are unable to establish proper relations with their fellow human beings. They themselves feel quite all right, but the reactions of other people to them are such that they finally suffer. In milder degrees of adaptation difficulties, the individual may feel that his lack of success in life, from which he suffers, is due to his own failings and his emotional attitudes. He seeks to change these attitudes. No one can be successful always. Difficulties may occur in everyone's life, such as the loss of one's beloved. The outward circumstances of life, because of the general political and economic situation, may become unbearable and cause the individual to suffer. He may feel that his suffering is out of proportion to the actual difficulties in his situation, and will therefore ask for help in these problems of everyday life. Finally, the individual may be brought to the physician by someone else. He may believe himself quite healthy, but those around him suffer more or less through his actions and do not hold this opinion. They believe something is wrong with him in the mental sphere, and therefore they insist that he get help from a physician. To this group belong children with mental deficiency or behavior problems, criminals, psychopathic personalities, and mentally ill persons. Thus we have five roughly divided groups of individuals who are brought to the physician either because they themselves suffer or because they make others suffer, i.e., individuals with (1) a physical complaint, (2) a mental complaint, (3) a complaint of lack of success, (4) complaints due to the ordinary difficulties of human life, and (5) complaints of others.

In the first group we find patients afflicted with the so-called organic diseases or organic deficiencies. A person who has lost a leg, for instance, needs a prosthesis, exercise, advice, and help for mental and physical adaptation. Many persons who complain about physical ailments are not what we would call organically ill. We have learned that every mental problem reflects itself in the physical sphere. It may take a form resembling an organic disease without being identical with it. There are at least some organic diseases that originate in the psychological sphere. In most of these cases the patients will complain, not about their psychic conflict, but about their physical ailment. In some cases the organic complaint, having originated in the psychic sphere, may be only occasionally corroborated by so-called physiological changes. The patient who complains about a physical ailment which is purely organic in character professes by the mere fact that he goes to the physician that he suffers and needs relief. He seeks not only help by physical agents but the aid of the physician as person to person.

In the second group of cases we find neurasthenics and patients with obsessional neurosis who complain about the disturbances in their psychic processes, such as a lack of concentration, or about their obsessions and compulsions as such. Depersonalization cases may complain about their lack of interest and their inability to feel. It is, however, rare that the complaints are restricted to the psychic sphere. Patients of this type almost invariably complain about physical signs like fatigue, constipation, tensions, and pain. Many of the cases with complaints about difficulties in their psychic life are organic cases. Obsessional symptoms in encephalitic cases are common, and as my own investigations have convinced me, careful examination, even with our present imperfect methods, will often reveal signs of an organic process or of an organic inferiority in obsessional neurosis. The difficulties in concentration may be due to an arteriosclerotic process, or to a beginning general paresis. Depersonalization signs may be connected with a true depression, which, I believe, has at least strong organic components. Also the schizophrenic, who suffers from a disease which is organic in the same sense as a depression, might complain about the change in his mental activity.

The third and fourth groups of our patients have not always gone to the physician when they needed help. They previously went to the priest or minister, or they sought moral guidance. Many of the individuals of this type are not free from physical symptoms, especially at a time of stress. In some of these cases an organic disease may be a partial cause of the maladaptation.

In the last group we may expect to find a comparatively large number of individuals who are organically ill.

Even such a casual survey gives us the impression that most of the persons who suffer, suffer in body and soul. Furthermore, the border line between a psychic and a physical ailment would not appear to be very sharp.

Human beings are social beings. They have social contacts of various types. The child is at first dependent upon his mother and the persons who nurse him. Social contacts with other children are limited. When the child grows older he may develop contact with siblings and the other children in the neighborhood and school. Then contacts with teachers and other grownups are added. The grownup has relations to persons of both the same and the opposite sex. We may talk about friendship and love. He has social relations to his family, to the social group in which he moves, to his professional, racial, and political circles. He lives in a complicated system of social interrelations. These are rather obvious and trite observations. My own investigations have revealed that the social character of human experience goes even further. We build up the image of our own body only in relation to others. Even when we perceive and are interested in objects outside of ourselves, we are addressing ourselves to others. The lonely dreamer and the philosopher in seclusion dream and philosophize before and for an unseen public.

The relations to other human beings may be roughly divided into two groups: the social relations in the narrower sense, and love relations.

The social relation can be one of equality. The one individual is interested in having the other exist as an equal to himself. It is a relation of give-and-take. It can be one of superiority and inferiority. The individual still remains interested in the existence of the other person, but he does consider himself superior or inferior to the other person and does not wish to have this relation reversed. The give-and-take relation may still be present, but the giving may express either the superior or the inferior attitude. Usually, the superior person will maintain his superiority by giving. The relation between parent and child is one of the relations in which superiority is inherent in the situation. The same is true for the situation between teacher and pupil. The relation between employer and employee almost always belongs in the same category.

This relation may be one of aggression and submission. The aggressor may even have a tendency to a partial or total destruction of the other person, but he is still desirous that there be a sufficient number of counterplayers present who can be subdued. The subdued person might be gratified in his submissive role. We usually believe that a severe degree of destructiveness in the relationship between two persons also involves libidinous attitudes. We then speak about sadomasochism.

If a state of equality is attained, it cannot be a lasting one—it cannot be maintained. It is more or less of an ideal around which social relations move. At best it can be but a point of passage in a dynamic relation.

In all social relations the existence of the other is not only physically necessary but meets the inner psychic demands. Destructive impulses against the other, although present, are a phase in a social process in which interest in the existence and mental and physical integrity of the other plays a leading part. However, the seriousness of destructive tendencies should not be underrated.

Biologically and psychologically, the love relationship between two human beings is different from other social relations. In the love relation one individual professes his basic incompleteness and wants completion by the person of the other sex. A system of activities is co-ordinated to the erotic relations between two persons. In the basic love relation between man and woman there is no difference in the activities between the two sexes. There is merely a difference in the phases of activity. Whereas the man is more active in the first phase of the love relation in general and of intercourse in particular, the woman is more active in the second phase of both. The dynamic equality between the two sexes may be changed into a relation of superiority and inferiority, aggression and submission (sadism and masochism).

In social and sexual relations human beings offer gifts to each other. These may be objects, or service, or erotic gratification. The actual satisfaction of physical needs, regardless of how they serve the maintenance of the body or sexual satisfaction, is but a small part of our life. We do not live only in the narrow presence of actual sensual experience. The range of our activities extends far beyond the horizon of immediate perception, in space as well as in time. We need not only actual gratifications but promises of future gratifications as well. This future gratification also transgresses the space of the immediate present. Humanity has elaborated a sign system for such gratifications. Such a sign system enriches our world in an almost immeasurable way. In this sign system, language and words play the most important part, but the system is in no way limited to the spoken and written word. I shall point to the function of money in social life.

Sentences and words may thus become signs for any type of gratification in social and erotic relations. When a sign is actually functioning, the value diffuses from the object into the sign, and the endearing word of the lover becomes a value in itself, irrespective of the fact that it promises the pleasures of intercourse.

The tool of psychotherapy is language as a sign system. The physician who treats a patient by physical methods introduces substances into the patient which change his body function directly. The surgeon actually cuts the human body. The physician plays the part of a physical agent in a more or less direct way. So do massage and physiotherapy in general. The psychotherapist has no immediate access to the body of the patient and to his gratifications. The influence he has on the patient is merely due to the words he speaks. What is the power behind those words? Two persons who speak to each other are in a social relation which in the widest sense of the word includes the erotic.

On the basis of the previous remarks about social relations we conclude that the following relations between the physician and the patient are possible. We speak here primarily about the psychotherapist, but since patients go to the physician because they suffer, it is obvious that the psychotherapeutic relation is inherent in every relation between physician and patient.

(*a*) Physician and patient are fellow human beings. There is no fundamental difference between them. The physician merely has more knowledge in a field of experience in which the patient happens not to be so well versed. In compensation for the advice, the patient gives money to the physician as he would give it to anyone else who serves him. Relations between physician and patient are mostly not of this type.

(*b*) The patient wants to go to an outstanding physician. The mere fact that the patient chooses the physician gives to the latter the superiority in their relation. The patient, especially when he comes with psychic problems, wants to find a leader in the physician. Human beings need a leader whom they admire and who takes a part of their responsibilities. In one type of leadership the leader is merely expected to have superior insight. If the patient expects such leadership, the relation between the two will be a relation of superiority and inferiority, and in their discussion common sense and reason will prevail.

(*c*) Since the discussion between patient and physician circles around the moral problems of life, it will sooner or later become apparent that purely from the point of view of reason, the physician is not greatly superior to the patient after all. Sooner or later the patient will have to add faith to his relation to the physician if he wants to get a sufficient amount of consolation out of this relation. The physician himself will eventually be compelled to demand faith from his patient, unless he discharges the patient in disgust as some practitioners do when they see that the patient cannot avail himself of the physician's advice. We may suppose that this elementary faith (not based upon reason) very often enters the psychotherapeutic relation without the knowledge of either patient or physician. The method of persuasion as developed by Dubois is, as we shall later see, far from being a method based upon common sense. When faith enters the relation, the superior-inferior relation between physician and patient is obviously still more emphasized, but seemingly a new element has been added. The relation becomes similar to that between the adult and the child, or better and more specifically, the relation is more like the one between parent and child. In such a parent-child relationship, sexual elements are almost invariably present in addition to the social elements. Furthermore, a sign (word) coming from the parent has a much greater value.

(*d*) From this relation to the complete surrender of the patient to the physician is only a short step. The physician does not only become a father, but he also becomes a father endowed with magic powers. The sexual element entering into this relation will be more or less primitive. Since the physician is so far superior in this relation, reasoning obviously becomes unnecessary, and the physician has to direct the faith of his patient. He may become a mystical leader, or he may use the more definite technique of suggestion and hypnosis. When the faith of the patient in such a relation is blind, the physician himself is no less blind. He is called to take over a leadership by reason or faith; and according to the whole situation, he cannot know where he should lead the patient. The physician ultimately will become discontented with his role as a fellow adviser who does not know what to advise, and as a rational or mystical leader who does not know where to lead.

The modern approach to psychotherapeutic problems stresses the necessity of gaining insight into the patient's personality and conflicts. In this respect, Janet, Freud, Jung, and Adler are of the same opinion. A full social relation to other human beings is only possible on the basis of a general good will and the acknowledgment that they are fellow human beings. In order to respect them, we must know them; or in other words, we must acknowledge them as specific and distinct personalities. Psychotherapy, therefore, has the task of not only establishing the relation between the physician and the patient, but of finding out methods by which better understanding can be had of the problems of the patient. Only then is a full relation between the patient and his physician possible. There is the underlying conviction that suffering due to psychic reasons is dependent on conflicts which the individual is not only unable to solve, but is not even aware of. The psychotherapeutic process therefore must reveal the personality and the conflicts not only to the physician but also to the patient himself. The approach by reason and faith is much less dependent upon theoretical assumptions than this type of psychotherapy, which Fritz Wittels has called "unveiling." The problems of this psychotherapy are:

(*a*) What method is there to uncover the conflict underlying the neurosis? (*b*) How can we bring the patient to understand his conflicts? (*c*) How can one bring the patient actually to use his insight?

(*a*) The method employed is necessarily based on uncovering new material. This new material can be obtained by a discussion directed by the underlying assumptions of the physician, as in individual psychology. By a more or less direct questioning, the facts of the life of the patient have to be elicited and grouped into an order which gives them a new meaning. The search for details which could lead to such a rearrangement will indicate the method of interpretation of dreams, of the mistakes in everyday life, and of seemingly unrelated events of life. Such an approach is basic for Adler's individual psychology and for Adolf Meyer's psychobiology. Psychoanalysis uses the method of so-called "free association." This method is based upon the assumption that when the individual is relieved from the necessity of logical thinking and reports everything going through his mind he will necessarily, under the pressure of emotions which tend to expression, bring forward basic material. Mistakes of everyday life, and dreams in which a partial liberation from the fetters of logic and repression is already achieved, will be particularly valuable material in this respect. This method assumes that the so-called logical and conscious thinking hinders important parts of psychic life from expression. This method therefore tends to a liberation of deeper layers of psychic life and emphatically stresses the emotional character of these deeper layers. This methodological principle is common to the classical psychoanalysis in the Freudian sense as well as to the Jungian type of analytic procedure.

(*b*) If one considers the process of insight preponderantly from the logical side, no special problems arise concerning the insight of the patient. The results of the physician's investigation merely have to be communicated to the patient. Those who use psychoanalytic procedures believe that insight is only possible in connection with emotional re-enactment of previous conflicts. If hypnosis is used for the recovery of forgotten material, the re-enactment becomes more or less a matter of course. Whereas psychoanalysis stresses the emotional re-enactment with the physician as the central figure, Jungian analysis stresses the emotional experiences in connection with emotional experiences belonging to the common racial background. The products of the so-called "collective unconscious" then acquire a particular importance.

(*c*) Whereas the methods which emphasize intellectual insight sooner or later have to appeal to the good will of the patient to make use of the insight which he has gained, psychoanalysis in the Freudian sense is optimistic in so far as it supposes that reliving the emotional conflicts means immediately that the individual will be able and willing to control his conflict. Other types of psychoanalysis require a further educational, synthetic process in order to direct the individual to a better use of his freed emotions for further tasks.

The first method puts the stress on the assumption that psychic life is determined by the events of the past, and the unraveling of the past is the paramount issue.[1] The second method believes in an inner drive towards the future which has to be helped.[2]

It is clear that all the methods which propose to reveal something to the patient are not concerned with his present situation only, but also with his past. Childhood thus becomes the hunting ground for modern psychotherapy. Freud has been most consistent in this respect. Adler and Jung, although agreeing with this general principle, either are not so interested in the specific details of the past or believe that the appeal to the community spirit or the collective unconscious is more fertile. The psychotherapist in these three systems plays a part which is less dangerous than the one he plays in the methods in which, as a leader by faith and reason, he is less interested in the individual problems of the patient. He is either a wiser older brother representing society (Adler), or the psychagogue of the collective and creative unconscious (Jung), or merely the disinterested catalyst (Freud).

A critical evaluation of these methods is, of course, not possible yet. We merely point to the dangers involved in every one of the attitudes basic in psychotherapy. The wisdom of the older brother and of the psychagogue may tend to crush the individuality of the patient. The social or mystical leader may become too convinced of his superiority. The disinterested attitude in classical psychoanalysis introduces an element of aloofness which is not a true expression of the psychoanalyst's countertransference. His disappearance behind the protection of the method inflates his ego.

[1] The first method, or the genetic approach, has been summarized by Heinz Hartmann and Ernst Kris in "The Genetic Approach in Psychoanalysis," *The Psychoanalytic Study of the Child* I, 1945. It is also discussed by Otto Fenichel in *The Psychoanalytic Theory of Neurosis,* 1945. [L.B., Ed.]

[2] The second method, which is also referred to as the cultural approach or the interpersonal approach, has been presented by Erich Fromm in *Escape from Freedom,* 1941; Karen Horney in *New Ways in Psychoanalysis,* 1939; and Harry S. Sullivan in *Conceptions of Modern Psychiatry,* 1947. Finally Clara Thompson has summarized the contributions to both approaches in *Psychoanalysis, Evolution and Development,* 1950. [L.B., Ed.]

One cannot deny that all systems discussed reveal important aspects of the total problem. But psychotherapy must at any rate unravel the conflicts of the present and bring them into the proper focus. It also must, guided by a similar point of view, unravel the conflicts of the individual's past and return as far back as possible into the early childhood. The individual must be seen in his relations to the actual community and to the more mystic community of human beings. It should see the individual as suffering because of his past, and yet aim into the future. The individual needs the guidance by the older brother, by the mystical leader, but he also needs the impersonal representative of his own total past and that of the community. Finally, the individual has also to reach an acknowledgment of his own inner independence and has to recognize the relativity of leadership of any type.

The psychotherapeutic relation between the physician and his patient thus becomes a mirror of possible social relations between two human beings, in which the physician is no less affected than the patient himself.

Psychological processes occur in an individual who has a body, and they have an influence on the physiological processes going on in the body. They must therefore be of a nature partially identical with physiological processes. We know, thus, that they are experienced and have a physiological character; they are in connection with the physiological processes going on in the brain. On the other hand, they are influenced by physiological processes in the body in general as well as in the brain. No psychological experience is without a physiological value. The special problem arises, What are the empirical correlations between psychological processes and physical occurrences? This problem is of great interest for psychotherapy. If psychological processes influence the body, psychic conflicts may lead to transitory or permanent changes in the body—in one word, to disease in a "physical" sense. The scope of psychotherapy will have to be extended to organic diseases. Such an influence undoubtedly exists, and therefore the question arises, What diseases have been provoked by psychic processes? and the question which is not quite identical, What diseases can be cured by psychotherapy? At any rate, psychological processes are physical agents.

Sleep is correlated with a physiological mechanism which has its center in the posterior wall of the third ventricle. All kinds of organic processes taking place in this region provoke sleep disturbances. The details can be found in the papers of Poetzl and von Economo and in my book, *Mind: Perception and Thought.* Experiments in hypnosis have shown conclusively that sleep can be provoked by psychological methods. It is easy to suggest sleep. Hypnosis and sleep have common basic trends. Everyday experience shows that the sleep function is altered under emotional stress. August Forel has justly emphasized the central importance of the wish to fall asleep. The wish to fall asleep is a physiological agent acting on a specific part of the brain. The psychological sleep theory gets further confirmation by the experiments of Pavlov, who has shown that dogs become sleepy when, in a delayed conditioned-reflex formation, the animal has to wait too long a time for the food which has been promised by the signal. It is true that Pavlov's interpretation is different. My own experiments have shown that the readiness for psychogenic sleep can be increased by drugs affecting the sleep centers.

Another instance of the physiological influence on psychic processes is obvious in the so-called Berger rhythm of the brain. This consists of electric waves which can be inducted from the occipital lobe when the individual is in a state of rest. Under the influence of optic experience or psychic concentration, these electrical phenomena are diminished. Hypnosis influences it, too (cf. the papers of Adrian, Adrian and Matthews, and Davis and Davis).[3]

The psychogalvanic phenomenon is due to changes in the secretion of the sweat glands. It is a good indicator of psychological processes. Vasomotor phenomena on the skin, wales, and hemorrhages have been provoked by psychic influences. The psychic influence seemingly acts as well on the blood vessels as on the tissue itself.

E. R. Jaensch was able to mix the color of objects merely represented in eidetic images with actual colors. He and his school have made a great many experiments of a similar type (cf. Heinrich Kluever).

The suggestion of dizziness provokes phenomena which correspond to organic changes in the function of the vestibular apparatus. It is controversial whether this is merely an influence on blood vessels or whether one deals with an influence on nerve centers. Vomit-

[3] See also the works by Margaret A. Kennard, Hans Strauss, and Sidney Rubin and Karl M. Bowman on the effects of psychological processes on the electroencephalogram. [L.B., Ed.]

ing, due to an influence on vagus centers, can be provoked by psychic influence.

The metabolism of an individual can be changed by psychological influences. The basal metabolism may be increased up to 40 per cent through suggestion. Rage and fear will increase the blood sugar and the output of adrenaline.

Changes in the function of the thyroid under emotional stress have been repeatedly reported. The observations of Agnes Conrad at least suggest a strong psychogenic component in exophthalmic goiter. I have observed two cases in which psychogenic factors were obviously important in the outbreak of the disease.

The calcium content of the blood is dependent upon psychogenic factors, although this factor is not clear in every patient. According to Russian experiments, antibodies can be produced in the conditioned-reflex experiment. The conditioned experiment, seen from the psychological point of view, is a habit formation. Heilig and Hoff have provoked changes in the phagocytic index by suggestion in hypnosis. They have also provoked herpes zoster in the same way.

It is well known that the pulse rate increases under a corresponding suggestion. It is more difficult to obtain a slowing down of the pulse rate, but such experiments have been reported too. The blood pressure, according to widespread experience, is dependent on psychological factors. The experiments of Wundt and his school, among others, have shown conclusively that the blood-vessel function varies according to psychic activity. It is less interesting, from our point of view, whether these blood-vessel changes correspond to every shade of emotional activity or whether they merely indicate psychic activity and tensions. The blood-vessel changes can be general or can be directed to specific parts of the body with corresponding suggestion.

Changes in the rhythm of breathing occur, as psychologists have shown, under the influence of any emotional attitude. Benussi found characteristic symptoms in the breathing curve when persons were lying.

The psychogenic secretion of saliva varies according to the food offered. The whole secretion in the gastrointestinal tract is dependent upon psychic influences. It has been proved for the stomach secretion as well as for the duodenal secretion. The influence of psychological factors on the gastrointestinal motility has been studied by X-ray examination.

Psychological factors play an outstanding part in the function of the sex organs. For this point, erection and orgasm due only to psychic factors are proof. The urorrhea and the secretion in the female genitals under the influence of psychogenic sexual tension belong in the same category. Vaginal fluor may be influenced by psychogenic factors. Forel has conclusively shown that psychic factors influence menstruation.[4]

The effect of psychological attitudes on allergic factors is proved by clinical experience, although this influence seems to be limited. I have myself seen an asthmatic attack subside under hypnosis, and I have observed an allergic skin disease which disappeared with the progress in the psychotherapy of the patient.

This is merely an enumeration; but it is not necessary to offer details, since the books of Oswald Schwarz and H. Flanders Dunbar review the whole literature. I furthermore point to the studies of Wiss, De Jong, and Weinberg.[5]

We are merely interested in the general problem that there is a psychic influence upon every organ of the body. This influence is a double one. Although it is not very probable that the different types of emotions express themselves in a characteristic way in every organ, it is more than probable that every emotion finds a specific expression if one considers the changes in the different parts of the body as a unit. This is an influence which expresses the general attitude of the individual. Besides this general effect, changes occur in specific parts of the body with specific problems that concern these very parts of the body. One may suggest, for instance, the disappearance of a specific wart. In the experiments of Ernst Weber, the volume of an arm increases towards which specific attention is directed. The intention to move the arm has the same effect. It is furthermore obvious that psychogenic influences are directed towards specific parts of the body when the complexes and emotional attitudes point in this direction. The differentiation between a general emotion and the specific complex directed to a specific organ should not be taken in a too schematic way. An emotion is always in connection with a situa-

[4] Important contributions to the psychology of women, the psychology of the menstrual cycle, and related subjects have been made by Helene Deutsch, Therese Benedek, Viola Klein, and Mary Chadwick. [L.B., Ed.]

[5] Psychosomatic studies have been summarized by Franz Alexander, Thomas M. French, Weiss and English, Leland Hinsie, Smith Ely Jelliffe, and C. Alberto Seguin. [L.B., Ed.]

tion in human life; it is never a general emotion. Such a situation must have been specific in content, and we may expect that the psychical reactions connected with a general emotion would be different, according to its content. In one of my observations, for instance, severe vasomotor attacks occurred after a patient had witnessed the death of a nephew by an automobile accident. The vasomotor phenomena were particularly apparent on the face and in the arms. The attacks lasted two to three hours, and the temperature rose to 100.6° F. In hypnosis the traumatic scene was revived; the vasomotor phenomena appeared in full strength. The spontaneous attacks did not carry the memory of the accident with them.

One cannot separate the ideational and emotional parts of a situation. Hans Hoff and his co-workers succeeded in changing the quality of the urine, not by a suggestion that the urine should be different, but by suggesting that the individual had been drinking a great amount of cold water. A suggestion and a mental process become efficient only by the way of specific representations which are in connection with the situation. I have called these "key representations," and in order to influence a specific organ one has to find the key representation which fits this organ. This is merely an expression of the general principle that we live in specific situations.

We have to differentiate between the direct influence of psychic processes on the organism, as described in the preceding pages, and indirect influences of the psyche on the body. Psychogenic motives may, for instance, increase the rate of breathing. With the increased rate of breathing, the acid-base relation of the blood changes, and tetany occurs. This is a psychogenic tetany, but not in a direct way. An individual may, for psychogenic reasons, turn ten times around his longitudinal axis. Nystagmus will occur, but this is not a psychogenic nystagmus in the ordinary sense. After all, the most important effect of a change in the situation consists in the change of our attitudes and in the actions which may ensue. Is that not also a psychogenic influence, with far-reaching consequences in the organism? When a man sees a naked woman and gets an erection, is that psychogenic or organic? We should not separate the two. We should see the organism living in specific situations and changing with the situations. The question is not to determine which processes are psychological and which processes are physiological. All attitudes of the individual are attitudes in which the body participates as a whole. So-called psychological processes are always physiological processes of a specific degree of complication. There are some physiological processes which have no psychic reflection, so far as we can ascertain. It is our task to find out which physiological processes are connected with psychic experiences.

Chapter 2

THE PSYCHOLOGY OF ORGANIC SYMPTOMATOLOGY[1]

It has been mentioned in the first chapter that a patient with an organic disease does not come to the physician because of a change in his anatomy and physiology, but because he suffers. He has complaints, and we may call these complaints also symptoms. A symptom in this sense is not the increase in the blood sugar, or granulated casts in the urine, or changes in the color index of the red blood corpuscles. If one calls these physical changes symptoms, one should at least be aware that such a symptom is, in its structure, fundamentally different from symptoms like fatigue, palpitation, weakness, pain, and difficulties in breathing. Symptoms in this sense are not so different in the so-called organic and in the so-called psychogenic cases. The suspicion may arise that in the so-called functional case there may be some organic change which we cannot find with our present anatomical and physiological methods, and that the so-called organic case may not be as independent of psychological processes as it may seem at the first sight. At least suffering is the common bond between the two. Since the symptom, in our sense, has a psychological character, it has to be at any rate in connection with the other psychic experiences.

[1] Reprinted, with minor changes, from the *Psychoanalytic Review* 24: 264–76, July, 1937, where it appeared as "The Psychotherapeutic Approach to Medicine." I am indebted to Dr. Smith E. Jelliffe for permission to reprint.

As a human being, the sick person has his psychological problems, and if there is an organic manifestation it cannot remain isolated from his other psychic experiences. The mere fact of suffering makes the individual more dependent upon other human beings, and he justly expects to receive more consideration and love. Feelings of guilt play a very important part in human life. We not only fear punishment, but owing to attitudes in early childhood, we feel that we should be punished. With our infantile self we expect punishment for whatever has been forbidden to us by the parents and their substitutes. Freud was inclined to believe that the feeling of guilt was merely in close relation to forbidden aggressive impulses. I think this formulation is too narrow and that we may feel guilty, too, because of our sexual drives and actions. When a person suffers from organic disease, there is no need for further punishment, and he may be relieved from his feeling of guilt.

Human beings are always in dynamic relations with other human beings in the fight for superiority. The person organically ill may attain a superior position in the family which he would not have obtained otherwise. He gets this superiority without strife. His other efforts in life become futile and unnecessary. He no longer needs to strain himself in the struggle for his position in society. Nobody demands any more of him, and neither does he of himself, to be successful. I emphasize that this psychological attitude comes with the organic diseases even if the individual has no particular tendency to utilize the organic disease. Organic disease serves, at any rate, a variety of psychological functions. The sick individual cannot help remaining an individual; according to his psychological structure the psychological function of the organic disease will vary, and different sides of this function will be emphasized accordingly. An organic disease may thus become a source of neurotic behavior. According to the discussion of the previous chapter, the organic process itself may be influenced by the psychological processes, culminating in a specific attitude towards the disease. The psychotherapeutic approach in medicine should, therefore, be neutral concerning the question of whether a symptom is organic or not. We are here concerned with symptoms of body ailments. It is worth our while to keep in mind that they show only a limited variety. The following table will orient us concerning the basic symptoms of body ailments as far as they are important from a psychotherapeutic point of view.

(1) Symptoms of the surface of the body:
  (*a*) Swelling or addition to the image of the body
  (*b*) Mutilation or subtraction from the image of the body
  (*c*) Change
  (*d*) Loss of integrity, as bleeding

(2) Symptoms of the openings of the body:
  (*a*) Occlusion, as constipation, difficulties in breathing, absence of sweating, absence of menstruation
  (*b*) Excessive discharge from the openings, as vomiting, diarrhea, excessive menstruation, hyperhidrosis

(3) Symptoms of the senses, as impairment of sensory intake or perception

(4) Symptoms of the inside of the body:
  (*a*) Increased heaviness, general or localized; fullness; densification
  (*b*) Diminished heaviness, general or localized; cavities; emptiness
  (*c*) Change in density of tissues or fluids, as solid, liquid, or gas

(5) Symptoms of motility:
  (*a*) Diminution by paralysis, weakness, fatigue, general and local
  (*b*) Increased motility, such as fits, cramps, twitchings, tension, restlessness, general and local

(6) General symptoms:
  (*a*) Anxiety
  (*b*) Dizziness
  (*c*) Nausea
  (*d*) Pain
  (*e*) Inhibition
  (*f*) Fatigue
  (*g*) Weakness
  (*h*) Restlessness
  (*i*) Tension

According to this table, the general symptoms and the motility symptoms have close relations to each other. Every one of these symptoms can occur in the course of an organic disease as well as by psychogenesis. If one of the symptoms occurs from an organic point of view, it will carry with it specific psychological attitudes. The pain experienced in angina pectoris is connected with anxiety and a fear of sudden death. Patients suffering from this disease generally develop a very close attachment to those whom they love. They do not want to be separated from them in space, and death means to them sudden removal from the beloved in space. If the anginal syndrome develops on a psychogenic basis—the so-called pseudo-angina pectoris—we find a similar psychological attitude as a causal factor in the formation of a neurosis of this type. Anxiety, fear of death, and unwillingness to be separated from the beloved ones are no less outspoken in the psychogenic case. In the organic case as well as in the psychogenic case, we should be aware of the life situation of the patient, of his earlier experiences, of his love relations in early childhood and in later life. Our basic approach to the organic case as well as to the psychogenic case must be based upon this insight.

I have no doubt that angina pectoris is an organic disease, in the ordinary sense. Cardiologists assure us that angina pectoris has something to do with the stress of modern life. They are not very specific about just what the stress of modern life is. They seemingly mean the problems of modern life, and not muscular effort or nutrition or other physical agents. They have offered no conclusive proof for their contention. To be sure, Felix Deutsch reports about the successful analysis in an angina pectoris case. We shall hear later that the successful psychological cure of an organic case does not prove its psychogenesis. The organism may have merely reacted to the additional stress of the psychogenic influence and gained its equilibrium after the stress was removed. The organic factor of the lability of the equilibrium may remain.

The whole question of the psychogensis of organic diseases is in a rather unclear state at the present time. Organic medicine, in a very great number of cases, is not able to explain why a disease has overcome the individual at a specific time, under the specific conditions of the case. In the majority of cases, medical psychology is also unable to explain why the psychic conflict has expressed itself at this particular time in this specific way, and in this specific organ. It is in vain, therefore, if one tries to explain the organic diseases merely from the organic or from the psychological point of view. The question can only be decided on the basis of a careful investigation in both directions. The importance of organic factors in angina pectoris cannot be denied, even if it were only the age factor. We have no definite proof that anatomical changes occur in pseudoangina. Functional changes are obvious. There are changes in the pulse rate, contraction of the blood vessels, and even changes in the blood pressure. Cases of death by sudden fright have been reported. I do not think that we have convincing evidence that this is possible in an otherwise healthy organism.

A. A. Brill holds to a different opinion, quoting experiences in primitive people. We are more interested here in the fact that specific emotions have an influence on the psychological mechanism of the heart. We also have the suspicion that this influence is comparatively small from a quantitative point of view. The conclusion is allowed that a symptom concerning the heart can originate from the individual problems of a personality, or, as I put it, from the center of the personality. It progresses from this center to the body. As near as the body may be to ourselves, it is not so near to us as our own inner life. I consider, therefore, that the body is in this sense the periphery of the personality (ego circle). In the psychogenic case we therefore have to deal with a movement which goes from the center to the periphery. We may call such a movement centrifugal. If the symptom starts in the body and changes the attitude of the individual, we speak about the movement going from the periphery to the center of the personality, and call it a centripetal movement. In my book *The Image and Appearance of the Human Body* I have dwelt on these connotations in detail. We have to perceive our body. We build up the picture of our own body in space. I call this three-dimensional picture of one's body *the body image.* A symptom in the sense characterized above changes one's body image. The table of possible symptoms which I put at the beginning of this chapter is based upon this conception of the body image.

An organ can therefore be affected by psychological as well as by physiological processes. I have spoken about the principle of the two-way passage. Human problems of a specific type have, therefore, specific relations to specific organ systems. The disease of a specific organ system due to organic causes is liable to provoke specific psychological attitudes. Hence, when we approach the table of physical symptoms and ask for the meaning of every symptom, we should come to a general understanding of human problems.

It is through the surface of the body that we perceive ourselves and others. This perception of the outline of the body is the basis for one's attitude of self love towards one's body (narcissism). The problem of beauty is a social problem of the first order. We should know in every patient why he or she thinks himself or herself handsome or ugly. Organic and psychogenic skin diseases touch on this point. In one of my cases, for instance, the beginning of an acne around the sixteenth year changed the whole aspect of life. The general integrity of the body is symbolized by the integrity of its surface. The psychogenic aspect of skin diseases has been discussed by Klauder and myself.[2] There is a strong psychic reaction to mutilation and wounds in any part of the body. The reaction is stronger when parts are affected which have a social and an erotic value, like the face, the breasts, or the sex parts. The problem of castration thus links up with the wish of keeping the body intact as an integrated unit. All experiences of this kind reach back through their roots to early childhood. They are arranged in strata which we have to unearth if we wish to come to their complete understanding. We should never forget that the way in which we appreciate our body is dependent on how others appreciate it. The love we give to ourselves is based upon the love others have given to us. We may formulate the following questions for the patient: Are you beautiful? What do others think about your appearance?

Lauretta Bender has studied the psychic consequences of actual abnormalities in the body structure, especially those concerning size. In the treatment of neurosis one very often sees that children have suffered very much either by being considered too small or too tall. Changes in their relations to others and to themselves have followed.

The openings of the body provide us with more qualified sensations than the other parts of the body. They are, accordingly, psychologically more active than the rest of the body. They are erotic centers. The mouth as well as the anus has, of course, other important functions. It is a vital problem for every human being to keep the

---

[2] See also O. S. English, "Role of Emotions in Disorders of the Skin," *Archive of Dermatology and Syphilology* 60:1063–76. [L.B., Ed.]

openings intact. The fear of mutilation concerning the opening is continually in the foreground of human experience. This is another type of castration fear. Openings may be made in the body by force. Every wound is an opening. The individual then comes into a passive position. One can push something by force into openings. However, the individual may want to receive something in his openings. There is a voluntary and enforced passivity and submission concerning the openings of the body. Castration may lead to a forced passivity. Body openings can substitute, in a large measure, for each other. They are interchangeable. Children find their way to their openings partially by their own experimentation. However, parents and nurses, because of their own interest, may reinforce the importance of the one or the other of the openings. Such an overemphasized opening, for instance the anus, may then take over the functions of other openings, as of the genitals. I have observed a patient with a carcinoma of the rectum who developed, after a proctoscopy, a delusional and hallucinatory picture in which he feared that he might be forced to anal homosexual relations.

We then come to the following questions: Which openings of the body are of particular importance for an individual? Does the individual want to be passive concerning these openings? Does the individual fear to be forced into passivity through the openings?

It cannot be emphasized enough that one's own body and the bodies of others are in a continuous interrelation. The problem of openings and the problem of protrusions are very closely linked to each other. An individual who emphasizes his or her protrusions, such as nose, penis, finger, toe, may want to be active and to push the protrusion into the opening of another person. We come to the following questions: Which protrusion is of particular importance for an individual? Does the individual want to be active with the protrusion? Or does the individual feel like doing away with the protrusion?

Occlusion may impair the function of openings. It impairs the intake and the output; the occluded individual is not able to receive. The individual may wish to be occluded or may resent it. Occlusion may impair the female genital intake. This is one type of female castration complex. One may desire an excessive intake by the openings. The problems arise of sexual and oral greed and of the general desire of taking the world in. One may want to take in, either to keep or to give out. One may wish to push out in order to get rid of something—as in vomiting, for instance, in pregnancy. One may want to give out in order to give away and to give to others. Alexander and his co-workers have recently formulated similar problems in connection with gastrointestinal disturbances. They speak about tendencies to reception, to excretion, and to retention. The reception may be passive or aggressive taking. The elimination can be giving away or can be aggressive elimination. Cases of ulcer of the stomach show, for instance, a strong passive-receptive and active-receptive tendency. We add, therefore, the following questions: Does the individual want to take or give? Through which opening? What does the individual wish to put out of his system? Of course we have to ask again: What are the early experiences in which these tendencies manifest themselves? How are they linked up with later experiences? And which part do the attitudes of other persons play in it?

The symptoms of the senses can now be easily understood. The chief function of the senses is to take in, and the occlusion motive is the principal one concerning the senses. As far as the senses have a receptive function, they may symbolize any other opening. Many of the sense organs are connected with distinctive parts of the surface of the body which also serve decorative principles, as the eye and the ear and the nose. The sense organs also belong, from a psychological point of view, to the surface of the body. They are, accordingly, carriers of intensive self-love (narcissism).

The inside of the body is, according to my previous formulations, chiefly perceived as a heavy mass, not different from any other heavy mass. Whatever leads to an organic or psychogenic weakness of the muscular apparatus will make it insufficient in relation to the heavy mass of the body, and the apparent heaviness of the body will increase. Fatigue and paralysis will have certain effects irrespective of the organic or psychogenic origin. Since depression is to a great extent based on a fight against the individual's aggressive and sadistic tendencies, the individual inhibits his aggression so completely that weakness and fatigue result. Depression will thus increase the apparent weight of the body. Elation, with its free output of muscular energies, will decidedly decrease the apparent weight of the body. Whatever may influence the muscle tone will also change the apparent weight of the body.

The vestibular apparatus is one of the important regulative organs concerned with the apperception of the body weight. Its stimulation decreases the apparent weight. In the organic sphere, the vestibular apparatus is stimulated when there is a discrepancy in the data coming from the sense organs or when an organic process hits this spot of the body. In the psychological sphere, the vestibular apparatus answers easily when there are any conflicting instinctual drives. Serious conflicts will therefore influence the apparent body weight, the psychic conflicts acting on the physiological functions of the vestibule in the broadest sense. We then come to the following questions: Does the individual dare to permit his impulses to go free, or does he inhibit them because of his feeling of guilt? Are there conflicting inner drives? Why is the individual depressed or elated, and what are the tendencies behind it? Has the individual feelings of guilt, or is he self-confident and optimistic?

The mass which psychologically constitutes the inside of the body image is generally experienced as rather equally distributed and follows the laws of gravitation. When we stand upright, the density of this mass is greater at the base of the skull, in the lower part of the abdomen, and in the lower part of the legs. When we lie down, the mass is chiefly in the posterior part of the head, at the back, and around the calves. Emotional problems change the density of the body. When there is too much taken in, the stomach may feel too heavy. The fullness of the stomach may be organic or psychogenic. This links up with the problems of the openings of the body. What has been taken into the body can be food as well as feces or the penis. Local increases in density have a symbolic significance. They are due to a symbolic intake. Something sticks in the body. How does it come in or go out?

Local emptiness or lightness is a deprivation concerning the inside of the body. Something has been taken away. Something has been cut out. This links up with another facet of the castration complex. The following questions arise in the individual case: Does the individual want his body enriched by something coming from another individual or from another part of the outward world? Does the individual want passivity or activity? Is the person afraid of incompleteness inside of the body? Is he afraid that something inside the body may be destroyed? These problems link up with those of masculinity and femininity—i.e., to take the dense penis into an empty space or to take the dense child into the uterus. Does one want to have the food or the feces inside? The problems of the experience of local density in the body are thus linked with the general human problems of taking and giving in the sexual (genital) sphere and in the gastrointestinal sphere. The human problems corresponding to these symptoms are, therefore, very similar to the problems concerning the openings of the body. The local densities, increased or diminished, are the result of what is going in and out through the opening.

It is very difficult to treat the problems in connection with motility as a separate entity. It has been mentioned that individuals who are afraid of their aggressiveness inhibit their activity in general. If the inhibition is not completely successful, and the drives still demand to have at least some expression, restlessness may follow. Thus motility is associated with the general aims of the individual. Paralysis and weakness, as well as fatigue, express the unwillingness to act. A hysterical paralysis of the arm may be a self-punishment and a warning concerning a sexual action which either has been committed or was intended. Increased motility of all kinds will very often correspond to a partial satisfaction of drives. The hysterical fit very often corresponds to strong wishes for sexual intercourse. Tensions in the muscles correspond to sadistic attitudes which have found only an incomplete expression. Epileptic fits organically determined are very often connected with the expression of severe aggressive and sadistic tendencies. We may ask: How much sexuality do you intend to allow for yourself? Do you allow yourself masturbation and sexual intercourse, in reality and in phantasy? How often do you dare express your ill will and aggressiveness towards other persons? Which parts of your muscle system do you use especially in love and aggression?

Modern psychological theory and modern psychotherapy stress the importance of anxiety for the understanding of normal development and for the understanding of the problems of neurosis. Many analysts consider neurotic and psychotic symptoms as only defense reactions against anxiety, which thus becomes the cardinal problem of disease in the psychological sense. Freud advocated the belief that some types of anxiety are due to immediate toxic influence. The toxin might be furnished by incompleteness of sexual gratification. It is difficult to reconcile the modern point of view with this old formulation of Freud's. We might be inclined to believe that some organ systems have closer relations to anxiety than others. Ludwig Braun stresses the relation of the heart to anxiety. He seems to consider anxiety as a sensation originating in the heart. I am inclined to believe that we deal, at any rate, with a general personality reaction. According to the newer formulations of Freud, anxiety is a danger signal indicating a danger coming from inside or outside. His paradigm for the outside danger is the castration. But also the inward danger originates from sexual drives which could lead the individual into situations which ultimately lead again to castration.

In my opinion, the castration fear is only one of the many expressions of the fear that the integrity of the body might be violated. Maybe it is its foremost representative. However, the basic complex is the fear of being dismembered. Anxiety, therefore, sums up the dangers which may threaten on the outside of the body, the inside of the body, and its openings. It is understandable that the organic threat to such an important organ as the heart finds its reflection in the psychological sphere in anxiety. Freud believed previously that he knew the energies from which neurotic anxiety came. He thought it was transformed sexual energy. He later became skeptical about his previous assumption. All psychic processes are connected with energies in the sense that energies are physiological entities. Since at least many processes of anxiety are connected with sexual problems, I do not see any fundamental difficulty in assuming that so-called sexual energies participate in the phenomenon of anxiety. Since the problem of dismembering transgresses the sexual limits, I do not believe that sexual energies alone enter this process. I am not inclined to believe that anxiety and fear are fundamentally different from each other. As I have stated on another occasion, the object of fear is circumscribed and clear-cut, whereas the individual is not quite aware of the object of his anxiety. The newer formulation of Freud is progress in so far as it stresses the danger situation and the reaction of an individual in a situation. It is obvious that organic disease must lead to situations of fear and anxiety, since every impairment of the body and of the body functions is experienced as a threat of further impairment. Chronic heart disease and decompensation manifest themselves very clearly with difficulties in breathing, the genesis of which is not our concern. The individual is impaired in the important matter of intake of air. There is the danger of occlusion and suffocation. Every organic disease and every organic impairment of function carries with it specific fears and anxieties.

Anxiety is very often, though not always, connected with the fear of death. Death means, then, deprivation, to be unable to keep the body together, to take something in or to push something out. We come, therefore, to the general questions: What are you afraid of? What is your attitude towards death? Are you afraid to die?

Death means, of course, not only mutilation and deprivation in the narrower sense, but also to be removed from those whom one loves. It is an interruption of object relations. It is a bereavement, even if one's own body is intact, either to have one's loved ones die or to be removed from them, even if it is not by death but by separation in space. The following questions arise: Are you afraid to be alone? Are you afraid to die alone? These fears reflect basic tendencies of our relations to love objects, and we have to ask: What do all these fears mean in relation to father, mother, and other love objects? I have discussed in detail the question of angina pectoris and have emphasized its organic character. It provokes a specific attitude of anxiety of the same structure as an anxiety based upon psychogenic motives. Psychogenic anxiety, although not the cause of the disease as such, doubtless can provoke a single anginal attack. The data are insufficient at present to proceed with a general theory, but the suspicion is aroused that those psychic situations may gain an influence on the course of an organic disease which correspond to the psychic attitudes provoked by the disease. The enormous motor discharge provoked by the organic process of the epileptic attack leads, as mentioned, to sadistic attitudes. Situations of anger very often provoke epileptic attacks after a latency of a few hours.

Dizziness is the psychological sign of a sensual or moral disorientation in the world. Do you know what you want to do? Do you think you act in the right way by following your instincts? Are you sure that you have homosexual interests or not? Dizziness is a danger signal as important as anxiety. It is the first sign that we are no longer sure what to do. Dizziness is, from a merely organic point of view, a sign which may occur in the beginning of almost any organic disease. It is possible that psychogenic factors, indicating the feeling of insecurity in this world, participate. Psychogenic dizziness can be found in almost every neurosis, especially in the beginning.

Nausea is the beginning of an attitude of rejection, of course primarily concerned with the intake into the gastrointestinal tract, but in further development it is an attitude towards any kind of intake. It is connected with the feeling that one cannot keep what has been ingested and that one is helpless and weak and unable to satisfy one's cravings concerning the openings. The weakness expresses the attitude that muscular effort is useless or impossible, since the individual rejects the intake or is unable to take in. The following questions arise: What are you striving for? What is your aim in life? What do you live for? Is it worth while, what you can reach? Are you satisfied with what you have? Do you want to give up whatever you may have?

In order to reach something, in order to get satisfaction, we need action. Action in human beings is based upon the system of striped muscles and the complicated apparatus in the nervous system which is the basis for action. To reach a goal we must handle objects. We must get hold of them and master them. These objects are animate or inanimate. Action is mastery of objects and contains in itself a component of destruction. When we move an object from one place to another, we disturb the peace of the object. Acting, we shall become superior. Exaggerating, we may say that acting in itself contains a tendency to blend with destructive and sexual elements and thus to become sadistic. The best instance of this is the hyperkinesis in encephalitic children who grow destructive by the increase in motor impulse on an organic basis. We want to be strong to be able to fight. If we feel thwarted in our ability to act, we may become weak and submissive.

The following questions arise: Are you strong? Do you want to be strong? Do you want to be superior? Do you have confidence in your superiority? Can you stand being in an inferior position? Are you cruel? What do you want to reach in life?

Weakness means giving up or being forced to give up in these respects. It is, therefore, a sign that the individual is not able to handle any of his problems. Weakness is paramount in every severe organic disease, but it is also the expression of any neurotic disturbance in which the individual feels that he is no longer able to exert his power, or that he is morally no longer entitled to do so. The complaint of inability to act is thus closely connected with conscious and unconscious feelings of guilt.

Fatigue is psychologically very closely allied to weakness. Organically it occurs when the power of the individual has been overtaxed. We have reason to believe that fatigue from overwork is easily and quickly reversible unless a definite organic process is going on.

Otherwise, in functional cases it is the sign that the individual no longer feels equal to his tasks. He confesses in this way that his aims are not worth while and that he should resign. When aggressiveness and sadism have become too strong, the individual will often feel that he should check himself. Fatigue thus becomes a symptom in the sadistic neurasthenic and the depressive case.

The following questions arise: Have you been too aggressive in pursuing your aims? Are you able to continue to be aggressive? Is it right that you were aggressive and that you are aggressive? I have used the term "sadism," indicating that the problem of aggressiveness and submission, superiority and inferiority, activity and passivity, link up with the problems of sex, masculinity and femininity. The ideology of our civilization is based upon the wrong assumption that masculinity and activity are identical and that femininity and passivity are the same. Human beings therefore live with the fear of being too feminine and too passive when they are men. The fear of castration is closely linked with the fear of being too passive. In the female, fear of being active may be the expression of the fear of not being feminine enough and losing the psychological and anatomical possibility of receiving. The questions arise: Are you active or passive? Are you courageous? Can you be passive and receptive with good conscience? Must one fight? Must one feel masculine (if a man)? Must one be feminine (if a woman)? Do you have characteristics of the other sex? Are you afraid of having characteristics of the other sex?

I have always felt that the correction of the wrong ideology concerning masculinity and femininity is an important part in every psychotherapeutic approach, and that the courage of being passive and of confessing to one's own passive side is a necessary step for a deeper adaptation. The general problems of restlessness and tension have been discussed previously.

Pain is not merely a local sensation, but an impairment of the activity of a total body. It therefore sums up the dangers threatening the body and the inabilities of individuals to master the situation in which they are. It is thus a central point in which all the complexes, fears, and attitudes of the individual find their expression.

The questions arise: Are you afraid of pain? What do you do in order to escape pain? Do you want to inflict pain on others? In which situations do you suffer mental pain?

Human beings are not sums of organs, but there is a unit—the organism. The reflection of the organ systems into the psyche is, after all, only a partial view of the problem. Personalities as such have goals and aims in life and are driven by desires and instincts. Different systems of psychotherapy see individuals driven by the force of their past experience—as, for example, psychoanalysis—or attracted by goals and aims before them. Human beings go into the future but picture the future and develop their aims through the past. The following questions arise: What do you live for? What is your idea of a good time? How much money do you need a month in order to be happy?

The problems of human nature are: (1) the problems of social aims and adaptations crystallized in the attitudes towards money; (2) the problems of strength, force, superiority, and aggressiveness; (3) the problems connected with sex, expressing themselves in the questions of masculinity and femininity. The attitudes towards death express all our goals and aims and instincts.

The fundamental problems of human beings are never seen clearly by themselves. Every one of these problems is surrounded by a system of verbalized ideas in which tradition and individual history are summed up. Instinctual difficulties lead to ideologies which, for their part, are the form in which the instincts are pressed. Words have to fortify these ideologies, especially when the words are only incompletely understood, as is usually the case.

There is no difference in this respect between the cases who suffer from organic and psychogenic disturbances. If we want to understand the psychology of the organic case we must see him as a person with his problems, we must understand the reflection of the organ systems into the psyche. We may help him then in his attitude towards the disease, and in some cases will be able to change the symptoms which are in a sense defined as dependent upon the personality. In a small number of cases we might even be able to influence the organic process as such and to change the course of the disease. The influence of the psychological process on the single manifestation of the disease may occur even if the basic process has not fundamentally changed.

Our approach has, so far, been very one-sided. We have studied organic and psychogenic symptomatology merely from the point of view of the body, or better, the body image. But suffering is not only related to body suffering; it is also mental suffering. In the final analysis, as the above discussion has shown, both must be identical. Mental problems are not only mental problems but find their expression also in the body image. Organic problems are not merely organic problems but find their expression in the psychic processes too. It is well worth while approaching the problem of mental suffering. Our subsequent discussions will, therefore, deal with the symptomatology as far as it expresses itself in mental suffering.

Chapter 3

THE SYMPTOMATOLOGY OF MENTAL SUFFERING

FRANZ BRENTANO has stated in his *Psychology from an Empirical Point of View* that human beings not only have sensations, feelings, and thoughts, but also know when they experience, and when they feel, and when they have sensations and thoughts. Self-observation thus becomes one of the fundamental characteristics of experience. Theodor Reik has added that the function of self-observation is in connection with the fact that we see ourselves with the eyes of others. He ascribes the function of self-observation to the superego in the psychoanalytic sense. The superego originates by the identification of the child with the parent. It is certainly true that when self-observation has become dominant, the patient sees himself in the way others have seen him before and would be likely to see him now. However, every experience is socialized in itself. We are continually experimenting not only with our experiences concerning the outward world but also in order to bring our inner experiences into a coherent context. We compare each experience with other experiences. We live in different levels at the same time. The term *inner experience* has aroused many controversies among psychologists and philosophers. It is used here in a very simple sense. We are partially directed straight towards the world of objects and partially towards processes going on in ourselves, such as sensations, phantasies, representations, thoughts and feelings. We call these latter processes inner experiences.

The tendency towards the outward world, however, is also present in these inner experiences. The process of self-observation is a process of great activity. We see ourselves with the eyes of almost everybody with whom we come in contact, and we make an effort to react to a unified view of ourselves. We try to see ourselves with our own eyes, quite in the same way as we know very little about our own appearance and have to construct our body image very often with the help of a mirror to find out what we are. We are never completely satisfied, we try again and again to find out what we are as persons with inner experiences.

Self-observation is not merely self-criticism; it is a much more general function. We are never theoretical observers of ourselves. We observe ourselves in order to find out how far we are capable of action and success in the outward world. Furthermore, we want to know whether we are able to get the love, admiration, and esteem of the other person. We measure ourselves concerning our ability to perform the tasks of life. It is astonishing how much and how many things we demand of ourselves. We continually exert checks and controls over ourselves. We ask what we should eat and how much we should eat. We require of ourselves that we should work, write letters, study, read certain books, sleep longer or shorter hours, save money, and so forth. There are innumerable tasks in the course of a day which are not only demanded from us but which we demand from ourselves.

It is a matter of experience that any particular degree of aggressiveness and any strong demand for love change the function of self-observation. Aggressiveness turns into self-observation and self-criticism when its direct outlet is prohibited. Every individual asks himself two questions: Am I lovable? Can I be successful? If individuals overemphasize these questions to themselves, they will sometimes feel that they are supremely attractive and superior and will, from there, plunge into the misery of feeling unlovable and inferior. There will be wide swings between an attitude of exaggerated self-appreciation and an attitude of self-depreciation. These swings are present in some degree in everybody. We do not always feel completely satisfied with our achievements in regard to our inner and outer experiences.

This process of testing ourselves is closely related to our actions, and self-observation plays an enormous part in judging the efficiency of our actions. It is understandable that success and failure very often determine the appreciation we give to ourselves. The discontentment in one's self manifests itself in what Janet has called "sentiments d'incomplètude," feelings of incompleteness and insufficiency concerning our psychic functioning. In the so-called depersonalization cases these feelings of incompleteness reach a pitch. They extend over the whole realm of psychic life. The patients complain that they are unable to think, to feel, and to imagine. Furthermore, they complain that their perception is incomplete and unsatisfactory and finally they depreciate themselves as a whole and call themselves automatons and dolls.

Lilian S., for instance, says that previously she had felt important when she was talking, now she feels unimportant. She thinks that others are important and clever. In her childhood she admired her father and he seemed important to her. A.A., suffering from a severe social neurosis, would very much like to be important, brilliant, and clever in conversation, but he always lags behind his ideal for himself. When others talk, they seem to be important and clever. Gertrude Stein, in her novel *Americans in the Making,* emphasizes justly whether her Americans feel important and have an important feeling in themselves. She further asks whether these people feel important in the one or the other sphere of life—as, for instance, one may feel important in religion, or in business.

Indeed, we make general demands of ourselves and then view our shortcomings, but we insist that we be capable of specific tasks. We may ask that we be capable of observing correctly, of seeing clearly, or we may seek the capacity for a rich phantasy life. We may desire to limit our exuberance in daydreams and phantasies. There may be a desire to be educated, clever, and brilliant, and we suffer when we fail in this respect. Very often specific demands concerning one's emotions are raised. One of my patients, Edna, demands from herself that she always love her children with a deep love. The complaint of not being able to love fully is one frequently encountered in early depressions as well as in depersonalization cases. One may also complain that one loves too much, is too dependent upon a person. The individual may regret his own jealousy. One may not only be sad, but complain that one is sad. Many people feel that they are not good enough. They want to have nobler feelings. They want to direct their thoughts and tendencies.

There is suffering if a thought cannot be eliminated from one's thinking. We then speak about obsessions. The individual suffers either because these thoughts or imaginations do not fit the situation and hinder him in enjoying his mode of existence, or because they are an impediment in the performance of a specific task. We shall hear later that the power of otherwise seemingly indifferent thoughts to disturb is bestowed on them by strong emotional drives for which they substitute. There are many such drives in the individual which are not tolerated, and one suffers because of these drives and impulses which are not approved by society and by the part of the psychic organization which represents the society.

The sex drives are rather complicated in their nature. Indeed, one needs a rather strong constructive effort to come to an appreciation of a love object from a physical and mental point of view as well. Sexuality has many part functions. We may mention the oral and the anal ones, which have to be integrated into the total pattern. This integration is not always completely successful, and the individuals become impatient with themselves. They disapprove of their sexual drives in full or in part, are unable to change them, and suffer by their continuous presence. They may be made discontented by the force of the sex desires or by the special direction they are taking. They may also be discontented because their drives are too weak or even absent. A., for instance, during periods of impotency complains bitterly that he has no sex feelings at all.

Emotions, feelings, drives, have a tendency to become full actions. This is indeed their real meaning. I have shown elsewhere that the customary division of experiences into sensory experiences, emotions, and actions has only a limited value and is basically artificial, since we are continually acting. Every obsession and every drive has in it an element of action which becomes a compulsion when the individual refuses to act in the direction of this drive or disapproves of the act when it has been performed.

Obsessions and compulsions are indeed very closely related to each other. Compulsions can be classified in three large groups. The one type of compulsion consists of indifferent acts which merely hinder the individual in the performance of the tasks he has put before himself. The individual may feel compelled to count the number of windows, or may feel the urge to look again and again to see whether a door is actually closed. Obviously, as in obsessions of the same type, these tendencies or actions have gained their influence from another source and are merely substitutes. In the second type of compulsion the individual reacts to his unpleasant feelings and thoughts and tries to relieve them—for instance, in the compulsion to wash one's hands again and again. Compulsions of this type are almost exclusively in connection with dirt and fecal matter. In the third group the individual feels compelled to sexual and aggressive acts of which he disapproves. The purely sexual compulsion is rarer. One of my patients suffered from the compulsion to perform cunnilingus on her daughter. The contents of compulsions are mostly of an aggressive type. The one individual wants to curse God. The other individual wants to kick people in their genitals. The third one may want to cut other people to pieces. Edna feels the urge to kill her children. In the chapter on obsession neurosis, more details will be given.

It is obvious that the individuals suffering from difficulties in any part function of psychic experience do not merely disapprove of this part function, but disapprove of themselves as a whole and as responsible carriers of this part function. One should keep in mind that individuals do not suffer in the final analysis from a mysterious change in the fictitious entities of sensation, imagination, thought, feeling, and action, but that they suffer for their actions as a person in a situation. The difficulties arise from actual situations and attitudes. Even when the individual experiences a general incompleteness in his attitudes, this incompleteness has arisen from specific problems. The partial incompleteness of experience which has been characterized above originates in the same way from specific situations, although the individual may not be aware of it. Whenever the individual blames himself or suffers from an insufficiency in one of his psychic functions, he also objects to himself as a person.

When the individual blames himself for his sexual drives and actions, feelings of guilt originate. Aggressiveness leads also to feelings of guilt. Late in his life, Freud held the opinion that feelings of guilt originate only from aggressive impulses. This formulation is too narrow. Feelings of guilt appear whenever the individual has impulses or commits actions against the moral code. This moral code either originates from society or is self-imposed. In the latter case, it is also social in origin. It is, therefore, a derivative of the fear of punishment.

Fears, of course, are devastating. There is tension and incompleteness of the situation in fear. When the punishment is received, the fear is relieved. The tension no longer exists. Furthermore, if the punishment has not led to a complete annihilation, the individual may be again secure and get approval and love from those who have punished him. The individual may even wish punishment in order to be relieved of his tension and have the situation completed. Freud and Reik have justly spoken of a wish for punishment of which the individual may not even be aware. Fear and its counterpart, anxiety, in which the object of fear is not clearly defined, show clearly that inner processes cannot be understood unless one sees them in relation to the outside world. The individual who fears or is in a state of anxiety has not merely the fear and anxiety, but is aware of it and suffers because of their presence.

Suffering, in connection with one's relations to other human beings, deserves special interest. One of the symptoms is shyness. I illustrate this by the report of a woman patient who, according to the opinion of the author, was not only better-looking than the average, but also endowed with a superior intelligence.

"I think that what I fear in social situations is not that people will not agree to an overevaluation of myself, but rather that they will confirm my low evaluation. I seem to hope that I am not really so bad or that at least I can get away with it, but I am always somewhat afraid that I will be found out. The trouble is, I have not the least idea what could be found out. Up until the last few years I think the difficulty appeared almost exclusively in larger social groups where the purpose of gathering was fun. When there was something for me to do, that is, where there were some prescribed patterns of my behavior, I had little trouble. Important interviews about scholarships, jobs, and so on, scarcely worried me at all, far less than they do most people. I felt little embarrassment in making family visits in connection with my husband's business and could conduct a rather delicate interview with some skill and almost no self-consciousness. Meeting that same woman a week later on a purely social footing, I would feel familiar insecurity and not be able to find the appropriate nothings to say. Even now, I am not bothered in situations where I have any conviction that I am right. I have several times put on a fearless and skillful fight when I felt sure of my position, but I really do not feel sure of my position. I have the underlying conviction that I am not a good teacher and that my methods are muddled and my personality uninspiring; therefore any deviation from the expected I interpret as an indication that my shortcomings have been discovered. I have the same feeling of my handling of that particular problem but not about my previous work.

"What worries me now is the fact that this lack of self-respect is becoming so pervasive. Last summer especially I felt that I had nothing at all to do. Frank (my husband) loves me. I did think that he was unreasonable in many of his positions . . . and on the whole I am a 'nice' girl. I mean I have not deliberately hurt anyone else. I don't make much trouble and I am sympathetic and generous. Lots of women, worse off than that, expect their husbands to love them. Evidently there is something wrong with my attitude towards myself. It could be, I suppose, à la Adler, I have set my goal too high, that it can never be achieved and that my mechanism for handling the situation is blaming myself before anyone else has the chance. It is a poor mechanism, though, because I do it not only with other people but with myself and get no satisfaction at all out of it, and anyway, this high goal should correspond to a deep sense of inferiority about something and I can't figure out what that something is. It seems to me more likely that instead of trying to preserve my self-respect by this mechanism, I am constantly punishing myself. What for? This absurd fear of being found out must indicate a profound sense of guilt.

"One thing I am afraid of, so much so that I can hardly bring myself to write it down, is that all this indicates a complete absorption in myself and that I am a God-damned narcissist and really love only myself. I have thought at times that I don't really love Frank but only the response he calls forth in me. I have thought that another man who offered the same satisfactions would do as well, but when I try to describe these necessary satisfactions I find that I have painted a pretty accurate picture of Frank himself and that the chances of my ever meeting his twin are rather remote and I have even here really been fearing a shadow. Can love be anything but one's own response to a person? Actually I am quite willing to give up my interests for his and I think I do honestly want his happiness quite apart from my own.

"In my dealings with other people, I find that I have frequently the feeling that I wouldn't dare to be nice to them. It actually seems to me a presumption to greet people cordially, send them little presents, etc., that I might be making advances to them which they would rather not have to answer. The question that seems to me important about this narcissism business is whether I really am narcissistic or whether I am using this fear, too, as a punishment for myself."

This is a rather clear report indicating the close relation between social shyness and depreciation of one's self. It is also interesting in so far as the patient, well versed in modern psychology, uses the ideology and terminology of psychoanalysis in the service of self-depreciation. The term "narcissism" deserves special attention. It has been devised by Freud to indicate primarily the love of one's own body. The theory was based on the wrong assumption that the individual knows about his body before he knows about the outside world.

Since I have dealt with the problem in detail on other occasions, I repeat merely those points which are of importance in connection with our practical problem. My own investigations have convinced me that the narcissistic person is in no way self-sufficient. On the contrary, narcissism is built on the influx of love from the love object. The child demands, needs, and receives this love from his mother. True narcissism would therefore be a certainty of obtaining a sufficient amount of love, which will protect against danger. When an individual is sure of such a love, he has every reason to be contented with himself. Narcissism is, therefore, self-assurance, based upon satisfaction and security in relation to other persons. The difficulties arise only in the later stages of development, when the individual makes such excessive demands for love that he does not care by whom he is given this love, and his relations to other people are leveled off. This patient, too, needs appreciation by everybody. She approaches others in a state of submission which of necessity later on has to lead to compensatory aggression. The patient speaks, furthermore, about the feeling of guilt. The importance of guilt feelings should not be underrated. But Freud and the new psychoanalytic literature had almost forgotten that guilt feelings are not the only feelings which indicate that the individual is discontented with himself. There are many ways in which human beings can feel that they are not equal to the tasks which confront them.

It is obvious that shyness and social insufficiency, subjectively experienced, are of very great importance in the symptomatology of neurotic suffering. Whenever there is any incompleteness experienced in one's own person, it must, since our psychic life is so thoroughly socialized, be felt in relation to other persons. "The social neurosis" is indeed of a practical importance which has not been sufficiently emphasized until now. It appears in every form of social intercourse. It may appear in an intensified form when the social character of the function is emphasized, as in public appearances for public speaking, or on the stage. Stage fright is merely a pregnant expression of social shyness. In stammering, the same problem finds a motor expression in speech, which is a communicative and socializing function par excellence. It is immediately obvious that all symptoms of subjective suffering do not remain merely in the subjective sphere, but find an outlet in motility. The complaint of not being lovable sums up many important problems of suffering.

I have merely attempted a description and classification of complaints as far as they pertain to inner experiences, in contrast to the complaints which concern the body image. But inner experience and experience concerning the body belong close together. We might venture the assumption that whenever an individual complains about himself as a person or about one of his functions, physical symptoms will occur. Indeed, in the social neurosis a wealth of somatic symptoms appears. Stammering, for instance, in which organic changes may play some part, can be considered a physical as well as a psychological symptom. Tension and restlessness have been mentioned under the symptomatology concerning physical experience. They could have been mentioned as well under the symptomatology of inner experiences.

We return to the symptomatology of social neurosis and shyness. Here we find blushing and sweating, which are doubtless somatic manifestations. Tremors and shakiness are common. Depersonalization cases do not complain only about the incompleteness of their experience, but they complain in addition about somatic changes. Hypochondriasis is, indeed, always connected with depersonalization.

In patients who complain about incompleteness of their sex experiences, somatic expressions in the form of impotency, premature ejaculation, spermatorrhea, and prostatorrhea are common. In obsession neurosis, symptoms of the gastrointestinal tract are not uncommon. No experience pertains merely to the psychic side of life; experiences are psychic and somatic. One has talked about conversion when somatic symptoms occur under emotional difficulties. The term has been created by Breuer and Freud. In their opinion psychic energies which cannot be lived out in the normal way, since the traumatic scene is repressed and forgotten, are diverted into other pathways and there provoke symptoms in the somatic sphere. Later on, Freud substituted for the original idea of the trauma, which provokes a hypnosis-like state and forgetting, the theory that the forgetting is due to a psychic defense. He substituted for the traumatic scene in general the psychosexual trauma as the origin of defense mechanisms and repressive tendencies, and conversion was now defined as a diversion of psychosexual energies into somatic pathways. The term has proved its usefulness. As to its interpretation I may point to the discussion in my book, *The Image and Appearance of the Human Body*. I do think a broader formulation is advisable. Psychological attitudes are psychosomatic attitudes and express themselves in the experiences of the body. Psychological conflicts and difficulties of psychological adaptation find an expression in the somatic sphere which may be more imposing. Since in every psychic conflict continuous experimentation is going on in the psychological as well as in the physiological sphere, conversion symptoms always have a history dating back as far as the history of the psychological conflict and are the result of a previous experimentation with one's own body. The conversion symptom thus becomes an accentuation of a general principle of psychosomatic experience.

Neurosis does not result only in suffering but also in failure in one's relations to other persons and to the world.[1] Neurosis is, in this respect, similar to sickness. Almost all neurotics complain that their neurosis hinders them from having the success to which they are entitled on the basis of their intellectual and human values. The patients afflicted with hysteria behave exactly like patients with somatic diseases. They complain that their illness hinders them from doing what they could otherwise do. They mostly complain not so much about difficulties in their thinking and emotions as about difficulties in the physical sphere. Captivated by their illness, they are hindered in their achievements.

Patients with social neuroses complain that their shyness, blushing, and sweating hinder them from social contacts, and they feel

[1] Reprinted from Paul Schilder, "Success and Failure," *Psychoanalytic Review* 29:353–72, 1942. [L.B., Ed.]

that they fail in their total adaptation since they fail in their relation to others. Success means for these patients poise, social graces, and friends. They crave the superficial admiration the man gets who is entertaining at a party. Alan did not want to be only a social leader and brilliant conversationalist but also a great success with women. Every woman whom he desired should give in without making much trouble. She should love him to the utmost as long as he desired, but there shouldn't be any difficulty if he wanted to end the relation. The girl shouldn't suffer too much but should continue loving him. He was extremely unsuccessful in business and had lost a great amount of money. In his daydreams he was a great builder, erecting houses and becoming rich. Although he had a rather large income he was not satisfied and would like to have spent more and to live in greater luxury. He suffered from shyness, was continually concerned with the suffering of himself and others, and was masochistic from earliest childhood. To escape his suffering would have meant success to him. He was convinced that his intellectual and personal endowment was far above the average but was not manifest because of his neurosis. These are typical features of a social neurosis.

The situation in stammerers is very similar. All these cases make excessive claims concerning their intellectual and personal endowment. They are afraid of failure and get the attention which they can't get by work and action in the neurotic symptom, which assures them that all the others are interested in them as sufferers.

In the obsessional neurotic cases the neurosis makes work and success difficult or impossible, and the patients are very well aware of this fact.

In most of the neuroses the failure adds to the fascination of the neurosis. The failure keeps one dependent and in an infantile status. One is not tempted any more to brave other dangers, and the definite annihilation is averted. One is punished by one's failures and the feeling of guilt is alleviated by this punishment. The neurotic accepts failure as a lesser punishment in order to avoid the greater dangers of complete annihilation.

Failure occurs when the problems of the present and of the future are dealt with from the point of view of problems of childhood. Rigidity occurs—reality is tackled from the point of view of whether it offers fulfillment of childhood wishes or escape from them. In this case the father plays the paramount part. The patient is still subjected to him. The person who fails submits himself to the superior force and clings to submission although it may be connected with suffering. It is characteristic for all these patients that they give up without any real struggle and without any real trial. They are either too convinced of their own capacities so that trial seems to be unnecessary or they are convinced that the will is thwarted anyhow. There may be an attempt to cover the basic wish for inactivity and suffering by mechanical and rigid activity.

These phenomena have very close relation to what psychoanalysis calls moral masochism. Fenichel has justly mentioned that compulsive actions are very often combined with moral masochism. One might be inclined to say that failure is the result of the wish for punishment. Such a formulation is superficial in view of the complicated facts mentioned before. Fenichel writes: "The moral masochist who exposes himself to punishment by fate gets in reality beaten by his father which in turn is a transformed expression for being the object of intercourse for one's father." Freud previously mentioned character types who answer with neurotic illness when they have success.

The cases mentioned have no neurotic symptoms, or only unimportant ones. They fail in their social endeavors. Failure is, in this respect, a perversion in social function. The individual who fails without having neurotic symptoms in any higher degree considers the suffering as the effect of circumstances and of the aggression of others. He does not blame himself, and a feeling of guilt is not present on the surface. There are at least some cases in which the feeling of guilt is also particularly weak on the unconscious level.

The neurotic as well as the individual who fails without having neurotic symptoms are bound by early childhood experiences and have given up experimentation prematurely. However, the neurotic gets some primitive satisfaction out of his symptoms and out of his suffering. He continually strives for gratification, although he strives to get gratification in an infantile manner. The symptom is a gratification in itself. It is in the sphere of the symptom where the experimentation has stopped. The individual who fails may derive masochistic satisfaction from his failing. However, he also stops his activity partially because he derives a great deal of satisfaction from the love his superego gives to his ego. It is really not necessary for him to act in an efficient way. His arrest is an arrest in social functions.

Failure, like neurosis, is the product of specific constellations in early childhood which come into appearance in connection with the situations of later life. One can say with certainty that the attitudes of the parents in which exaggerated admiration is combined with outbursts of aggression and severity are particularly dangerous. These different attitudes may be found in one parent or may be distributed between the two parents. It seems that if the parents fail in establishing an atmosphere of confidence, which allows the child a free experimentation with judgment and action, the chances of successful performance of the individual in later life are further diminished. Adaptability is only possible when the individual retains a curiosity for the world and is not chiefly interested in admiring his own capacity.

When failure is established one should consider it an illness which should be treated like a neurosis or, better, like a perversion. In the majority of cases it is useless to expound to the individual what he should be. The analysis of the present situation alone is useless, and the patient has to come to an insight into his early family situation. He must find out why he wants to suffer and why he thinks he is perfect enough so that he doesn't need any action by which he can prove that he is capable of mastering the world. In the majority of severe cases it is necessary to analyze for a long time before the patient gets a grasp of the banal possibilities of everyday life.

It is obvious that we are discussing only mental symptoms, but every ailment of one person, be it organic or psychogenic, necessarily influences the lives of other persons. It changes the attitude of the sick person, has an influence upon his capacity to work, and necessitates a change in the attitude of those who are around him.

The same is true about any mental suffering of a person, since the change in the attitude of one person necessarily influences the community.

The symptoms about which other people complain are those in the sphere of perception and intellect, of emotional attitudes, and of actions. This division is schematic since behavior is the common denominator of all disturbances.

In the sphere of perception the individual may be clouded in his consciousness. Hallucinations are perceptions which are not acknowledged by the community and therefore lead to a behavior which is disturbing to the community. Delusions are convictions unverified by others, originating in the private world of an individual and firmly rooted in his personality structure; they are outside of the process of social experimentation which leads either to a correction or at least a diminution of their dynamic value concerning behavior. It may sometimes be difficult to draw a sharp line between delusions and religious, moral, political, and social convictions. We know that everybody builds up intellectual structures, ideologies, which are also rooted in the life history of the individual and have become crystallized and comparatively stable. Still, ideologies do not have the rigidity of delusions, and far from belonging to the private world of an individual, they are shared by smaller and larger groups and are, very often, the connecting link between the members of such groups.

In the so-called intellectual sphere the lack of judgment and disturbances in the memory function, as seen in mental deficiency, general paresis, senility, and Korsakoff syndrome, may impair, more or less severely, the social usefulness of an individual.

In the emotional sphere, a lack of drive and loss of interest may appear on the surface of the mental picture in schizophrenics. Psychopathic individuals may offer similar pictures. We have reason to believe that emotional indifference in all these cases is merely on the surface and that the individual is overwhelmed by difficult problems. This is also true in a great number of so-called psychopathic individuals who do not obviously suffer in their attitudes but seem to suffer merely by the reaction of society towards their social futility or dangerous behavior. This is the problem of the criminal as well as of the pervert.

The drives of an individual, dependent on organic and psychological factors, may be excessive. If connected with elation we find manic pictures which, in their milder states, lead to actions in the sexual and social sphere which are disapproved. In the severe degrees of manic excitement, defense reactions of the community become necessary, by which the individual feels impaired. Similar considerations can be applied to the more aimless drives of encephalitics.

One may consider the criminal also from the point of view of acting in the wrong way. It is more difficult to understand the asocial behavior of the schizophrenic, whose drives are either merely exaggerated or diminished but mostly show a qualitative aberration.

It has been said about the person who makes others suffer that suffering, although not manifest, is experienced by him. The suffering either is based upon somatic sensations, or is mental suffering due to unsolved problems or to the observation that one's mental processes are changed. In addition, there very often is the suffering inflicted by the disapproval of society and by the measures of society taken against those whose behavior is of no social value. Obviously we deal in this group either with psychopathy and crime or with mental deficiency and psychosis.

It is obvious that the psychotherapeutic approach, so far as it is possible, cannot be identical to the one in which the individual himself desires relief from his suffering. In cases in which the organic factor is not paramount, the individual may be brought to a level of behavior by which he avoids the social counterreaction. Although convinced of the justice of his delusional or asocial claim, he may be brought to understand that it is wiser to yield the point. Experience has proved that such an approach is very often ineffective. I have mentioned that there are indications that in many of the cases who do not seem to suffer, suffering of which the individual is not aware may be present. The psychotherapeutic procedure would necessitate bringing the suffering into the foreground of consciousness. The individual would have to feel sick before we would be able to help him.

Is the lawbreaker really sick, and is he a problem for the physician or for the educator and lay penologist? [2] Generally we consider as sick only persons who suffer. However, this connotation has to be enlarged immediately since a person might not know that he is sick and his suffering might be postponed. Furthermore, there are deformations and physical shortcomings which merely impair the appearance or function of the individual without provoking direct pain or suffering. We would not hesitate to consider such individuals as sick. There exists furthermore a comparatively large number of cases of mental illness in which the patient does not experience suffering or feel ill. Cases of this type have, of course, difficulties in providing for themselves. They have difficulties in the community; they offend others who take revenge, and they would perish if no special

[2] The next six paragraphs were taken from Paul Schilder, "The Cure of the Criminal and Prevention of Crime," *Journal of Clinical Psychopathology* 2:146–61, 1940.

help were given to them. Sooner or later physical discomfort would be the natural consequence of their behavior even if they had not become ill physically, as would happen in a general paresis case.

The so-called criminal certainly does not suffer directly from his criminality. He is not ill and he suffers primarily and consciously merely from the counterreactions of the community. He is in this respect like a psychopathic individual, if one uses these terms in a larger sense. We are accustomed to find in the noncriminal psychopath indications of difficulties in early life, and we consider his psychopathic action and shortcomings as comparable to neurotic symptoms, the difference being that the psychopath does not fight against his infantile strivings, which are nevertheless of symbol-like meaning. The neurotic does fight against the infantile tendencies which are about to break through. This is particularly true concerning sexual perversions, which are in most of the cases punishable by law. The assumption that a thief also has to be considered a sick person obviously conveys with it the meaning that his stealing does not merely imply the wish to get the valued object or money but has a meaning beyond that, which we call symbolic. The fact remains that the majority of criminals do not show any suffering in the ordinary sense, and furthermore mental illness is comparatively rare among them. S. H. Tulchin and others have also shown that there are no major deviations in the intelligence quotient, though E. Glueck has a somewhat different opinion. One sees that the idea that the criminal should be treated is therefore based upon rather complicated assumptions.

It is furthermore necessary to keep in mind that the term *criminal action* does not mean a specific action of an individual but means merely the attitude of the community in relation to a specific action. In other words, criminal action is an action which the law punishes. It expresses a specific relation of an individual who commits it to society. This formulation makes it clear that the problem is, in its major aspect, a sociological problem and can only be understood from the point of view of the individual's relation to society. It is, for instance, spurious to say that aggressive criminals might have been of a particular social value in a society which honors aggression also in peacetime. Such a formulation neglects the fact that it is always a particular type of aggression which is approved, and it is the capacity or incapacity to adapt which lies at the basis of the difficulties.

One may try to seek the basis for the difficulty in adaptation in the biological difference between the criminal and other human beings. The attempt of Lombroso's to define this difference failed. Newer attempts have tried to solve the problem from the point of view of heredity, especially from the point of view of the study of identical and nonidentical twins. There are, indeed, a comparatively large number of identical twins in which both twins are criminal, whereas there is no discordance in nonidentical twins. This method of study is not quite reliable since the great similarity between identical twins induces them to identify themselves with each other much more readily. Studies in which the one twin has been reared separate from the other do not exist. Those who consider that criminality is chiefly due to hereditary factors would have to put the emphasis on eugenics and the prevention of the procreation of serious criminals. However even if one puts emphasis on the hereditary factors in crime, one would still have to consider that it is obviously not the crime which is inherited but the capacity to become criminal under specific circumstances. Even under these circumstances therapy of the criminal should become valuable. Even the criminal in whom heredity plays an important part is a human being who is under the influence of emotions and reacts to the environment.

However, it has become more and more probable that hereditary influences are of minor importance for the crime problem. It is good to keep in mind that the majority of criminals are neither neurotic nor psychotic. In the Clinic of the Court of General Sessions in New York City[3] 1.6 per cent of the total felons convicted in 1937 were insane. Mental defectives were 3.07 per cent of the entire group. There were 197 psychopathic personalities in the total of 2,698 cases, and neurosis was diagnosed 114 times. The majority of criminals were normal from a psychiatric point of view unless one considers the repeated crime itself a sign of mental unbalance. But such a formulation would only substitute one term for another.

The definition of the term *psychopathic personality* changes from author to author. Lauretta Bender, for instance, considers that the psychopathic personality results from emotional deprivation in the infantile period in children that have been kept in institutions until they were two or three years of age. The child does not have an op-

[3] See *Report of the Psychiatric Clinic, Court of General Sessions, N.Y.C.*, 1936, 1937, 1938, by Walter Bromberg; see also Bromberg's *Crime and the Mind*, 1948. [L.B., Ed.]

portunity to form early object relations owing to lack of parents and parent substitutes. Similar pictures are sometimes produced by head injuries and encephalitis which damage the brain. Others include among psychopaths individuals with constitutional abnormalities of the emotional life, who show, for instance, a tendency to dissociation. Generally we are inclined to talk about psychopathic personalities in individuals who give in to infantile drives or their modifications. They do not suffer directly but suffer by the reactions of society to their infantile behavior. The criminal is merely akin to the psychopathic group in so far as he does not suffer directly but merely by the reaction of society. It cannot be doubted that criminal action is to a greater extent determined by childhood experiences or, in other words, by the unconscious. The criminal act in this respect can be understood as a neurotic symptom in so far as it serves a more primitive drive. At the same time it shows some adaptation to society. There is some capacity to form groups, and furthermore there is the capacity of acting so that one may at least partially escape the consequences of one's actions. An enormous number of crimes remain unsolved.

At any rate, we come to the conclusion that besides the suffering which is fully experienced, a hidden suffering exists. Even in cases of general paresis there are hints that the individual is aware of the decline in his faculties and suffers severely because of it. This has been found by myself,[4] as well as by Ferenczi and Hollos. The general paretic case brings the mental decline in connection with his syphilis and with sexual misdemeanor in general. All the fears connected with masturbation are revived. Fear of castration and of mutilation are dominant and are overcompensated for by an exuberant feeling of sexual and intellectual capacities. Even in far-progressed cases, this mechanism is obvious. When the general paresis case experiences an exuberant feeling of physical health and mental well-being, he obviously overcompensates for his knowledge of his miserable mental and physical state.

I have made similar observations in persons dying or suffering from severe illness. The problem of physical and mental health arises. The individual seemingly does not intend to give in to suffering and

[4] See David Rapaport, *Organization and Pathology of Thought* (Columbia University Press, 1950), for translation of Paul Schilder's *Studien zur Psychologie und Symptomatologie der progressiven Paralyse,* 1930.

disease. There is a wish for health, and if this wish is strong enough, the individual experiences health. The mechanisms involved in this striving for health will be discussed in the following two chapters.

We have made a preliminary division of symptoms into those based upon the physical and mental suffering of a person and those which make others suffer. We have reached the understanding that whenever there is physical suffering, there is mental suffering and a mental change is present. We have seen, furthermore, that mental suffering always expresses itself in feelings concerning the body and in physiological or even anatomical changes in the body. Whenever there is suffering, the individual tries to escape this suffering. He tries to be cured and defends himself psychologically against the experience of suffering. It seems that in patients who are sick and who make others suffer, a hidden knowledge of their illness exists although they may appear to be successful in hiding this knowledge from themselves. There is, therefore, a connecting link between these three groups. They merely present three sides of the same fundamental problem.

Chapter 4

SOMATIC HEALTH AS AN EXPERIENCE [1]

ONE GENERALLY takes it for granted that the person who has no disease should feel healthy and that the person with an organic lesion or dysfunction should feel sick. One is inclined to consider the experience of one's own health as an immediate reflection of the physiology or pathophysiology of the body. An individual who has lost one leg and walks with a prothesis or with crutches is not sick. Whenever there is a stabilized defect, either in form or in function, the organism adapts itself psychologically as well as physiologically. The feeling of health is the expression of stabilization in the psychophysiological organism.

Lower organisms, in which the possibilities of regeneration are almost unlimited, react to a considerable loss in the material of the body by melting the remaining material into a diminutive picture of the intact organism, even without food. When the egg of an echinoderm is divided in half, a complete embryo develops. Lizards regenerate their tails. When one leg of a dog is amputated, the adaptations are adaptations in function and attitude. They occur when the contact with the ground is lost. The loss of each leg necessitates a different adaptation. Walking, trotting, and galloping are possible with three legs (Bethe).

[1] Reprinted with minor changes from the *Archives for Neurology and Psychiatry* 37:1322–37, June, 1937. I am indebted to the editors for permission to reprint.

The new equilibrium of the organism is reached, therefore, either by growth and regeneration or by a change in the function and attitude. The experience of health is the expression of such adaptive tendencies in the psychological sphere. The psyche tries to maintain it even when a severe organic disease exists. Psychiatrists and neurologists have always been very much interested in the fact that disease and suffering occur out of the individual problems, and one has even considered organic disease as an expression of tendencies to fall ill. One has, however, overlooked the fact that there exists not only a psychogenic disease but also a psychogenic health. The problem of physical health has never been studied in its psychological aspect.

Even the completely healthy person is aware of continuous sensations coming from various parts of the body. One is fatigued, has a little pain here or there, a little headache, some disagreeable abdominal feelings and some itching. In order to experience health one must either co-ordinate the smaller sensations into a unit or make the attempt to remove them completely from the field of consciousness, and to forget about them. The vegetative system offers a great number of sensations which might impair the feeling of well-being: hunger, thirst, the urge to urinate and defecate, and finally the smaller stimuli arising continually in the genitals. The experience of health can, therefore, be maintained only in a continuous dynamic interplay. When this dynamic interplay is disturbed by inner conflict, the small stimuli acquire another dynamic significance. Although this is unquestionably not the only source of so-called conversion symptoms, it is a contributing factor.

If serious disease threatens the individual he still tries to maintain the experience of health by minimizing the organic discomfort or by completely neglecting it. Far-progressed cancer cases clearly show this tendency. A sixty-one-year-old workman with carcinoma of the stomach says: "I was operated upon about eight months ago for a tumor. I had pain before. Everything I ate went through me. Now nothing will go through me. My bowels are not all right. I had pain. I vomited always. I did not think it was dangerous. It got worse. I don't know why. I came into the hospital to be cured. They gave me a spinal anesthesia. I was not afraid at all. I had confidence. When they give me a physic now it tears me to pieces. Otherwise I have no pain. I thought I had an ulcer but I know now it is a tumor. It feels like a growth. When I get well I will go to work again. I am pretty weak now, although I eat fairly good." When asked what he enjoyed most in his life, he says going out with a lady friend on Saturday nights. If three wishes could be fulfilled for him he would wish to be strong, to go to work, and to have a few more good years. "I have suffered enough." The patient says he feels much better now, "although I had a bad day today." He has a sister whom he likes very much. He is not married. During the last few years he has had no lady friend. He has a hopeful attitude, although a slight apprehension breaks through occasionally.

The attitude of this patient is fairly typical of the attitude of patients with severe organic ailments. One would expect that the patient would know that he has a malignant growth. But he does not acknowledge his physical disease fully. He minimizes his symptoms and deceives himself about his physical weakness. He wants to maintain the experience of health again, at heavy odds, and is partially successful. The psychic organism maintains its integrity better than the physical organism. In so far as he does not allow himself to know how sick he is and how badly he feels, we have the right to speak about repression. The repression would use narcissistic libido as one of its mechanisms.

This connotation does not fully explain the facts. The organic disease and the symptoms produced by it are in their very nature not a personal concern of the individual who is deeply moved only by his moral problems. Organic disease lies not in the center of our personal life but in its periphery.

I have spoken about the circle of the ego (*Ichkreis*).[2] We know from immediate experience whether we are touched in the core of our personality, whether the experiences are near to the nucleus of the ego or not. Our problems, emotions, feelings, and attitudes in this respect belong closer to the nucleus of the ego than the experiences relating to the outward world and to our body. Not all sensations are at the same distance from the hypothetical center of the ego. Pain, sexual excitement, and anxiety are in the center of the personality. The individual is completely in them.

[2] The term "ego" is not used here in the psychoanalytic sense, but in the sense of general psychology. If one tries to correlate the connotations, one would probably consider the psychoanalytic ego nearer to the periphery of the ego circle than the id. [See M. Sherif and H. Cantril, *The Psychology of Ego Involvements,* 1947.—L.B., Ed.]

Some parts of our body are nearer to the center of the ego than others. It makes a great difference which part of the body has to be operated upon, and case studies of postoperative psychoses show that mutilating operations will provoke more psychoses than non-mutilating ones. Operations on genitals, breasts, and eyes threaten parts of the body which are nearer to the center of the ego than others. In schizophrenia and neurosis the complexes lie in the center of the personality. The experiences of organic brain lesions, as, for instance, general paresis, arteriosclerosis, head injury, concern material which is rather impersonal. It has nothing to do with the vital problems of the personality. In organic brain lesion, the psychological experiences are in the periphery. Cases with organic diseases are generally much more objective towards their disease than psychogenic ones. It is as if the organic disease were not so much one's personal affair.

A thirty-five-year-old case of nephritis, who subsequently improved, said that he never really felt sick but merely had difficulties in breathing. He felt that he would recover. He did not even worry when he became blind from retinal hemorrhages. He knew that he would go to the hospital and it would be the task of physicians to cure him. The difference in attitude is particularly clear in cases of impotence. The case with organic impotence has an almost heavenly patience in relation to this occurrence. The organic disease is in the periphery of the personality. The psychogenic disorder occupies its center. When one studies the history of the conversion symptom one sees at first that the individual is very much concerned about his problems. He is worried as a person. After he has succeeded in developing the conversion symptom he cares less for the conversion symptom than one would expect. Hysterical hemiplegias are almost as happy as organic cases. The problems have wandered from the center to the periphery. In accidents, for instance head injuries, an organic disease starts in the outward world and in the body, and not with the problems of the personality. The individual merely becomes secondarily impressed by the disease. I believe that many organic diseases belong in this category and that in almost all of them such an extraneous factor participates. In these cases the experiences wander from the periphery to the center. Psychic life is a continuous movement of experiences wandering from the center to the periphery and back. The body and the organic disease belong in some way more to the periphery than to the center of the personality.

Not only in carcinoma and nephritis are such attitudes to be found. We meet the same attitude in the organic heart case, unless pain and anxiety come into the foreground. In a sixty-four-year-old man of Jewish extraction, coronary occlusion was followed by a period of memory disturbances with confusion and confabulation. At the time of the examination the patient was clear, oriented, talkative, jocular, euphoric, and even showed some memories of the time he was confused. He reports that his disease started with difficulties in breathing. "I could not get air. I certainly thought I would die. Who would not be afraid?" The patient talks without sign of real emotion and is rather objective. "I felt only a heartburn; I had no pain. I felt so bad I wanted to die. What could I do any more after sixty-four? I can't work, I can't make money. I have nothing to live for. I want only that my wife does not go to charity. My wife should have support. I can't sleep. I struggle to get well." The patient is very much at a loss when he is asked in what way he struggles to get well. He says merely that one has to go to bed very early in the hospital.

Many other cases show this attitude in a still more clear-cut way. It is not necessary to increase the material, since Fahrenkamp has shown in an extensive study that organic heart cases show, in striking contrast to the objective findings, little or no consciousness of disease and consequently no insight. Complaints, such as shortness of breath on exertion, are minimized or dissimulated. On the contrary, in heart neurotics we usually find a marked subjective experience of illness (*Krankheitserlebnis*) referred to heart or circulatory system (cf. Flanders Dunbar's book).

A particularly striking instance is given in the attitudes of patients with cerebrospinal meningitis. It is rather typical that cases with cerebrospinal meningitis, when they recover, remember hardly anything but headaches, which they do not object to very much. They never have any feelings that they have had a severe organic disease.

A nineteen-year-old girl, for instance, who was feeling ill three days before admission and complained of a headache and vomiting, did not talk at the time of admission. The somatic picture and the spinal-fluid findings were typical for meningococcus meningitis. Her stupor and drowsiness subsided, and twelve days after admission she answered—to the question "How do you feel?"—"Pretty good. I don't know what happened to me." Also in the subsequent days she remained clear, felt very healthy, minimized the headaches she had had, and had no idea that she was seriously ill.

Another case, a man of forty-two, was found sitting on a doorstep in a stuporous state. His employer had found him groggy. In the hospital he proved to be clouded, stuporous, and lethargic. It was a case of typical cerebrospinal meningitis. He improved after a week. His final attitude towards his disease was reflected in the following remarks: "I don't know how I got here; the last thing I remember is when I left for work. They told me to go home because I wasn't able to work. I was just dizzy—dizzy all over. Sure I had a headache." He had an amnesia for the stuporous period.

One might object to the last few instances and emphasize that organic toxic changes are going on in the brain of the meningitic cases. There is no denial of this fact. The attitudes are not merely created by the toxic factors. It is a general but very often neglected principle of psychopathology that organic and toxic changes do not create the problems and attitudes of the individual but bring them more into the foreground of consciousness. The organic influences on the brain sensitize in different directions, and it is probable that the wish to be healthy is helped by the majority of toxic influences of various kinds, which is in itself an important problem. The euphoria and optimism of the tuberculosis case which has for a long time been in the center of medical attention is, therefore, merely a specific expression of the general problems of the psychology of organic disease. The increasing feeling of weakness, the mechanism of neglect, and minimizing and repressing of the organic disease become insufficient with the progress of organic disease and the more severe impairment of function. A more elaborate defense is needed to retain the experience of one's own health. A seventy-year-old woman with extensive carcinoma metastases, who is mildly disorientated but so composed that she can be kept in the medical ward, although very weak and unable to get out of bed, feels very happy and does not realize she is so weak and that she is unable to get up. She is deeply attached to her son, who visits her about twice a week. "I am happy, very happy about my son. He gives me food, he visits me. I have no pain, I am not sick; I can eat." When asked about her relatives she says, in a deprecatory manner: "My poor sister was very sick. She is in heaven. I have no parents; they are dead." Thus the patient very readily acknowledges disease and death of others but she herself escapes into the infantile state of oral satisfaction. It is a variation of Descartes' statement: "Cogito ergo sum." It reads: "I eat and therefore I exist and am healthy." Felix Deutsch reports about a dying heart case who also regressed to the oral level of libido but revived also an old love relation to her brother in her phantasy.

Cases of this type escape the suffering of organic disease by regression. The regression revives infantile love relations and finally goes to the oral stage.

In another group of cases, the mechanism of projection plays the outstanding part. Of course, projection is based upon regression. However, we deal here with such an important form of a primitive mechanism that an independent discussion is necessary. In an earlier study I observed a case of far-progressed tuberculosis, who heard the command of God that he take a fresh-air cure in order to recover. He was born again in order to rid the world of tuberculosis. He said that his brother, to whom he gave his name, was sick, but not he himself. He called himself spirit, savior, and Jesus Christ who saved humanity with himself. The projection mechanism is obvious here.

A fifty-year-old patient with carcinoma felt attacked and defended herself with violent aggression. Another patient, fifty-eight years old, with a cancer of the stomach, said that somebody wanted to murder her but she recovered from death and from tapeworm. Finally, immediately before death, she considered herself recovered and said she had saved the whole world.

The regression is here connected not only with projection but with narcissistic ideas of grandeur.

Regression to narcissism and projection is in no way limited to the most severe cases. Joseph Wortis has shown that in psychosis with heart disease the projection mechanism plays an outstanding part. The patients feel persecuted, followed, threatened, and sometimes they even feel that they have been beaten up. Wortis is of the opinion that one deals with an attempt to get rid of the anxiety by projecting it outside. It is easier to defend oneself against persecution than against disease. Patients maintain their feeling of health by the mechanism of projection.

Projection helps even against phenomena of pain. It is well known that when falling asleep, physical pain is projected into others. I have previously observed patients with gynecological diseases who referred their pain to beatings by a little man. The cases of pernicious anemia are of special interest from this point of view. L. Bender has pointed to the fact that patients with pernicious anemia very often refer their disturbance, especially the nervous complications, to hostile influences coming from the outside world. Pictures may occur which show a great similarity to paranoiac cases. A short time ago I observed a patient with pernicious anemia who, in the beginning of her illness, complained to the police that there was always a smell around of brewing hooch.

The literature on psychoses with pernicious anemia has been reviewed by Karl M. Bowman. The mechanism of projection is not the only mechanism by which pernicious anemia cases defend themselves. In the beginning of the disease, the feeling of weakness is very often overcompensated by phantasies of wish fulfillment, as in one case in our clinic, who elaborated a story that she is a daughter of the Czar, and completely neglected her severe paraplegia. The astasia-abasias of psychogenic type, not so rarely observed in the beginning, not only serve the tendency to make it clear to the others that the patients are sick but probably give the patient a feeling of consolation, since he feels that he has provoked these symptoms.

A fifty-four-year-old woman was brought to the hospital with the statement that she was suffering from hallucinations of smell and that she had the delusion that numerous airplanes contributed to the foul odor.

The patient who was irritable and depressed complained bitterly about her mother, who stated that the patient had made suicidal attempts. "It was a big stroke on her part; she was very vicious to me. It was her aim to put me out. She is a combination of a tigress and leopard; very obstreperous and very spatty. She wrecked my life. There is an irritating smell which burns my throat and swells my intestines. The airplanes give out a vapor as they pass me. They swell me up and pull all my bones out. I am very susceptible. These smells swell me up and stop my heart; they turn my ankles and pull them out of place. They are very big from poisonous gas. When the poison gas goes out, I can move my feet. I want treatment immediately. I had all my teeth extracted. My mother would steal my food. She is a racketeer. She has always been that way but I found it out two years ago." The patient was irritable and talkative but not confused.

She was also extremely irritable with physicians and nurses. The report of her mother is as follows: "There are no nervous and mental diseases in the family. She has always lived with me; she was very bright, a good scholar, and always wanted to learn. She was going to be a teacher. Then she got sick. Her nerves gave out and she was told to stop. Between seventeen and twenty she worked as a bookkeeper up to the time of an intestinal operation. The following year, 1917, her ovaries were taken out. She has been sick for fifteen years. She has been devoting all her time to irrigating her nose and throat. She used 150 pounds of soda in one month. Her nose was operated on three years before. She would leave her meals five or six times to irrigate. During the last six months she has been more cranky than ever. She says that everyone in the house is a spy and is trying to murder her. She complained that the people around put disinfectants in her room. She cusses and called me a thief."

Physically, the patient showed a high degree of emaciation, cyanosis, pallor, and argyrosis. There was an edema of legs and thighs. The tongue was smooth, glazed, but not inflamed. Sinus tachycardia and slight enlargement of the heart were present. The blood count showed 2,360,000 red blood corpuscles, hemoglobin 30 per cent, leucocytes 7,000, polynuclears 82, lymphocytes 16. The blood smear showed very marked poikilocytosis. The fingernails on both hands showed marked spooning, koilonychia. The glossitis and the type of anemia are compatible with the diagnosis of idiopathic hypochromic anemia, Plummer-Vinson syndrome. The congestive heart failure was accounted for by the severe anemia as well as by protein deficiency. The silver involvement was probably an associated pigmentation rather than a heavy metal poisoning.

After very stormy periods of paranoid excitement with shouting, accusations, etc., the patient's mental status improved markedly. She was much more agreeable and had lost her delusions completely. The mental improvement went parallel to the physical improvement under the treatment with blood transfusions, iron, liver, and diet.

This case of Plummer-Vinson's anemia is particularly remarkable for the clearness of the projection mechanism. The oral symptoms connected with the anemia are ascribed to hostile influences with gases (cf. Hurst's paper on this type of anemia).

I come, therefore, to the conclusion that the experience of health can be maintained by the projection mechanism. If the projection mechanism is incomplete, the discomfort of disease is experienced as the result of hostile influences. If the projection mechanism works more completely, the patient feels that not he himself is sick, but others. In the beginning his opinion on this point may be uncertain. Finally, not only their own disease is cured but the diseases of others as well. With the more complete projection narcissistic ideas of grandeur come more and more into the foreground.

One might ask why these elaborate mechanisms should be necessary in order to maintain the feeling of health, if organic disease is in the periphery of the ego. The experiences in the periphery of the ego, the sensations coming from the body, are in themselves not always at the same distance from the nucleus of the ego. Pain in itself has the tendency to progress from the periphery into the center and to fill the whole personality. Any physical change transgressing above a certain quantity will provoke an overflow from the periphery to the center, and the psychic mechanisms discussed above have as their aim to defend the center of the ego against the inroad from the periphery.

Two symptoms provoked by organic changes make defense necessary. The one is, as mentioned, pain of major degree and the other is anxiety. If the pain is not very great, as for instance in pneumonia, the individual may at the height of the discomfort go into a delirious episode. It is rather interesting that patients forget about pain in their delirium, and it is also characteristic that in the reports patients give, they always emphasize that they did not know about their disease and pain at the moment the delirious episode set in. I will present an excerpt of a protocol of a sixty-year-old woman who had just got over a lobar pneumonia. She talked continually and said: "Last year I hardly escaped pneumonia. This time I was hot but had no pain." (*Fever?*) "I had a cold." (*Would you not be afraid of pneumonia?*) "I could not stand pneumonia." She said she saw another woman strapped down with pneumonia. A few minutes later, however, she said in the course of conversation: "They told me I had pneumonia type 3."

Since it is known that the delirious pneumonia patient very often wanders out of his bed and endangers his life, it is obvious that the psychological defense might be detrimental to the patient. One comes to very similar conclusions regarding anxiety. It has been mentioned before that the case with heart disease defends himself against anxiety by projection. If the anxiety surpasses a specific degree, the defense becomes insufficient. It is probable that the acute onset of the anxiety contributes in making the psychological defense impossible. This is true in the angina pectoris case in which the feeling of anxiety is all-pervading. We are here not so much interested in whether anxiety is, as Ludwig Braun thinks, a sensation coming from the heart, or whether the anxiety is due to an edema of the brain stem and of the medulla oblongata, as Hausner and Hoff state. I have no doubt that central factors participate in this feeling of anxiety, which is connected with the conviction that one has to die. Not only did Hausner and Hoff find anxiety and the feeling of impending death and destruction in tumors of the fossa posterior but I have found the conviction of impending death with anxiety also in chronic encephalitis cases with vasovegetative phenomena. It is characteristic that the individual feels utterly helpless when this anxiety comes over him, and he is ready to give up completely. We may draw the preliminary conclusion that the physician faces the duty of helping the patient where the psychic defense is so utterly abolished. At any rate, intensive pain and anxiety are organic symptoms against which psychic defense is insufficient.

One might doubt the validity of the formulation that the individual is trying to neglect organic diseases and to defend himself against the knowledge of being organically sick, and might point to the fact that so-called psychogenic symptoms are often found in organic diseases. It is doubtful whether the term "psychogenic symptoms" is always used in a correct way. Human beings have to have attitudes, and these attitudes are psychic. A symptom is always a psychic attitude and not merely a reflection of prospective findings on the autopsy table. Individuals cannot help having problems, and these problems are a part of their attitudes. It is true that there are patients with organic diseases who not only have an exaggerated appreciation of their disease but demand the attention and pity of others. Pernicious anemia may develop conversion symptoms, but these conversion symptoms almost invariably are to be found at the time when the organic disease is not yet fully developed. In the Viennese Clinic we always suspected beginning multiple sclerosis when conversion symptoms were very outspoken. The complaint of the patient with organic disease is very often in an indirect proportion to the degree and severity of the disease. Psychogenic symptoms may also occur during convalescence.

I have among my observations a case of tuberculosis full of fear of death, and the complaint of dizziness, weakness, and inability to concentrate. The tuberculosis is completely cured now, and prior to the time of his illness he was very much interested in sports and narcissistic about his own body. He was much moved by the fact that his sister had died of tuberculosis.

In another case, a severe neurosis consisting of the fear of getting infected with bacteria followed a herniorrhaphy which was not completely successful. The patient was an athlete with extremely increased narcissism, whose life was shattered when it was clear to him that he could not excel as a baseball player any longer.

A thirty-six-year-old patient who had recovered from acute nephritis, in which the blood pressure rose to 180, complained that his chest and arms had flattened out and felt that his whole breathing apparatus did not belong to him. He felt that there was no blood in his arms and face. He felt also that his penis looked smaller and thinner. The patient was at the time at a rather unexpected height of his career. His complaints came after the organic disease had passed.

It is interesting to see how the appreciation of organic disease varies according to the general state of mind. A woman patient, fifty years old, acquired a rheumatic heart disease in early childhood. She occasionally had attacks during which she could not breathe and felt that she would die. She then felt her heart enlarged as if it smothered the windpipe. For the most part she was not aware of feeling very much except weakness. After the death of her mother in 1926 she had a nervous breakdown. At that time she first became conscious of her heart disease. For the last two years she has had no attack, but in connection with a sinus trouble which made irrigations of her nose necessary, she developed the idea that she had a terrible disease and was telling it to everyone. She thought that her finger was rotting away. A religious ring on her finger turned black. At this time she first felt that her heart was very bad. The more depressed she became, the less she felt about her heart. Finally, it was as if her heart had turned to stone and wouldn't give any sensations. At the time of the examination the patient was rather happy and contented. She had no sensations concerning her heart. At a later time during observation the complaints concerning her heart varied according to her moods.

It would be easy to cite many more instances. It is clear that the experience of health and disease is dependent not merely upon the so-called organic findings but also upon the problems of the individual. The fact remains that there is a tendency to maintain the experience of health even in the face of severe organic disease and that severe organic diseases are not the basis for conversion symptoms. Organic symptoms of minor degree may be the nucleus of conversion symptoms or may be used according to the general attitude of the individual. Organic symptomatology of severe degree is never without relation to the problems of the personality.

I talk about the experience of health, but one might very well say that there are many components in this feeling of health. There is the general feeling of vigor. Wilson has very well described the psychic attitude of the multiple sclerosis case, but he was not interested in the problem from a general point of view, and has therefore failed to emphasize the point that the attitudes of multiple sclerosis cases are merely a specific expression of what is going on in every organic disease. He speaks about eutonia sclerotica. There is the happiness, euphoria sclerotica, and the conviction that whatever may be experienced in the way of discomfort will not be lasting. I want to emphasize that these three experiences go together. They are a unit although the one or the other may be outstanding. Wilson has pointed to the importance of the psychiatric findings in multiple sclerosis. He finds that in the phase of serious organic disability patients retain the experience of health, and he is inclined to find an organic explanation for this fact. He believes that a lesion of the thalamus opticus has such an influence. I have emphasized that this attitude is a general attitude of the case who is organically ill. It is true, however, that the multiple sclerosis shows this phenomenon in a particularly strong degree.

We come to the conclusion that the lesion of certain parts of the brain might help the psychic attitudes which neglect the organic disease. For reasons I cannot discuss here I am inclined to believe that it is not the lesion of the thalamus opticus but a lesion of the periventricular gray matter which has such an influence. Since no definite proof is possible at the present time, we have to be content with the general statement that the noncortical lesions might help in the experience of health.

We are on safer ground in discussing the psychic attitude of cases with sensory aphasia. It is typical of the sensory aphasia case that he shows a great amount of drives and impulses, not only in the sphere of language but also in the total field of motility. His euphoria is very outspoken. He often overlooks his defect completely, especially in the beginning. In the later development the patient may experience difficulties in finding words, but he will not be disturbed by it. He will remain decidedly optimistic, and will retain the feeling of health. I reproduce a protocol of a case of head injury. It is of a man forty years of age, who has no remembrance concerning the accident and no insight into the fact that he is sick. He has difficulties in understanding and also in finding words. Several days after the accident the pain asymbolia which was present in the beginning disappeared.

When the patient was asked, *"Are you happy?"* he said: "Well, no, I could be happier. There is something I would like to know: how to be happier." (*In what way are you not happy?*) "For one reason because laying here and not making steps forward, I am not happy." (*Are you sick?*) "I am not really sick. I am recovering from a road that means more significance." (*Are you sick?*) "Not really sick, not now. I am healthy. I feel strong and I wish you the same identical thing. That's all in happiness is to seek and find happiness in life but trouble is to get established so as not to seek. It does not make any difference what people you come in contact with, white or colored. I will never ignore any colored race but interview them. It is all cycles of business, commercialized. Undoubtedly I may be wrong in this."

When he was shown a key, he made a sucking motion and said: "Maybe it's good luck stone I am kissing. I have a ring with a flowery design like that. There is no asking towards. Let's talk about something else." (Shown key.) "It might be luck, I suppose." (Shown key.) "It looks like a key." (Shown handkerchief.) "Handparchef or handerchief." (Shown pen.) "A tool piece of your own. I am just jumping at the analysis."

It is remarkable that patients of this type keep their euphoria and their optimistic attitude in spite of the headaches they experience at the same time. It is also characteristic that the patient names a key a good luck stone.

It would be easy to increase the number of instances. One may find others in my paper "Psychic Disturbances after Head Injuries." I emphasize that, of course, these psychic attitudes are in no way restricted to the sensory aphasia cases which occur after head injuries. Every lesion of the Wernicke region provokes the same picture with the same characteristic psychic attitude. The attitude is, therefore, due to the local lesion of the brain.

The importance of these findings comes into a better focus if one compares the attitude of the sensory aphasia case with the attitude of a so-called motor aphasia case who is moody, depressed, and has the feeling of being sick and a normal or exaggerated consciousness of his deficiency. I have also studied a group of cases in which motor aphasic signs, increased sensitivity to pain, and exaggerated mimic expressions and gestures are in the foreground. Although these patients have a full insight into their defect, they are euphoric and have the general comportment of well-being.

Paraphasias and syntactic errors may clear up and the general attitude of euphoria, the feeling of health, may remain. There is an undoubted relation between the Wernicke region and the experience of health. I have observed cases in which pictures of this type occur in head injuries without definite aphasic signs.

It is interesting in this connection that, according to my previous formulations, there exists a center in the supramarginal gyrus, the lesion of which impairs the appreciation of pain. Other parts of the parietal lobe have something to do with the appreciation of defects, and a local lesion may prevent an appreciation of defects. It is the merit of my teacher Gabriel Anton to have pointed to the general importance of this fact.

Since I have discussed this problem at length in *Image and Appearance of the Human Body,* I only point in a general way to the importance of the parietal lobe for the construction of the body image and for our appreciation of our own health and disease.

Many phenomena in organic diseases of the brain in which the lesions are more or less diffuse thus find their explanation.

One will understand better, for instance, how patients with head injuries, and those without sensory aphasia, are so often not concerned about their head injury. Even the retrograde amnesia of head injury cases can be better understood on the basis of the general theory of the experience of health. I come, therefore, to the conclusion that the experience of health and disease, although an attitude of the personality, is dependent upon the function of specific senses in the brain, among which the Wernicke region is the most important one.

It would be easy to extend the discussion into the field of psychiatry, but these remarks are chiefly devoted to the problems of organic disease which is not accompanied by psychosis. Suffice it to say that in organic brain disease the experiences and disturbances are, as would be expected, in the periphery of the personality in the sense defined above. In contrast, the psychosis in which no gross anatomical lesions are found is in close relation with the center of the personality.

Are these mere theoretical discussions or can we deduct practical conclusions? I think that the knowledge of attitudes of organic and psychogenic diseases is of primary diagnostic importance. We have also to understand the specific attitudes connected with specific organic diseases. We shall then better understand the psychogenic pictures and their specific relations to beginning organic disease. We still lack a symptomatology of internal diseases from a psychological point of view. I think that such a symptomatology of internal diseases, evaluating the psychological structure of the pathological experiences of the organically sick, will be of indispensable value, not only for the diagnosis but also for the treatment of the patient. It is trite to say that every sick person needs psychological help. We can be more specific since there is the tendency of the organic case to forget about his organic disease or to minimize it. We have to lead him back in this respect to reality. It is indispensable in the treatment of the organic case to bring the patient to an appreciation of the reality of the disease. Nonappreciation of the disease and the experience of health are in many of these cases dangerous, as in the pneumonia cases who in their delirium lose an appreciation of their illness and act accordingly. The adaptation of the patient to his disease has to be an adaptation based upon insight. Even when he has insight into the nature of the organic disease he will keep it in the periphery and adaptation will be possible, unless there is pain and anxiety. Both symptoms call for the physical help of the physician.[3]

The other part of the therapy will have to be a causal and not a symptomatic one. We only have the right to let the patient maintain

[3] It would be very interesting to study morphine from the point of view emphasized here. The drug does not create anything new but merely reinforces the psychological tendencies which drive to painlessness and ease.

his experience of health in the face of serious physical ailment, if he is incurable. Then he should be allowed to project his ailment and regress to a state of narcissistic bliss. This is also the answer to the problem of euthanasia. Incurable illness leads the individual away from the experience of health and well-being. It is true that the individual regresses deeply. However, he still lives fully, and there is no more reason to kill the physical sufferer than to kill a child. The psyche maintains the experience of health even in the face of death.

Chapter 5

PSYCHIC HEALTH AS AN EXPERIENCE

INDIVIDUALS ATTEMPT to maintain the experience of health even when threatened by serious illness. We may expect that human beings will no less tenaciously cling to the experience of psychic health. We consider ourselves as healthy when experiences come and go in a freely flowing manner and when we feel equal to the tasks put before us. We want to feel assured of ourselves in our relation to the inanimate world, in our social relations, and in our love relations. We desire the capacity to construct, to destroy, and to construct again. To be able to live in a full world and have complete experiences is our wish. Such an experience of psychic health, closely related to the tasks of our life and its purpose, expresses itself in the feeling of happiness and contentment.

Difficulties repeatedly arise when a sudden change occurs in the outward situation which is physically or psychologically damaging. We speak about a trauma. Now changes are going on continually, and every change puts a new task before us. A world which would not offer any difficulties would be empty and meaningless. A trauma merely necessitates a more thorough adaptation. We speak about trauma in the physical world when an event disrupts the unity of the body image. We have dealt with this problem in the previous chapter. Physical traumas which do not kill immediately put new problems before individuals. The trauma does not, therefore, remain merely in the physical sphere, and it has to be seen from the same angle as organic disease in general. The defense reaction against the trauma may develop in the psychic sphere. The individual may forget the accident, but his forgetting, as in the cases of head injury, very often has a purely organic meaning. The psychogenic forgetting of an accident develops out of the individual problems which are not so rarely brought to a head by the accident. Freud has developed a complicated theory that organisms defend themselves against the trauma by warding it off before the full intensity has penetrated to the inner core of the organism. The unused energy manifests itself later on, by repetition. To be sure, the observation is correct that many people dream about their accidents and these dreams very often are more or less photographic repetition of the traumatic scene. However, the careful study of any one of these cases reveals that they revive the past situation, which was impressive, whenever they feel threatened by a danger in their actual situation. They use the past experience as a warning and as a consolation, since they have survived. Because of their dynamic value, traumatic scenes have a greater tendency than the average to be kept alive, with all their intensity, and to offer themselves rather readily for use in the present situation.

One of my patients who had been gassed during World War I revived the whole scene whenever he was threatened by an actual difficulty. So, for instance, in a hallucinatory scene which he had before he was to be operated on for appendicitis, he shouted so loudly he had to be brought for psychiatric observation, and he thus escaped the operation, temporarily. But he reacted similarly when in danger of not getting compensation. No mechanical tendency to repetition (repetition compulsion) exists. However, it is true that we are likely to keep in our mind situations to which we could not completely adapt and which are unfinished. We try again and again to arrive at some new adaptations, and in the course of these attempts the unfinished scene may reappear. Quite in the same way as no mechanical association occurs, mechanical repetition of traumatic scenes does not exist. We may concede that the availability of any memory material undergoes changes which are in part dependent upon the rhythmical functions of the organism, and not only upon the psychological situation. According to this discussion, we are not even justified in the assumption that the physical trauma, with all its suddenness, is merely an accident. It is in relation to the previous adaptation of the individual.

This is even truer in the case of the so-called psychic trauma. A psychological situation becomes traumatic only in connection with our attitudes. It is true that some psychic situations may exist to which an adaptation may be particularly difficult, especially for the child. But even then we may expect that in a majority of the cases the child will have been repeatedly exposed to this difficulty and also will be afterwards. In this sense, there is some truth in the statement of Alfred Adler: "We do not suffer from the shock of our experiences—the so-called trauma—but we make out of them just what suits our purposes. We are self-determined by the meaning we give to our experiences and there is probably something of a mistake always involved when we take particular experiences as the basis for our future life."

Adler stresses self-determination too greatly. The individual and the situation cannot be separated from each other. We may call situations of particular difficulty traumatic situations. It is well known that Breuer and Freud at the beginning of their studies put great emphasis on the trauma as the cause for a subsequent hysteria. They even postulated that an organic hypnoid state follows the traumatic event which is responsible for the act of forgetting. Freud only later on gained the insight that the forgetting of the traumatic scene was not merely due to a physiological change, but was the result of a psychic defense and this was responsible for the repression. The further fate of the theory of psychic trauma was variable. Freud came to the conclusion that only sexual traumata have a pathogenic effect, and considered psychic traumata of later childhood, as seduction by the father, as the cause of neurosis. Later on he found out that many of these traumas were merely invented by the patient. The theory of the sexual trauma was therefore dropped, and the psychosexual development in the earlier childhood was considered as the basis for the later neurosis. But in his paper on the history of an infantile neurosis, Freud came to the conclusion that the primal scene (Urscene) of sexual character could be found in the early history of the patient either by direct associations, or by reconstruction, and this scene had to be considered as the basis for the neurosis. The psychoanalytic literature concerning this point is unfortunately very meager and unconvincing. Specific experiences of this type can be found only in the minority of cases. We are furthermore entitled to believe that such early scenes, even when their existence can be established with reasonable certainty, are merely early crystallizations of problems which are not simply confined to this one scene.

We can sum up by saying that traumatic situations do exist. Situations in everybody's life are changing, and during this change situations must occur which are more difficult to handle. We are entitled to call these situations traumatic, especially when they occur rather suddenly. Tasks before which individuals are placed are never simple. Even the simplest object sets us conflicting tasks. There always are tendencies to follow different trends in handling any situations in life. By doing something we neglect many other things; and as previous discussions have shown, we come to a full appreciation of a situation and of the outside world merely by the fact that the conflicting tendencies imposed upon us by the different sides of reality force us to give attention to the various aspects of objects and situations. The trauma is, therefore, merely one particular point in the series of events which consists of conflicting tasks before which reality puts us.

Modern medical psychology speaks justly, accordingly, of the importance of the conflict, but has made the mistake of considering the conflict merely from the point of view of what may go on in ourselves, and has talked about the inner conflict. Paradoxically, one might say that an inner conflict does not exist. We are always directed towards real objects and real situations, even in our phantasy life and in our daydreaming. We always have purposes and want to solve tasks, and the inner tasks are merely the reflections of the tasks we have in relation to the outside world. Conflicts are not in the air. Human beings live with other human beings in an atmosphere of reality. Conflicts are conflicts concerning situations, and the term "inner conflict" is justified only when we want to point to a specific side of the conflict.

When a situation becomes very difficult and the individual feels unable to master it and is unable to acknowledge defeat, he will seek to preserve his self-esteem and his feeling of psychic health by defending himself against this difficult situation. We speak, following Freud, about psychic defense. One should consider psychic defense not merely from the point of view of gross psychic pathology. It is in close relation to the constant necessity we have of forcing into the background one or another experience which is incompatible with the task we intend to solve. In order to construct, we continually reject parts of the material which the situation offers us. If we do not, we may get lost in the insignificant details and never reach our goal.

The psychic defense may simply lead to the forgetting of material which impairs our psychic well-being. We may then speak about repression. Repression is, therefore, the type of psychic defense which leads to the forgetting of material threatening the well-being of a person. The fact as such is obvious. We forget scenes in which we did not play a very advantageous role. Sexual experiences one has had in one's childhood with one's brothers and sisters are very often forgotten. If one studies cases of this type carefully enough, one finds that these forgotten scenes are never really forgotten. They are present but pushed aside. To one's astonishment, the patients very often will say that they knew these things but did not want to tell them. There is no real forgetting, but merely different degrees of awareness. This is particularly obvious with cases of hysterical amnesia, as for instance in the cases called amnesia victims where it is easy to demonstrate that the patients always knew who they were and what they had been doing.

Repression in this sense, leading to complete forgetfulness, is a comparatively rare occurrence. In the majority of cases, the individual starts to reconstruct the past till it becomes acceptable. There are various ways of reconstructing the past. The memory of a situation in which one has been defeated is changed until one is convinced that one has played the role of the hero. In one of my head injury cases the patient reported at first that he had been frightened by several persons and had beaten them up. In reality he had been run over by a truck, which he remembered later. This was an organic case and his memory disturbance was on an organic basis, but we are accustomed to see the psychological mechanisms becoming particularly clear under such conditions. We may change the situation merely in phantasy, and find the fitting repartee, which would have silenced our adversary, long after he left us. It is easier to reconstruct in our phantasy.

The instances given pertain to a reconstruction of the situation with the use of extant material. Very often the individual goes back into the past when the situation becomes too difficult. We then speak about regression. One of my patients, a seventeen-year-old girl who wanted to escape sex at any price, took refuge in fairy tales which she had enjoyed in early childhood. Her favorite story was that of the Sleeping Beauty. She was particularly impressed by the prince cutting the hedges with his sword, an obvious symbolization of the sexuality which she wanted to escape. Psychoanalysis correctly speaks of the return of the repressed material in a more acceptable form. One may go back to actual experiences of childhood which have been more satisfactory: for instance, the infantile love of one's father or mother. Old thoughts may be revived, and even old ways of thinking may be of new importance.

Such an early way of psychic life is materialized in the mechanism which is called projection. It is usually defined as pushing parts of our own experience which pertain either to the body or to our psychic experience into the outward world. This definition is too narrow, since it neglects the fact that the body and world are always coordinated with each other. They are always present, and a continuous effort is going on in order to find out what belongs to our body and what belongs to the outward world. We are never quite sure which experiences have originated in ourselves and which are the experiences of others. In childhood the activity which is necessary to ascertain one's border lines necessarily has to be greater. In projection, a new construction takes place which determines what belongs to one's self and what belongs to the outward world. Hallucinations are the clearest expressions of this process of projection. The hostility one feels against the love object may appear as the hostile act the love object commits against oneself. One of my patients felt that the people around him made remarks about his homosexuality, which upset him very greatly. But he had strong homosexual trends against which he fought so vigorously that they appeared only in dreams. In one of his dreams, for instance, he felt that he had been raped through the rectum. He shoved the individual away and took out of his rectum a twisted rope a yard long.

We have learned that the dream world as well as the world of the paranoiac and schizophrenic is built according to the individual's emotional problems.

The projection has its counterpart in appropriating parts of the outside world to oneself. We then speak about appersonation. This process of rearrangement between the outside world and ourselves takes not only isolated parts of the outside world into ourselves, but even whole persons are taken into ourselves and made a part of ourselves. Very often we try to get rid of failures in previous stages of our development and make them a part of the outside world by what we may call self-projection. This is particularly well seen in some cases of homosexuality in which the love objects represent abandoned stages of one's own development. We are continually putting ourselves in the places of others and others in the place of ourselves. There is a continuous stream of persons going into our ego and forming there either a part of our conscience or forming a part of the self which we do not want to be. Such images of persons who have wandered into ourselves may be easily projected again into the outward world. We know that the identification with the parents and love objects plays the paramount part in this process.

But this effort to rearrange our experiences does not lead immediately to projection. We may try to devaluate our experiences by feeling that they are impersonal acts; we then speak about depersonalization.

We may also call our own impulses obsessional or compulsive. We may finally commit automatic acts which we pretend not to understand. This latter instance leads us into the field of conversion, where a psychic conflict is no longer experienced as such and the somatic change appears instead. We have dealt with the problem of conversion in detail above.

We may experience further, instead of the conflicting situation, hypochondriac sensations in any part of the body.

We are entitled to say that in many of these attempts we deal with a return to more primitive types of reaction and, therefore, with regression.

All so-called primitive types of experience show evidence of a larger use of symbolic thinking. Since I have dealt with this topic in detail on another occasion, only a few remarks are necessary. When we are not capable of a specific solution in thinking or in action, we must content ourselves with a more general type of connotation and actions based upon them. Indeed, thinking in the early stages uses the single case as a pattern for acting in any similar situation, and by a process of experimentation a specific type of acting and thinking is reached. If the experimentation is incomplete and not sufficiently guided by the actual situations but by the wishes of the individual, a connotation or a picture may be chosen which is only correlated to the connotation which would lead to the correct action. We call such results of an incomplete experimentation *symbols* when we are vaguely conscious of the relation of the correct connotation to the substituting picture. We speak of symbol-like pictures when the individual has succeeded in keeping the relation of the picture to the real situation out of his mind.

Symbols thus are the expression of a deficiency, of an incompleteness, or better, are an incomplete stage of experimentation. Children, indeed, seem to have symbolic thinking. On closer inspection, the similarity between the thinking of children and symbolic thinking is not a very deep one. The child is, in truth, experimenting in a progressive way, and it overcomes its insufficiencies in the further process of development. The adult who uses symbols may be trying not to be forced into a full insight of the situation. Of course, he may go back to this more general and less definite type of thinking when he feels that his thinking has become too rigid, that he has to start and to try all over again. Indeed, in our thinking and in our actions if they remain useful we have to give up the rigid forms. The charm of symbols in art and poetry is owing to the fact that their indefiniteness promises a new development. Symbolic thinking is very often reached by regression when the individual is too much afraid of the consequences of clear insight into a situation. Symbols are in this respect, also, inexact signs and do not permit a correct action, but they contain a greater readiness in several directions.

The process of differentiation leads not only to unified connotations and actions, but also to more or less coherent attitudes and emotions. If the individual is afraid of such a commitment, his unified attitude is given up, the situation is split up into different parts and so into different emotional directions. One speaks then too mechanically about ambivalence, meaning that there are emotions which also contain their opposite. On closer examination, it becomes obvious that the so-called ambivalence occurs when the individual is not capable of coming to a full unified attitude towards the situation. Therefore, in seeing sometimes this and sometimes the other side of the situation, he vacillates between love and hate. Such ambivalence may be considered again as regression.

In catatonic states the individual goes back to primitive motor reaction. In the so-called automatism to orders, the individual chooses the simple expedient of giving in completely to what the other says.

In catatonic negativism, the individual answers to every approach with defense, and expresses these attitudes in the muscles. It is not always possible to see a connection of these primitive reactions to earlier stages of development. But the general principle remains that when the individual tries to escape from a difficult situation and goes back to a primitive one, the reaction occurring is very often in its essential points identical with, or at least related to, the stages of development in childhood and to the behavior of so-called primitives.

Many patients feel overwhelmed by a situation and give up every effort. One may see this in cases of hysterical stupor, especially in persons accused of serious crimes. Some neurotic cases simply go to bed and stay there, as I have observed in a patient who, after a psychic trauma, spent several years in bed till she finally died from tuberculosis. Similar mechanisms can be seen in some hebephrenics and in some catatonic stupors. The depressive stupor has a more complicated psychological structure and corresponds more to self-punishment and self-torture, but we are here more interested in the general problem of the results of psychic defense. We may summarize by saying that the individual either tries to neglect the difficulty in the situation or he goes back to more primitive solutions. It should not be overlooked, however, that the attempt of an individual to regain his psychic health by going back into the past or to primitive modes of reaction is never merely an effort to go back. There is a constructive effort even in the attempt to organize the experiences on a deeper level of organization; and furthermore, when this organization is reached the individual still may attempt to regain an adaptation even to more complicated situations.

It is obvious that the term "not being adapted to the actual situation" is insufficient. It characterizes merely one part of the situation. We want to know what are the reasons which make an individual make use of the defense mechanism. Why should the individual adapt; what happens if the individual does not adapt? He may suffer physical damage and the consequences described above, or he may react with the painful experience of anxiety, guilt, insecurity, and the feelings of insufficiency.

The danger lies in the situation with which the individual is confronted. We have, therefore, to understand the danger situations. The danger may originate from nature, in its widest sense. Weather, flood, an earthquake, scarcity of food, famine, wild animals, falling trees, precipices, and darkness may threaten the individual. Other dangerous situations arise from one's relations to one's fellow human beings. One may be attacked by them and has to fear their aggression. One may not find their co-operation and help, which is indispensable in the difficulties of life. One may be deprived by them of one's property. One also needs love and understanding in the widest sense. This is sexual love as well as the tender feelings which one expects from one's love object. The consequences by which one is threatened are deprivation of love, food, and support, and an encroachment into the integrity of the body. This may be either bodily harm, wounds, and mutilation, or restriction of one's free movements. Disease belongs, in this respect, to the dangerous situations. The child and the primitive very often consider disease as inflicted by hostile influences.

The world which we have immediately before us is comparatively narrow. The world consists of regular sequences. The beginning of a sequence is a sign. The world before us has, besides its immediate perceptive value, a sign function. Among the sign functions, words have a special significance. However, the sign functions are universal functions which expand the range of perception and put us into a world which is richer and more varied. This expansion is an expansion in space as well as in time. The radius of human activity is increased. One may gain some amount of security by heeding danger signals. One learns also about dangers which one would not otherwise have suspected.

One fundamental difference between the world of the child and the world of the adult lies in the greater reliability of the signs the adult uses. The sign function in the child is less extensive; in addition, since insufficient experimentation has taken place, the signs are not sufficiently differentiated. The child is also helpless against the actual danger situation and therefore needs a greater amount of love and support from the adult. One might suspect that the narrower world of the child must be experienced as particularly dangerous.

One might be inclined to say that danger situations are not situations in the outside world, but originate merely from the attitude of the individual. Such a statement is incorrect and neglects the fundamental psychological experiences. It cannot be denied, however, that how much of the danger situation is perceived and experienced depends upon our constructive efforts.

One may summarize the dangers of the child as deprivation of love, food, and support, and an encroachment on the integrity of the body.

In the course of an extensive scientific program, the workers in Bellevue Psychiatric Hospital acquired a definite dynamic and constructive approach to childhood problems.[1] The child is a growing organism with definite problems of maturation, as has been particularly emphasized in American literature by Gesell. Great stress, however, should be placed on living situations and emotional problems of childhood, as these are continually modifying the developmental process. The development of the child is seen, in accordance with the general principles of psychoanalysis, as an emotional interdependence between the parents, the surroundings of the child, and the child himself. Furthermore, human beings have social connections in general, and therefore particular emphasis was placed on the psychology of the group, and group therapy was used not only in theoretical situations but also in the practical carrying out of treatment.

The development of the child is not merely a maturation process but also a continuous process of social experimentation by which, after trial and error, final construction is reached. This final construction is dependent upon basic principles of psychophysiological organization which, in the form of configurations and gestalten, determine the beginning, the continuation, and the end of the experimental process.

In "The Child and the Symbol," I have written that the child approaches the world in a continuous process of constructive experimentation which is determined by the maturation level and by individual factors of psychological development. One has not the right to call these products of experimentation symbols even when the approach to reality remains incomplete. These processes of experimentation come out in children's drawings, in the formation of concepts, and in the language products of children. Symbols and symbol-like pictures are signs which point to an unclearly seen referent. The incompleteness of the symbol-like picture has to be revealed

[1] From Frank J. Curran and Paul Schilder, "A Constructive Approach to the Problems of Childhood and Adolescence" (a survey of studies from the Children's and Adolescents' Ward in Bellevue Psychiatric Hospital, New York City), *Journal of Clinical Psychopathology* 2:125–42, 1940.

by specific methods. Symbols and symbol-like pictures appear where the experimentation process belonging to a specific maturation level is prevented by danger and threat. Symbols are, therefore, danger signals concerning the adaptation of the child to the world. The primary aim however is to go to the reality as such, and in the literature for children and puppet shows, the use of symbolic material is only justified when the immediate approach to reality would be too difficult. However, the symbol should not be a purpose in itself but a step towards the final mastery of reality according to the maturation level.

This agrees with a tendency in modern education not to make unlimited use of symbolism and fairy tales, but instead to help the child to adapt himself to the everyday-life surroundings in which he lives. From a similar viewpoint, I have doubted the usefulness of Lewis Carroll's *Alice in Wonderland* for children.

Symbolism is therefore only a passing phase in the adaptation process of thinking in the child. This process was studied in connection with the attitude and concepts of children towards death by David Wechsler and myself. It is difficult for the child to correlate the conventional religious ideas with his own experiences. The connotations and judgments derived from adults are taken by the child as a part of his immediate reality. The child is merely interested in reality. In general the child finds it hard to incorporate conventional, metaphysical, and religious conceptions into the bulk of his experiences; and he only succeeds in doing so when he decides to accept the conventions without analysis, however contradictory to experience they may be.

In a similar study, David Wechsler and I also asked children what they thought about the interior of their bodies. Many workers have considered the experience of one's body as the mechanical summing up of single experiences. This point of view, in our opinion, is no longer justified, as the experience of one's body is built up by continuous experimentation and interchange with other human beings and forms a specific experience that is the body image.

In reply to the question "What is the inside of your body made of?" the typical answer was that it contained food just eaten. This indicates the concrete nature of the child's thinking. Two of the children said they were under their skins and inside their bodies. Now it is one of the paradoxes of our bodily experiences that our sensations relate to the surface of the body, and yet we do not regard this as our body proper.

In German and English alike there are phrases which suggest that we can strip off our skins, i.e., "jump out of our skins." It seems, then, that sometimes we think of our skins as our most intimate possession—i.e., "to save one's skin," or life. At other times it is merely the envelope of our true self and what is inside of us. However, in the deep infantile strata of our minds we are not perfectly certain whether there is anything inside of us except what is crammed into us from the outside, i.e., food.

It should be stressed that the child is not merely aggressive but that he has genuine and lively interest in the well-being and existence of those about him. Lauretta Bender and I made an investigation into the psychology of aggressiveness in children, based upon the clinical observations of eighty-three children between the ages of three and fifteen years. The problem of physical aggressiveness was studied. We considered violence to be an act which damaged the body of another person or distorted the body image by pain or discomfort. The children were not only observed clinically, but were subjected to a definite play situation, to a series of pictures depicting aggressive situations, and to a questionnaire on aggression.

We concluded that:

Aggressiveness finds expression more directly in younger children, in actions as well as in play, in words and in the description of pictures. Young children seek immediate satisfaction and are in immediate fear of punishment and retaliation. The narrowness of their world does not allow the co-ordination of a great number of facts. Good or bad in the adult sense is more or less an arbitrary decision of the adult. Deprivation of love or food increases the aggressive tendencies of children.

In all the children, there gradually emerges the idea of right and wrong, dependent on immediate advantages and disadvantages. The youngest age group express their aggressiveness freely, verbally and in play, but the older age groups are inclined to be inhibited, and often a play situation or other indirect method is needed by which they can unconsciously express their aggressiveness in the idea of punishment of others for their sins. Aggressiveness against a group is expressed more freely than aggressiveness against single individuals.

There is a process of gradual organization of aggressive tendencies into a socially accepted concept in which the attitude of the surroundings is of paramount importance. The psychological situation of the child leads to the final crystallization of his aggressive attitudes.

In the youngest children there are no discrepancies between their actual behavior and their answers to questions. In the older group, however, the verbal morality is usually higher, while the aggressiveness finds expression in play and tends to become more or less unconscious and repressed.

Aggressiveness has close relation to motor drives and to instincts in general. It undoubtedly has foundations in the organic structure, and its variations may be constitutional. Organic processes influence the general output of energy. The hyperkinetic child shows increased aggressiveness. The aggressiveness on an organic basis is mostly diffuse, whereas psychic trauma leads to an aggression in relation to specific situations.

The above-mentioned studies in aggressiveness clearly indicate that emotional factors and impulses are very dependent upon organic factors and especially on organic motor problems. Several papers dealing with this problem have been published.[2]

Play concerning posture, which children love so much, is often not handled in the right way by the adult. It is obviously correct to let the child experiment with any posture and action. It is justifiable to rock the child, to raise it in the air, and then to let it drop, provided that the danger situation does not become overwhelming to the child. It should learn that after experimentation and danger it can regain security with the help of others. It may finally learn to rely upon its own capacity of regaining postural security. It should never be brought into a panic of equilibrium or, more generally, into a motor panic. Furthermore, it should not be thrown into postural situations which it resists more than necessary. It should not have the feeling that motor restrictions which are lasting are imposed upon it.

It appears that the motor training of a child is a preliminary step in every education and carries with it important emotional and libidi-

[2] Much of the work on the problems of the organically brain-damaged child was subsequently summarized by Lauretta Bender in "Organic Brain Conditions Producing Behavior Disturbances," *Modern Trends in Child Psychiatry,* edited by B. Pacella and Nolan D. C. Lewis (Grune and Stratton, 1945), and in "Psychological Problems in Organic Brain Disorders in Children," *American Journal of Orthopsychiatry* 19:404–15, 1949. [L.B., Ed.]

nous implications. We may suspect that mere knowledge on the part of the parents will not be sufficient in order to handle the problems of equilibrium in the child in a correct way. The parents will need, besides their motor equipment and their will to help the child in its motor expression and security, an emotional inner balance. Equilibrium is not merely a motor and vestibular problem but also a moral one. The normal development of postural reactions has been studied by Joseph Teicher.

Both pattern formation and motility have an important part in the play of children. The form of the organism and its motor possibilities determine the play of children. Rotation of the total body around its longitudinal axis and circular movements of outstretched limbs are of special importance. The motility adapts itself to the plane on which the play takes place. The play starts with the formation of foreground and background. The child undertakes a continuous experimentation concerning the geometrical qualities of lines, angles, and clusters. In the three-dimensional game, the child is particularly interested in whether something can be put into something else. Further experimentation concerns gravitation, push, pull, and momentum. The experimentation with space and mass (geometry and physics) is based upon the instinctive drives of children and, therefore, dependent upon their individual emotional problems. The definite form of the play is adaptable to the biological situation.

Lauretta Bender [3] stresses the continual interplay between the emotional and the intellectual problems of the child and emphasizes that almost every activity of the child must be considered from both angles. The emotional life grows out of the family situation and reflects the psychosexual organization directly or in a symbolic way. There are four important principles which have been contributed to the understanding of the emotional life of the child by the Freudian school. These are: (1) the theory of infantile sexuality; (2) the development of the superego in early childhood; (3) the development of the Oedipus complex in early childhood; (4) the psychoanalytical interpretation of the emotional symbols in the unconscious life of the child, which may be expressed by means of his play, his dreams, his drawings, etc.

[3] These problems have been discussed more fully by Lauretta Bender in articles on aggression, hostility, anxiety, etc. See bibliography. [L.B., Ed.]

The superego is built up in the child by its relationship to those who administer to its physical needs, family or parents, and especially in the early stages to its mother. If the care is interrupted at too early an age the pattern becomes shattered and the child's personality and superego become arrested at the infantile level, and he may develop into what is known as a psychopathic personality in adult life.

Frank J. Curran, working with boys of twelve to sixteen who were patients on the Adolescent Ward in Bellevue Hospital, has studied the psychotherapeutic problems arising at the time of puberty. With the exception of the sexual problems, there are no specific problems of early adolescence. The same types of neurotic and conduct disorders seen in younger children are also present here, but certain problems are more clearly brought into prominence at puberty. Symptoms of shyness or overassertiveness occur simultaneously with the rapid changes in voice and growth at puberty. Overt sex behavior, including exhibitionism, open masturbation, manipulation of sex organs of others, homosexuality and heterosexual experiences, occur frequently in association with puberty. In Children's and Wayward Minor Courts, the chief delinquency in girls is a sexual one, although the girl may technically be labeled as "wayward."

When children play doctor they investigate each other's bodies.[4] They put their fingers, straws, or instruments in every opening they can reach. Sometimes they are rather rough in this procedure. The psychoanalytical formulation that the interest in medical studies is based upon sadomasochistic and anal tendencies is basically correct although it is not broad enough. One might say that this interest is based on curiosity concerning the human body as a whole and an appreciation of the experience of suffering in oneself and in others.

One might raise the question whether individuals with such tendencies are not more exposed to psychological dangers than those who choose professions which bring them less in contact with sick bodies and suffering persons. However it is possible to find a psychogenetic basis for every choice of profession. Very often this choice is in close relation to infantile strivings and tendencies. Those who love the work they are doing derive a great deal of their energy from infantile sources and their work is none the worse for it. Generally we may

[4] Reprinted from Paul Schilder, "The Mental Hygiene of the Medical Student," *Medical Bulletin of Student Assoc., New York University College of Medicine* 4:68–70, 1939.

say that persons who choose their profession according to their own preference might be more in danger of being overrun by infantile tendencies if they do not get insight into these infantile strivings and learn to control them.

However, the medical student is not in a greater danger in this respect than the college student in general. Strecker, Appel, Palmer and Braceland have compared in two studies the mental health of medical students with the mental health of college students in general.[5] The estimates of the frequency of emotional maladjustments among college students vary between 10 per cent and 18 per cent. These disturbances are considered as sufficient to warp the lives of the students. Angyll and others come to the conclusion that from 86 per cent to 88 per cent of the students have more or less serious emotional problems. It does not seem that the occurrence of neurotic characteristics among medical students is greater. However, in the medical school of the University of Pennsylvania, slightly more than 46 per cent of senior students suffered from neurotic handicaps of major character. It seemed also that an impressive number of unstable personalities appeared to be rendered more unstable and insecure as a result of medical school experiences.

What can the medical student do for himself when he is beset by fears and anxieties? These fears and anxieties center about the problems of health, sex, physical efficiency, beauty, intelligence, mental efficiency, and problems of social contacts with others. Economic problems may play a more or less important part. We have surmised that the interest in the human body is one of the prerequisites for the interest in the study of medicine. It is not merely the riddle of the bodies of others but also the riddle of one's own body with which one is confronted. There will be particular pride in one's own body and a great love for one's own body. No wonder that one starts to doubt whether the body will fulfill all the functions demanded of it. The medical student hears continually about disease, and it will be easy for him to discover the signs of more or less insidious diseases in his own body when his feelings of security concerning his body once have been disturbed. Such feelings of insecurity may originate from overinterest in the functioning of one's own body, but they may come from any other insecurity in relation to human beings,

[5] Cf. also C. Fry, *Mental Health in Colleges* (New York Commonwealth Fund, 1942). [L.B., Ed.]

which is merely expressed in distrust in one's own body. When one has good human relationships with other human beings, one will also trust one's own body. And if there are real signs of disease then one will be able to let the physician who represents social and medical health take care of the problem. So we may formulate: Trust your own body!

Very closely related are the problems of strength and beauty and of the capacity for excelling in physical exercise or sports. In an interesting study, David Wechsler has stated that one may consider among 1,000 people only one on either end of the scale as "pathological." The other 998 can be considered as "normal," and the variability among those is much less than one would expect. Many people are induced by chance experiences to demand of themselves a specific size, appearance, and strength. They demand of themselves a greater dexterity than they will ever reach. They compare themselves continually with an artificial ideal and put before themselves tasks which cannot be solved by going forward step by step. When the ideal is too high and the individual falls short of perfection, feelings of insufficiency and inferiority develop, and one will give up too easily because one cannot attain an ideal which is beyond the reach. Even one's ideals should have a tinge of reality about them, and in all situations one should not feel that every striving is useless unless the final goal is reached. One should also enjoy one's way. One should examine carefully one's ideals. Very often they are built up around words which are only incompletely understood. With one phrase: do not trust your ideals. Very often hopes and fears center around economic problems. Without underrating the effects of economic insecurity, only those who fail to adapt in other spheres of life will come into danger of losing their equilibrium under economic stress.

The fears concerning the body and its function blend with fears and concerns about sex in its widest sense. One may not only doubt whether one is strong enough, but one may doubt one's capacity for proper sex function. One may furthermore be afraid that one is not masculine enough, when one is a boy, or feminine enough, when one is a girl. Fears concerning masturbation or homosexuality may creep in. One's sex appeal may appear to be low in comparison with others and become the object of great concern. I am of the opinion that one has also underrated in this case the range of normal possibilities and exaggerated the range of variability. In the long run every human being has a value not only as a personality but also as a sexual being, and this value will be appreciated if one does not put too many obstacles between himself and the other person. There may be an exaggerated fear of the dangers of sex (although one should know them well), and one may demand too much perfection from the love object which one may choose. This may be transformation of the fear that one might not be capable of experiencing full appreciation from another person. One should keep in mind that every person is capable of giving and receiving love and sex gratification.

Obviously not everyone can be the most intelligent one in the class. Some have to be more gifted than others; some have better memories; some have a greater capacity for continuous work. It is not always good for one to desire to outshine others. One might demand more and more from himself until finally he cannot fulfill his own demands and starts to blame himself. Maybe it is the best thing not to compare oneself too much with others. As mentioned, the range of human capacities is limited, and many people have more gifts than they think. These will appear when the individual thinks less about what he will be able to do and more about what are the things which could be of interest. One should tell most human beings and medical students especially that they should drift.

Of course, the medical student has to work—he has to study. If his secret ambitions and neurotic fears do not interfere, he will be able to do his work without being fatigued. Statistics show that fatigue is one of the great problems of students in colleges and in medical schools. I do not believe very much in fatigue as a physiological phenomenon. It is a sign that one is not quite sure about one's aim. When you are fatigued, ask yourself, "Where am I going?" I have never seen anybody who has been harmed as a personality by too much work. This does not mean that one does not have to follow the precepts of hygiene so far as they concern the body. However, when somebody works, blindly pushing forward, one should ask himself what it is that he doesn't want to see.

Most of the practical tasks of life can be fulfilled by everybody. Most of the students who come to medical schools have an I.Q. high enough to become useful physicians. It is difficult for anybody to say that he will be capable of doing more. There is no reason why one should not try, and if one thinks very highly of oneself, one should prove it to oneself and to others by actual performance. Trial will show that this problem can't be solved in a day. It usually takes years, and if success comes after a few years of trial and error, one may feel that perhaps it is still a small performance in relation to the ideal one has of oneself. Think of yourself that you might be the most gifted and the most intelligent person in your group, but try to prove it by your performance so that others believe you. Many people feel they would be geniuses or great men if they didn't become fatigued, if they didn't have so many sex urges. Very often one develops neurotic symptoms so that he can tell himself and others that he is only hindered by them from reaching his ideal level. Students should try to be honest with themselves, and this will be easier if they have friends and do not live in a world of their own.

Many human beings are afraid that they might not find love and admiration from persons of their own and the opposite sex. Most human beings are somewhat admirable and everybody is searching eagerly for persons who may allow him to give them admiration and love. If one doesn't hinder the other person, one can hardly escape being loved and admired. To be true, there is also hostility and aggression in oneself and others. It is good to know this. If one does, one will not expect to be loved and to be admired continually. One should allow oneself a good hate and should not shudder when he discovers such a good hate in others too. Only on the basis of conflicting tendencies which go through the whole realm of human emotions can one finally come to a social relation with others which is truly human. Companionship does not mean that one is free from hate, but it means that one can organize a human relation which appreciates one's own qualities as well as the qualities of others.

The danger situations of the adult are loss of money, position, and prestige; loss of love objects; loss of the integrity of the body, and disease.

When the individual feels insufficiency concerning the task which is created by a situation, fear and anxiety will appear. There may be the general feeling of insecurity and lack of orientation expressed in dizziness. There may be an insufficiency in thought, action, and emotion. Furthermore, the individual might feel sick. The feeling of guilt originates when danger is experienced as the consequence of one's own action. One immediately sees that human suffering in the somatic and psychic spheres cannot be separated from the danger situations.

Adler's approach stresses the outside situation. Freud's approach stresses the reaction of the individual. None of them can completely neglect the other side. Jung has seen a part of this problem. He has spoken of extroverted individuals and introverted individuals, the one directed towards the world, the other directed towards his own experience. The complication arises that the individual, according to his opinion, may become an extrovert in order to escape the suffering, and that one may become an introvert in order to escape the danger situation. In this complicated way he comes, for instance, to the conclusion that Freud is an extrovert and Adler an introvert. Skeptical of every sort of typology, I want to emphasize that the outward situation and the reaction of the individual are indivisible sides of experience. The different types of human beings, as far as one can ascertain the existence of such types at all, have merely different worlds before them and have different attitudes.

The attitude towards a danger situation is dependent upon the difficulty of the situation and upon the individual himself. It is characteristic of human existence that each has a biography, a life history. The patterns connected with, and developed in relation to, earlier danger situations will not remain isolated. They will be the basis for later reactions. Modern psychology therefore justly stresses the importance of early pattern formation. Since the possibilities of successful action are comparatively limited in the child, the attitude of the love objects of the child and of the persons who take care of it will very often have a decisive influence on the pattern formation of the child. Here lies the basis for the mechanisms which an individual chooses in order to escape suffering. A great interest of the parents in the child's body will increase the interest of the child in his body and will, later on, when difficulties arise, lead to hypochondriasis and conversion symptoms. A factual organic disease in childhood very often has a similar effect. When the child is punished for its aggressiveness or when its activities are unduly restricted, a feeling of guilt may come into the foreground which can easily be revived by later experience. When the child experiences a loss of love, anxiety may occur. This may occur also when the spoiled child develops such excessive demands that they can no more be fulfilled. This is only a very schematic description. In order fully to understand these problems, one would have to go deeper into the complicated sexual and social relations of the child to the persons around him.

The adult individual has a past, and in his present attitude of suffering and defense the infantile pattern will be used. Reading in psychoanalytic literature or in books on individual psychology, one would sometimes begin to think that the infantile patterns would be the only ones which are of importance. However, human beings are continually in a process of trial and error which never stops. Freud himself acknowledges the importance of the present but puts the chief accent on the past. According to Adler, one's style of life is laid down before the fifth year. The importance of actual life situations should be stressed more. The life style, the patterns and the configurations are not a dead past and their material is capable of reorganization in the actual life situation. It is true, however, that individuals who are overwhelmed by an actual situation do not dare to continue the process of experimentation in order to escape suffering, in the sense characterized above, and use defense mechanisms which lead back to the past. They neglect parts of the reality. They want to see the narrower world in which the primitive attitudes were successful.

Individuals who, in the face of difficult situations, try to escape the actual or threatened suffering not by an action or an adaptation which fits the situation, but by giving up the process of trial and error and going back to a narrower world, we may call neurotic, psychopathic or psychotic. The psychological defense mechanisms against physical and mental suffering have to be considered as preliminary adaptations on the basis of which a new attempt to gain contact with reality may occur. Psychotherapy attempts to hinder these preliminary adaptations from becoming permanent, and tries to lead the individual to new experimentation and adaptation. Very often it will be necessary that the individual substitute actual unhappiness for neurotic suffering before such adaptation will be possible.

Modern psychotherapy has very often stressed the idea that the neurotic and psychotic symptom brings satisfactions. For Freud, the symptom is a symbolic gratification of infantile sex desires. For Adler, the symptom serves the desire of the individual to gain power. But a neurotic and psychotic individual is still faced with the task of the outward situation and suffers continually from it. He also suffers from the symptom as such, which is always experienced as an expression of his incapacities. Even from the point of view of subjective experience, the symptom primarily means suffering. Psychoanalysts have felt it might thus satisfy one's wish for punishment in order to escape feelings of guilt. But such an argument tends to overlook the fact that suffering is the inalienable inheritance of human existence. It is deeply based on the anatomical and physiological organization, and it cannot be derived from the feeling of guilt. The latter points to another side of human experience: when we act we shall sooner or later also be hurt. And there is a deep reluctance in us to be hurt. One should not try to reduce the variety of experience to too simple formulae.

The following tasks emerge: We have to acknowledge fellow human beings as social units, and have to be acknowledged by them. One should be capable of having love relations and sex gratifications, of acknowledging the love-sex object as persons, and should be acknowledged by them. One should not be overwhelmed by the object reality.

Subjectively, suffering and unhappiness should be acknowledged as a necessary part of experience, which has to be tolerated. They should lead to a renewed attempt to change the social, sexual, and object reality till suffering and unhappiness are relieved. Organic disease, as far as it is not a regressive expression of psychic suffering, has to be considered as a part of the object reality. The full experience of physical and mental health—we may also call it happiness—can only be reached in this way. Since we are always confronted with new, difficult, and often even unsolvable tasks, happiness cannot be a static experience: it is a dynamic process which never comes to completion. Freud says justly that it is one aim of psychotherapy that the neurotic should be taught to stand displeasure tensions.

A case history may exemplify anxiety and guilt in relation to an extreme aggressiveness for which the patient fears retaliation. The patient, a thirty-three-year-old physician, has a rigid face and an enormous push in talking, so that an organic inferiority of those parts of the brain which are affected in encephalitis is at least probable. His increased drives may have an organic background. He has been in analysis for about fifteen months, with two other analysts. The present treatment has so far not been successful. His chief complaint is an all-pervading anxiety, a fear of death which hinders him from everything. He had to be revived at birth with great difficulty. He heard about it when he was four or five years old. It was probably a matter of pride for him that he had been born dead, and lived, nonetheless. His mother was sick after his birth. Two brothers and one sister are considerably older than himself. There is little material available about his earlier relations with father and mother. At four years of age he was afraid of thunderstorms and God. The thunderstorms might rush against the earth. He felt inferior and weak and was afraid to die. He felt that he would like to poison the bullies who had treated him badly. He was afraid to fight. In childhood he once dreamt that everybody in the family was dead in a coffin, he himself included. But the sister raised her head. It was merely a fake. He was deeply impressed by the death of his mother and his father. Eternity seemed very long to him and he became frightened. In puberty he had strong sexual wishes concerning his sister, with whom he slept. There were aggressive impulses against other boys. He heard about cannibals eating girls and was frightened. He was angry at God because He had killed his mother in a painful way.

The present neurosis started when he read about President Wilson's death. Wilson's physician had said to Wilson: "You have only two minutes to live." Wilson answered: "The machine is broken down." On this night a terrible anxiety started. He had strong sadistic impulses to slice a girl and to eat her up. He wanted to hit the analyst over the head. He liked profane language. He said, for instance, "I want to beat the sh— out of you." He liked the word f—. He had phantasies of biting the penis and eating it. His wife died in 1932 in childbirth. He feels that he, as the father, was responsible for it. He also feels responsible for the death of his mother, who was operated upon on his advice. After the death of his mother he had a compulsion to count. He had phantasies of knocking the wall out. "I often think about putting things into a meat grinder. It comes out like feces, all alike." He saw, at six or seven years, that his father's penis was very big. His brother made loud noises in urinating. He cannot differentiate between a dead and a living person. He is not sure that he should think of his parents as dirt or as decomposing masses. He also felt in this way while they were alive. Sometimes he complains that he will be distributed everywhere as a lifeless mass. "If everybody would be divided into particles, everybody would be alike." Sometimes in bed he feels that he is getting small, and gets frightened. He once killed a woman in an automobile accident but was exonerated. He says she bounced like a ball. Later on, he enjoyed the idea and felt as if he had raped with an enormous penis. In the further pursuit of aggressiveness he comes to the atom, to the point of final resistance.

In the course of the treatment he curses, shouts, makes threatening gestures, slams the door, stamps with his feet, says he would like to smash the chair on the physician's head, but always controls himself. He never is really aggressive in action and there is an underlying politeness behind all his curses.

There is not sufficient material available concerning his childhood. It seems that he felt weak and helpless as the youngest of the family and unable to express his drives, which, probably on an organic basis, exceeded the average. The combination of hyperkinesis, weakness, and educational forces repressing the hyperkinesis must dam up the impulses and transform them into sadism and aggression. In early phantasies and dreams he put all his adversaries and love objects to death. He transferred this attitude towards his wife. Since he felt tremendously inferior to his love objects as well as to other boys, his aggressiveness came out against both. It is debatable whether his accident is the expression of his sadistic impulsions, or whether his sadistic impulses did not reinterpret and use the accident, which, according to the investigation, was the woman's fault. The counting and using of obscene language become the substitute expression of his aggressiveness, which does not acknowledge differences between human beings any more. Cannibalistic phantasies, closely connected with anal phantasies, accentuate the aggression. He fears the retaliation of being dismembered, pulverized, and eaten up.

This is an individual overpowered by an external force. The feeling of weakness and helplessness is supplemented by the fear of the aggression of others, which is partially patterned according to his own aggressiveness and partially feared as retaliation. This is a type of anxiety which is not merely the fear of losing a love object and of being deserted; it is an anxiety in connection with violent aggressive impulses. One feels that one can gain at least some understanding of the situation in this way. His pattern is obviously taken from early situations. It has not been modified sufficiently by the experiences of his life. It may have hindered him from full love relations although his potency is intact.

The psychiatric pictures occurring in old age can only be understood if one takes the psychology of aging into consideration.[6] The psychiatrist observes that human beings between forty and fifty years of age start to think about the coming of old age. There is a gradual change in appearance; the hair may start to become gray, and there may be a feeling of diminished capacity for work. In women the menopause is generally considered as the end of one period of life and the beginning of a less desirable period. The individuals may feel that their erotic value is diminishing. If life has been satisfactory and there is a prospect of continued emotional and social security, they will feel that their value as a personality has not diminished and they can still enjoy the importance that their greater experience and social power bestow upon them. When later on the impairment of sensory functions and motor performances becomes undeniable, and when the decline in memory functions and creative mental capacities becomes obvious to the individuals themselves, they may be easily resigned to looking back on the experiences and achievements of their life spans. They may feel sure of their inner values in relation to their families or surroundings in general. We may expect that some individuals will be unable to stand their losses by age and may then revolt by complaining. Others will answer to the deprivation by giving up completely, and finally there will be a group who will try to find compensations in a phantasy world which may be an illicit revival of the past, and which may deviate in one or another direction from reality. We may speak about two phases in aging and call the first the phase of libidinous rearrangement, the second the phase of organic impairment.

Modern psychiatry is accustomed to view psychotic manifestations not as queer additions to the so-called "normal" personality but as specific aspects of psychophysiological developments which, in essence, are identical in the normal and the pathological case.

The physical disturbances connected with aging, especially with the menopause, may increase the strength of the feeling of general impairment. In milder cases this may lead to the picture of the so-called "neurasthenic, hypochondriac type" in which the connection with a specific difficulty is very obvious. In more outspoken cases, the anxiety in connection with the waning of the body and the libido is overwhelming, and depressive pictures result. There will be an

[6] From Paul Schilder, "Psychiatric Aspects of Old Age and Aging," *American Journal of Orthopsychiatry* 10:62–69, 1940.

overwhelming fear of death, which may finally lead to a desire for death. However, projections soon ensue, and the individual will experience the threat of annihilation from the outside. This threat may be directed specifically against the sex parts (castration complex), which are experienced as the essence of life, which is about to be taken away. These ideas of impairment of the body may be transformed into a general fear of being robbed. The idea of being robbed of money comes into the foreground. I therefore come to the conclusion that the depressive pictures of the involution are dominated by the fear of the impairment of the body function in general and of sex especially. They may culminate in a fear of death. Death is experienced in cases of this type as slow or fast dismemberment. This complex may be combined with acute anxiety or with inhibition. These primary fears and anxieties are met by two defense mechanisms. One is projection, as mentioned above. Depressive pictures of the involution often show this projection mechanism. However, the individual may also try to regain his lost youth in phantasies and in increased sex tension. This change however will be immediately followed by an increased feeling of guilt and by projections, and the sexual threat will then be experienced as coming from the outside. The persecutors of these cases may then represent the increased sex danger; however, they may also represent the danger of decaying sex. Furthermore, in some of my cases, I have gained the impression that the persecutors represent the endangered parts of the body, which have been projected into the outside world and retain their relation to the individual by coming back as persecutors. So-called atypical pictures may result from interaction between projection and reintrojection. Melanie Klein has stated that the dismembering motive plays an important part in the depressive cases. She correctly states that the depressive continues to care for, and about, the object. These worries are not present in the paranoid in whom the object, cut in pieces, becomes merely a multiplicity of persecutors, every piece growing into a separate persecutor. However, in the senile and presenile depression, the persecutor may indeed be a part of one's own body, which has become an independent threat. It should not be denied that in all these cases, relations to love objects persist. However, these love objects may not be appreciated in full, but only in part. We come very near to some of the formulations of Abraham, who attributed an important role to the tendencies of the depressive not to love the individual as a whole, but merely parts of him. There is no question that there is a continuous, complicated interplay between projections and introjections going on in these depressive cases. The introjections are identifications and appersonations. The projections throw either parts of the individual's body into the outward world, or parts of persons or total bodies previously introjected. There is no question that the enormous aggression of these patients, which is partially connected with the fear of decay, provokes feelings of guilt and a tendency to self-punishment, which may lead either to inhibition or to aggressive action towards the self. However, it cannot be the task of such a general discussion to go into details of the psychoanalytic theory of depressions. It should merely be stated that in involutional depressions, anxiety and fear of dismemberment play a greater part, in connection with the general characteristics of the coming age. This is particularly obvious in patients who, after several depressions in earlier life, suffer a new attack in the involutional or senile period. It is obvious that we also have to search in involutional depressions for the infantile determinant of the psychosis and, furthermore, for the constitutional and character problems involved. Titley has characterized the prepsychotic personality of patients with agitated depression as rigid, stubborn, overconscientious, and meticulous. "A rigid ethical code, proclivity for saving and extreme reticence, coupled with markedly sensitive and anxious trends, are recurrent throughout." It is interesting that not only the depressions of later age but also the manic states have a more chronic course (Wertham).

Although I have tried to characterize these pictures from a clinical and psychological point of view, I do not doubt that these psychoses have a biological background which is closely related to the involutional processes occurring in everyone.

One may generally state that the important characteristic of all these psychotic pictures is mental deterioration. Even the confusional states of the hypertensive show a difficulty in the perceptive and intellectual function akin to deterioration.

I have shown in my *Introduction to Psychoanalytic Psychiatry* that the memory disturbance is also connected with the breaking through of more primitive material. The stories which patients repeat are rebuilt to suit their emotional needs. They become the dominant figure and hero of every story. This is also true concerning the memory disturbances of the senile, which do not consist merely in distortions and condensations, but also allow the patient to live out many of his infantile strivings and desires.

We may generally say that we find in seniles not only a reversal to primitive forms of perceptive and intellectual experiences, but also a return to uninhibited emotions and infantile and juvenile desires.

Are these release phenomena due merely to the impairment of perception, memory, and judgment? Similar pictures may be found in senile patients who do not show very definite disturbances in the perceptive and intellectual spheres. We may assume that libidinous regressions are not merely in the so-called functional, but also in the organic, sphere (K. F. Scheid). The emotional factors in senile deterioration have only rarely attracted sufficient attention (Jelgersma). Old age is characterized by the increasing consciousness of decay and the fear of approaching death. Hall has given a dramatic description of this. However, there are forces at work which overcome aging and approaching death in a psychological way. Our patients say, "I think they all go backwards when they get to a certain age, but I don't." This patient answers the question "Are you strong?" with, "Not so extra; I go out once a week." The eighty-five-year-old L., who can hardly walk, says she feels healthy and doesn't want to get stout. In the colony where she lives an old man helps her in walking and brings her sandwiches. "Maybe he wants to make me." "He is not as old as I am; he is only seventy." "I don't want to be any younger; I want to live until God calls me." The patient complains that the nurses in the colony treat her badly and persecute her. A seventy-six-year-old woman says, "If you have something to eat, you are happy; if not, you are unhappy." She says one shouldn't think about death. "One has time enough to die." A sixty-five-year-old-man says, "I feel healthy and strong; I am happy." "I never think of dying; I want to live to about eighty." One may compare such optimistic remarks of demented patients with the remark of a fifty-five-year-old colored automobile mechanic who is well preserved and comes in merely because of drinking. "I always think of death; I am an auto mechanic; death lurks at every corner; I think especially of it when I am driving."

Generally speaking, the apprehensions and fears of the presenium and early senium are overcome by deterioration. These patients may feel happy and strong again, revive heterosexual wishes, or may at least feel gratified by oral satisfaction. The fear of being poor, of being robbed, or of being persecuted may persist and may act as a constant stimulus to escape into a state of greater happiness. The aging and senile person may even try to get renewed satisfaction in the sexual approach to younger people. However, in the majority of cases, this approach to youth will remain in the realm of daydreaming, phantasy, and confabulation. There are indications that these regressions follow the pathways through which the individual has gone in childhood, adolescence, and adult life. We may expect a revival of the Oedipus situation in all its variations. There are psychic compensations in senility. When the individual is no longer capable of enriching or maintaining his relations to the outside world, he regresses to infantile situations and looks from there to new possibilities. One may state that the senile still lives in a very real world. He has a definite relation to time and space, though the objective facts of time and space are distorted. Even when the senile regresses, he regresses differently than the schizophrenic. He does not go back to a magic world, but remains in a world which fulfills the strivings and desires he had in adolescence and manhood.

At any rate, the psychiatric study of senility shows with clearness that, whatever the difficulties of age and aging may be, there are compensatory psychological mechanisms which relieve the individuals from anxieties and guarantee psychological satisfactions.[7]

Only a short remark might be added. I have spoken and I shall speak about psychic mechanisms, following in this respect the terminology of Freud. There have often been objections to this term since there are no "mechanisms" in psychic life. However, the term is justified since many of these so-called mechanisms serve the individual's wish to take the personal character away from experiences, to make them mechanical, or to project them into the outward world. There is, therefore, no necessity to change the term *mechanisms* into the term *dynamisms*.

---

[7] See O. J. Kaplan, *Mental Disorders of Later Life* (Stanford University Press, 1945); E. V. Cowdry, Ed., *Problems of Aging; Biological and Medical Aspects* (Baltimore, The Williams and Wilkins Co., 1939); and R. Ginsberg, "Psychology in Everyday Geriatrics," *Geriatrics* 5:36–43, 1950. [L.B., Ed.]

Chapter 6

TECHNICAL TOOLS OF PSYCHOTHERAPY

THE PRECEDING chapters served merely the attempt to give insight into the fundamental aims of psychotherapy. They should not be considered as an outline of general psychology—a task which I approach in three other volumes [1]—nor as a general theory for the neuroses. We now proceed with a consideration of the tools which might be used in the psychological treatment of patients.

DISCUSSION

One may discuss with a patient whom one intends to treat by psychological methods his present situation and one may try to help him understand it. Such a discussion remains in the realm of everyday life, logic, and common sense. One may suppose that a person who sees the situation objectively, as the physician is supposed to do, will have a clearer understanding than one who is personally interested. One may also expect that a patient will talk more openly to the physician than to his love objects and friends. Furthermore, the physician is supposed to know more about human situations than

[1] *Image and Appearance of the Human Body; Goals and Desires of Man;* and *Mind: Perception and Thought in Their Constructive Aspects.*

many other persons. Moreover, he is supposed to have experience. Such a discussion will have to deal with the following topics:

1. The social and economic situations and the ambitions and disappointments connected with them; the profession and work, the relation to one's superiors, co-workers, and inferiors. Very often one will be able to point out that the amount of resentment and disappointment in all these directions is greater than the patient himself knows.

2. In the relation to one's friends, naturally many difficulties arise. Human beings are in a continual struggle with each other to gain superiority and to make the others subservient. Human relations in which one demands or receives too much admiration and subservience sooner or later lead to great difficulties. Even when there is a difference in age or in experience, the older and more experienced ones will incur the hate of the younger friend when insisting upon their superiority. Differences in the social status or in wealth may contribute to the tensions in such relations. In women one not infrequently sees relations in which one woman mentally participates in the chic, beauty, and sexual attractiveness of another who takes the erotic leadership. Similar relations in men may also occur. Such relations are unhealthy when the free stream of give-and-take is interrupted and one-sided. One sees here, immediately, that the physician in discussing even this simple problem is confronted with a fundamental problem of psychotherapy. He knows, or at least should know, much more about such relations than he is able to tell his patient, unless he takes the risk of upsetting the patient without having the possibility of helping him out of his problem through discussion only. In every psychotherapy, especially in the more superficial types, there is the great danger that the physician may use psychotherapy merely as a display of himself instead of considering the status of the patient. This problem will be met again and again. It is mentioned here merely from the point of view of the dangers involved in a procedure seemingly so simple.

3. Even the simplest discussion cannot avoid a discussion of the relation of the patient to his father, mother, siblings, and the family in general. The dependence of one member of the family upon the others should be considered in detail. It is obvious that the closer the family sticks together, the stronger the resentment is against the family and the less the patient is willing to see his or her own resent-

ment. Human beings have been educated to acknowledge in themselves only positive attitudes towards their families, especially their parents. They are frightened by every hint of disharmony. In our culture, only money problems make the inherent tensions in families more manifest. It is obvious that sex problems play an enormous part in this relation, but there will be hardly any opportunity in a simple discussion to touch upon these sex problems. Some patients come with a superficial psychoanalytic knowledge, and use psychoanalytic terminology which they do not understand in its full implication, even if a superficial and an intellectual understanding is present.

4. The problems of sex and love have to be discussed frankly and in an open way. One has the right to be skeptical about what patients tell at such occasions. The strength of drives is very often overrated. The bitterness inherent in many sexual relations, also in marriage, is very often not confessed by the patient and is not even fully conscious in him. The specific mode of intercourse should be discussed in every deeper psychotherapeutic discussion, but it is inadvisable to do so if the relation between physician and patient remains on a superficial level.

5. Even if the patient complains only about conflicts, it is advisable to investigate diseases and the attitude of the patient concerning them. The history of physical health is an important part in every psychotherapeutic approach, and one should always compare the health record of the patient with the health record of any other member of the family.

6. If the patient has children, one should investigate very carefully his attitudes towards his children. I have generally found that the reluctance for a discussion of this type is particularly great. Parents generally consider their children as their property. They want to mold their children according to their own complexes and usually are not very prone to acknowledge that children are human beings who have the right to live for themselves and do not merely exist for the satisfaction of their parents. Even when sexual motives and the attitudes of the parents towards children are as obvious as the attitude of gratification of one's own pride, a discussion will generally not lead very far. The chief difficulties in such discussions lie mostly in the fact that the patients do not want to see that they try to keep the other person subservient to their own wishes, and they do not acknowledge the other person as an individual.

ADVICE

Of course the physician is supposed not merely to discuss and listen; he is supposed to offer advice as a remedy. Two difficulties arise immediately. He should know that his advice is not based upon sufficient knowledge. He may rely upon his general experience and knowledge and his intuition—a dangerous procedure. The less the discussion goes into details, the more dangerous it is. The physician is in danger of overrating himself; he unwittingly becomes a party to the situation. The wish to help without sufficient insight is a form of superciliousness. If he is able to find the key to the situation and give good advice, the patient will very often not accept the advice. If there are somatic symptoms present which, according to the opinion of the physician, are not organically determined, he may reassure the patient in this respect. Even on the basis of the simple discussion he may increase the insight of the patient into the genesis of his symptoms. This procedure has a limited value. It is useless in cases in which the psychogenic symptom originates from the deeper layers. In the majority of these situations, the physician will not merely discuss the problems involved, but will appeal to his authority in the matter.

PERSUASION

Discussion is soon mixed with persuasion. This method, worked out in more detail by Dubois, explains to the patient, in a rational way, why he has his symptoms, and why it is unnecessary that he should have them. The physician appeals to the insight of the patient as an intelligent human being. One might, for instance, explain to the patient that his palpitations are not due to any organic heart disease, but that he is living under tension because of his difficult financial situation, that he should convince himself that he will be able to find some kind of solution, and that his apprehension is in no way justified; that he should tell that to himself and his symptoms will disappear immediately. Behind that stands the authority of the physician, very often not even conscious to himself.

APPEAL TO WILL POWER

Persuasion still has the advantage of appealing to the understanding of the patient and not burdening him with tasks which he is not capable of performing. One has very often appealed to the will power of the patient and told him he is not organically sick and should be able to overcome his symptoms. I do not deny that such an appeal might be successful in one or the other case. But whereas we have merely pointed to the incompleteness and dangers in the procedures mentioned before, we consider the appeal to will power as a theoretically wrong approach, which not only in the majority of cases does not help, but does damage to the patient by increasing his feelings of guilt and insufficiency. Persuasion is very much in danger of adding this appeal to will power to its otherwise also rather dubious method. The usefulness of the methods so far mentioned is limited. It is greatest in methods which involve helping the patient to understand his problems on the basis of a discussion of everyday events. It is less useful where advice is given to the patient based upon the discussion or where persuasion is used. The procedure of appeal to will power has decidedly the least value.

DISCUSSION OF THE PAST

If a discussion with a patient is carried on in the spirit of honesty and understanding, the discussion glides almost involuntarily back to the past. The problems of puberty, of the latency period, and finally the problems of early childhood emerge. The same problems which are present in the immediate situation are also present in the earlier situations; the problems of school and ambitions, the relations to friends, the relation to the family, and the sex problems. The problem of masturbation sooner or later makes its appearance, and finally one arrives at the border line of the important infantile period—around the fifth year. The scattered earlier remembrances, and especially the first memory, are very often indicative of basic attitudes of the patient, and the patient may even be brought to a partial understanding of his early memories. The value of such a procedure should not be overlooked, but it remains incomplete and unsatisfactory, and without using further technical tools the connection between the present situation and the past situation will not become sufficiently clear to the physician and to the patient. The picture may even be distorted and one-sided. I may recall that we do not discuss complete methods, but we discuss here merely the tools, and in a later chapter we shall try to come to an insight of how these tools can be used for a systematic approach. I may mention that in going into the history of early childhood it is very often forgotten how important somatic diseases in childhood are for the development of attitudes in children and in the parents.[2]

CATHARTIC HYPNOSIS

The progress of modern psychotherapy started with the employment of methods which brought forward material that was hidden from the patient. The method first applied in this respect was hypnosis. We are not concerned here with the psychological problem of the relationship between physician and patient in hypnosis. Neither are we concerned with the problem of suggestion in the hypnosis. We deal merely with hypnosis as a method to bring forward forgotten material, increasing in this way the insight of the patient and the physician. This method was used first by Janet, who brought forward by hypnosis the *idée fixe* which provoked the neurotic symptom by having remained unconscious. Breuer, whose experiences date further back, published his results with Freud several years later. According to their theory, the traumatic scene is forgotten and by being forgotten exerts a greater influence, which expresses itself in neurotic symptoms. Hypnosis makes the discharge of the dammed-up energy possible by bringing it to consciousness again—abreaction. This method starts from the symptom and forces the patient to remember where the symptom has originated. Freud quotes, for instance, the case of a young man who had hysterical attacks which were connected with an unexpressed rage against the employer who had mistreated him.

[2] In this connection, see Phyllis Greenacre, "The Predisposition to Anxiety," *Psychoanalytic Quarterly* 10:66–95, 610–39, 1941. [L.B., Ed.]

It was at first believed that deep hypnosis is necessary for bringing forgotten material into consciousness. In the famous case of Breuer and Freud such a deep hypnosis could be easily provoked. The patient brought forward, at first spontaneously, later upon insistence, earlier traumatic scenes and was relieved when such a traumatic scene was brought into the memory in an autohypnotic or hypnotic state and was transferred from there to a conscious level. Once she saw, for instance, all objects enlarged. In hypnosis she remembered that waking at the sickbed of her father during the night she wanted to know how late it was. Since it was dark she had to bring the watch so close to her eyes that it looked larger. The emotional tension of this scene expressed itself in hysterical macropsia, which disappeared when the tension was relieved by bringing the original traumatic scene into consciousness. Breuer and Freud make the important statement that the symptom disappears not when merely one of the traumatic incidents is revealed, but only when one has by a systematic procedure revealed the original traumatic scene. Generally it was necessary to trace back the symptoms through a series of earlier appearances to the occasion when the symptom appeared first. This procedure suffers from the disadvantage that the number of persons who can be brought into a deep hypnosis is limited. Freud substituted, therefore, superficial hypnosis of the patient, and later on he merely put the patient on the couch, laid his hands on the patient's forehead, and urged him to remember. Even this procedure proved unnecessary, and Freud substituted the method of free association for hypnosis and hypnosis-like procedures. This method relied upon the assumption that the traumatic experience, which is of an undiminished importance for the patient, will appear only if the patient does not hinder the free flow of his thoughts. It is probably the most important technical development in modern psychotherapy and will be discussed later in detail. It also involves another important innovation. In hypnosis, which tends to reveal forgotten material, the work is started with the symptom. In so-called free association, the patient is ordered to say whatever comes into his mind and need not fix his attention on the symptom. A hypnosis which brings forward forgotten material is called a cathartic hypnosis.

The method is used but rarely today. Only Frank and Bezzola adhere to it. When one studies their case histories, one will find that most of their patients were not in deep hypnosis and that the procedure is not very different from using free association. My own experience with cathartic hypnosis has been unsatisfactory. It is often impossible to gain new important material. It can be got much easier by other methods. Furthermore, the material brought forward in such a procedure is in no way reliable. I have observed a case who felt from time to time the irresistible urge to excessive masturbation. In a hypnosis which had all the appearance of a deep hypnosis, she remembered that her mother had pushed her finger into her, the patient's, vagina and she had tried hard to press the finger out. Later on, the patient—who, by the way, was uneducated—confessed that she invented the scene because she thought the physician would like it. The therapeutic results in Breuer's and Freud's cases were unsatisfactory in the long run according to the report of Freud in his *Gesammelte Schriften*. The possibility that cathartic hypnosis might give results should not be denied. The theoretical basis of the procedure is sound.[3]

HYPNOSIS CLEARING UP AMNESIAS

Hypnosis can be valuable in bringing forward forgotten material. In cases of hysterical amnesia, the forgotten material is available in hypnosis, as the investigations of Milton Abeles and myself show. Even when the amnesia occurs on the basis of alcoholic intoxication, the procedure might be successful, as the investigations of R. Stern show. This is not a cathartic method in the proper sense, since the material brought forward is not the traumatic material, but it may be useful in restoring the memory of the patient. The restoration of the contents of epileptic dreamy states by hypnosis has been of more theoretical than practical interest.

[3] This method was revived during World War II especially in the form of narcosynthesis with the use of intravenous barbiturates. See the Bibliography for the initial work by Roy Grinker with the war neuroses in North Africa in the Tunisian campaign, and the review article by Edgar R. Lipton, 1950. [L.B., Ed.]

REPETITION OF A TRAUMATIC SCENE IN HYPNOSIS

Traumatic scenes very often are not completely forgotten. They remain in the memory of the patient, but the patient does not react any more to the traumatic scene and he remains emotionally tense. One may occasionally revive such a traumatic incident to full strength and give to the patient the possibility of an emotional discharge. The revival of the traumatic scene, with or without the help of hypnosis, to be sure, is not alone sufficient. However, the patient will, with the revival, have the opportunity of coming to a better insight and to a better emotional adaptation to the traumatic situation. This method is, therefore, on the border line of methods which use hypnosis not for the recovery of material and abreaction, but for a more thorough education of the patient. This will be discussed later on.

FREE ASSOCIATION

As mentioned, the technique of free association, which we owe to the genius of Freud, has become the most important technical help in modern psychotherapy. The so-called repressed material of emotional value is in no way inactive. It is an experience which is incomplete and wants to be completed. It is an unsatisfied drive, an unfinished action, an open configuration. Psychic processes tend to the completion of the gestalt, the completion of the task, and the satisfaction of the drive. Unfinished experiences have, therefore, a greater dynamic value than finished experiences.

This is a psychological law which has been found to be true in the tachistoscopic experiments of Poetzl and his co-workers, in which the material that was not fully perceived had a determining influence on later dream material and associations. The experiments of the gestalt school show the efficiency of the same factors in perception and action. (Cf., for instance, the material collected in Lewin's book, *A Dynamic Theory of Personality.*) Psychoanalysis has collected an overwhelming amount of material in this respect.

When we use free association, the patient, lying on a couch, is ordered to say everything going through his mind. He is not to suppress anything. He is told that many of the thoughts going through his mind will seem unimportant to him. He has to say them. Many of the thoughts and phantasies will be disagreeable and may contain material for which the patient feels ashamed. He has not the right to keep it back. It is generally easier for the patient to bring forward material concerning himself than material concerning others, especially concerning the physician. The material may be frankly sexual, but there will also be material which, at the first sight, does not look sexual and still is painful to remember and report. The patient is also admonished that he has to report dreams and everyday-life mistakes which may have occurred during the day. In the beginning of the session, the patient is not asked any specific questions; he has merely to associate. It is the underlying theory that in the course of the free association, the repressed material will not only make its appearance, but that the patient will also recognize that the material appearing has an importance in the solution of a specific question and he will immediately experience the inner connection of the material appearing with his life history.

This material has been kept back by the repressing forces. The repressing forces are in connection with logical thinking. The logical thinking is the thinking directed to the community. It is conscious material in the analytic sense, that is, material which is socially approved and, therefore, also is approved by the patient himself. One usually employs the term "repression" in connection with these forces of consciousness, and the present psychoanalytic theory lets the repression originate from the ego, as the representative of the social functions of perception, action, and reality testing. The superego, the conscience of the individual, may direct the ego what to repress. I prefer to speak about the perception ego, since it is difficult to forget that the term "ego" has been used for generations to denote the totality of one's experience, equivalent to the term "person" or "personality."

Psychoanalysts, for instance Ferenczi, are well aware that we not only push aside material which does not fit our social existence, but also material which cannot be used for the present task.

The value of the method and its basic correctness are beyond question. The term "free association" is misleading in so far as the material coming forward is the result of definite strivings and tendencies. The individual wants to solve with one part of his personality the task demanded by a traumatic or difficult situation. He is hindered in doing so by stronger drives in another direction.

Freud interprets this fact by pointing to the causal determination of psychic life, and extending the strict laws of causality to psychic experiences. We may better understand the situation by saying that the tasks of life demand a constructive effort, and if such an effort has been interrupted, the task remains and is taken up again when the general situation permits it.

The difficulty in the practical application of so-called free association in psychotherapy lies in the fact that the general order given does not always help the patient to let himself go in the stream of his thinking. Very often he will not be capable of recognizing important material as such, and the analyst will have to give him an interpretation. If one reads psychoanalytic literature, one very often gets the impression that the patient merely has to lie down on a couch and talk and that everything else develops by itself. This is, of course, not so. The physician has to be active again and again and has to remind the patient of his task. The patient has again and again the tendency to escape the repressed material by bringing forward material which is unimportant.

One of my patients, for example, had been with another analyst for several weeks before he came to me. He had merely produced pictures pertaining to his early years in a country house. The pictures had no connection with his real problems, as the later analysis clearly showed. These are common occurrences. Sometimes the patient starts to enumerate objects in the analyst's room. Freud has said, too, that this occurs when the positive transference becomes stronger and the patient does not want to talk about it. If not told about it, the patient may go on for hours and hours. So-called free association might be, as in this case, merely an escape from really repressed material. The flightiness and the shallow and passing attention the manic patient gives to his surroundings are probably merely exaggerations of these same mechanisms. He wants to escape his deeper-lying problems.

It is, furthermore, quite frequently the case that a patient does not want to turn to infantile material. Very often he has to be ordered to do so. Particular difficulties arise concerning all material which pertains to the analyst, and the patient has to be admonished again and again not to keep it back. It is, also, acknowledged that patients do not find the interpretation of symbols for themselves. To sum up, a great amount of material brought forward in the free association is not in direct connection with the repressed material but is merely brought forward in order to hide the repressed material as much as possible. The analytical term for this occurrence is "resistance." The term has a double meaning. The individual resists bringing forward the painful material, and he also resists the efforts of the analyst and the analyst himself.

Resistance is, therefore, very often in connection with negative attitudes against the physician but is in no way identical with negative transference. The patient may resist from positive as well as from negative transference, and a hate against the analyst may bring forward invaluable material.

The so-called free association is, therefore, far from being an undirected process. When the patient comes to treatment, the situation already forces him into a specific attitude. In the further course of analysis the whole process is under the continuous direction of the analyst. This does not say anything new as far as the psychoanalytic practice is concerned. It is implied in the repeated statements of Freud that analysis is a process which works methodically with resistance and transference (the relation to the analyst). This implies that the whole process is under the continuous guidance of the analyst. I have heard Freud himself state, for instance, that it is important to force the patient to go to his early experiences when he wants to remain in the sphere of the material of the present, and that he has to be led back to the present situation if he merely concentrates his attention on the past. I have furthermore seen cases treated by Freud who had been told, at first, to remember what had happened in the first five years of their lives. It is, anyhow, an acknowledged part of analytic technique to tell the patient that he should start with giving his life history.

I want it to be understood that these are remarks which pertain not to the so-called active technique in analysis, about which we shall speak later, but to the so-called classical and passive type of analysis. Reproaches of analysts to the patient that he does not work well and does not make any effort are common, as I can state on the report of patients who have been analyzed by leading analysts. The so-called free association does not lead anywhere unless it is a directed process. Its direction comes from the human relation between the analyst and his patient.

A further difficulty arises from the fact that it is sometimes impossible to decide whether insight gained by the patient by free association or an interpretation given by the analyst is correct or not. In the long run, of course, only the patient can decide. However, Freud himself states correctly that the yes or no of the patient has less importance than the subsequent associations, after a preliminary interpretation is given either by the patient or by the physician. Among the analysts, Karen Horney has given the clearest formulation of this situation. I might, therefore, formulate free association as a mutual effort between analyst and patient to bring the conflicts and problems of the patient into clear appearance. Thus, it is a directed effort and is based upon a continuous inner activity of the analyst.

It should not be overlooked, however, that the technique of free association has taught us that we may go for long stretches without interfering too much with the activity of the patient. We have to wait until the patient has exhausted his possibilities and has definitely shown that he directs the stream of his inner activity in the direction of resistance before we are allowed to interfere. Furthermore, the activity of the physician cannot and should not express itself in arguing with the patient, but merely in interpreting and so giving to the thoughts of the patient a direction which may enable him to see and experience his real problems on the basis of true associations. Patients being analyzed very often complain that the analyst remains silent for a long time. That may be necessary; very often it is not, and it seems that present-day analysis is more inclined to break the silence in order to give interpretations—that is, directions. The fundamental problem of psychotherapy in general thus emerges from the problem of free association—namely, when shall we be active in interpreting and directing, and when shall we refrain from interfering with the activities of the patient? This problem can only be discussed efficiently after we have studied the relation between the physician and his patient. Freud himself demands from the analyst an attitude of free floating attention. This, after all, is also an active state.

PLAY TECHNIQUE

The process of free association takes place by words. Without underrating the importance of words, they are only one of the methods by which we express ourselves. Other actions may occur during the analysis. The patient may turn around at a given point. He may go to the toilet, he may sigh, etc. We are generally loath to interpret such actions unless the patient has given us associations pertaining to them. The word takes, then, the lead again in the procedure. Since the sign function of words is better elaborated and more reliable than the other sign functions, the analysis of the adult is based upon verbal material. Other actions are merely passing phases in this process. Somatic symptoms which may occur in the course of the analysis are sooner or later verbalized by the patient. In children the sign function of language is not yet elaborated, especially in children who are less than nine or ten years old. This date is chosen rather arbitrarily. In the child before the fifth year, the verbalization is still more incomplete.

Other techniques than the free association of language had to be devised. Melanie Klein uses the play technique with children. One may give to the child almost anything with which to play: paper dolls, rag dolls, dolls which can be taken apart, wagons, tin toys of all kinds can be used. Little blocks of wood or stone are very often useful. The child should have a choice between many toys, but the situation generally becomes obscured if the variety of toys is too great. It is usually better to use toys which do not move by themselves but which have to be moved by the child. Frequently the child accompanies his play with short remarks which elucidate the situation. Sooner or later one will have to interpret to the child what is going on. One may participate in the play and accompany one's actions with appropriate gestures. If the child is not very young it will usually be difficult to bring it to an insight into the situation without words.

Melanie Klein is very active in interpreting, and expressly advises such an activity. For instance, if the child in his play makes two cars collide, this is interpreted to it as a violent sex relation between the parents. Putting a toy into a box may be interpreted as the wish of the child to penetrate into the parent. The play technique which is used by Anna Freud and her co-workers with greater caution is certainly useful. There is the great danger of giving arbitrary interpretations to the child, and there are very few reliable criteria by which the correctness of an interpretation can be ascertained. The verbal acquiescence of the child is certainly no proof of the correctness of such interpretations.

One may try to put the child before more specific situations. One may put before the child, for instance, a porcelain doll and push it down three times, the child watching, and then put the doll before the child. Valuable material concerning the aggressiveness of the child may come out in this way; or one may put before the child a tin soldier between two cars and let the child proceed with the play. These are methods which Lauretta Bender, David Wechsler, and I used in the children's ward in Bellevue Hospital. If one wants to ascertain the attitude of the child towards sex differences, one may put sex organs made of clay on naked dolls and watch the reaction of the child. Very often material will make its appearance which otherwise would not have come out.

David Levy has used a more complicated situation, showing the child a doll with removable parts representing a mother nursing her child, which represents a sibling. Attitudes of sibling rivalry then make their appearance. It is important that one remains conscious in all these techniques of how much one has put oneself into the situation, and how much the experimental situation, and the play situation in general, forces the child into a definite verbal expression or play activity. At any rate, one sees here that the principle akin to free association is applied with a definite plan and direction of the therapist.

ASSOCIATIONS TO PICTURES AND PUPPET SHOWS

One may show pictures to children and study their associations and reactions. One may use artistic activities in the same directions. Methods of this type have been worked out by L. Bender. One may study the expression of drives of children by encouraging them to art productions and staging plays. One may study the way in which children continue stories, the beginning of which has been told to them. L. Bender and A. G. Woltmann have studied the reaction of children to puppet shows which were shown to a group of children. The group reactions of the children to the play, and later the individual reactions, were studied carefully. The same authors let the children work with clay. All these methods are in inner relation to the principles of the free association methods. They offer difficulties of their own. The principles of interpretation are sometimes difficult, but most of them, especially the puppet shows, give to the child a possibility of free expression which brings important material into the foreground, very often connected with a considerable emotional relief.[4]

OPINIONS OF CHILDREN

Obviously, one cannot make the child understand the principle of free association, but this is not necessary anyhow. The free talk of children inevitably brings the same material into appearance when the child is small and when it is not frightened by the attitude of adults. The opinions and the beliefs of children, so carefully studied by Piaget, have to be brought forward and can be utilized to understand the child's attitude and make it clearer to him. Many children like to tell fantastic stories, which open the way for a deeper understanding of their problems. It is obvious that most of the methods used in order to get children to express emotional material are difficult to handle; but if one does so, one comes to an undreamed-of understanding of the problems of children, which necessarily helps the children to understand their own problems and conflict situations. All methods employed with children serve basically the same aim as the principle of free association: they liberate the individual from the constraint of a narrow situation and help him to come to a clear expression of his drives and problems. He thus learns to understand situations from which he turned away previously because they appeared too difficult and dangerous. This leads, of course, to the understanding of one's self in relation to the situation.

[4] Lauretta Bender's *Child Psychiatric Techniques* (Charles C. Thomas, 1950) is a book which discusses the techniques used by the Bellevue worker in the diagnosis and therapy of children. It includes many of Paul Schilder's writings on the children's spontaneous art, play, and descriptions of pictures, etc. [L.B., Ed.]

DREAM INTERPRETATION

Dream interpretation in the modern sense is based almost exclusively on the work of Freud. We must, therefore, follow his reasoning very closely. According to Freud, dreams are wish fulfillments. This function of the dream occurs, according to Freud, openly in children. The contents are simple: the desire for food intake, or to go to places where the child is not able to go, is paramount. Similarly simple is the structure of dreams which fulfill an urgent need. The thirsty sleeper dreams that he drinks water and he can continue to sleep. The dream appears thus, as a protector of the sleep. Of course, when the actual satisfaction of the thirst is denied, the dream changes its character. The dreamer may drink salty water from an urn and finally awaken with the feeling of thirst. The wish reality is finally substituted by insight into the actual situation. The salty drink is on the way between the two. One may say that the salty water expresses, thus, the fight between two tendencies—the one, not to be disturbed in the sleep, and the other one, not to suffer by the thirst. Neither reality nor psychological problems are as simple as that. The urn expresses the interest of the dreamer in antiques. It is also perhaps a rather sinister hint. Without associations we would not know about the preference of the dreamer for urns, and we still do not know, since the water in the urn is salty, what the saltiness means. To drink salty water, anyhow, cannot be a wish fulfillment in the ordinary sense.

We must differentiate between the manifest content of the dream and its latent meaning. An old lady, separated from her grandchildren, dreams that one of them has to urinate. She puts her on the toilet, and awakens with the desire to urinate herself. This dream not only fulfills her wish to continue to sleep, but also makes it possible for her to enjoy her grandchild. There is no knowing how much she otherwise enjoys nursing the child, and maybe even enjoys this specific situation.

The picture of the dream serves, therefore, not merely one tendency, but several tendencies at once. One might say that every picture in a dream is the crossing point of several tendencies. One may call this wish fulfillment. One may also say that there are different goals in the individual for which he is striving. Freud would protest against this latter formulation, Adler against the first one. I consider these two interpretations as basically identical. The one expresses the problem from the point of view of the body, the other from the point of view of the outward situation. The last dream mentioned shows also very clearly that the individual solves her problem by projecting her urge into somebody else. Of course one might say, since the dream builds up a psychic reality without relation to the outward reality, that projection plays a part in every dream. The homosexual dream reported above is seemingly a fulfillment of the homosexual wishes of the patient. He wants to be used anally. Since he protests against it, the lover is changed into an attacking enemy. Since he does not want to think of the sex organ, he finds a piece of rope in his anus. We have found here instances of transformation and symbolization. One should not forget, however, that the patient is neither aware of his love for the attacker nor that the rope has anything to do with the attacker's penis. We cannot correctly speak of true symbols.

We come, therefore, to the preliminary conclusion that the dream transforms the contents of one's wishes so that they serve different purposes. This transformation may lead to symbol-like pictures. Furthermore, the dream is capable of transforming the inner reality into the outward reality and serves its general and special aims by a rearrangement between the two by projection. We may expect that when projection takes place, the individual may, in the dream, appersonate parts of the world to himself and may also use identification, taking other persons into the dreamer. One of my patients dreamed that he was prime minister in England, the youngest ever to hold the position. The minister of foreign affairs had to be appointed. He wanted to appoint a leader of the opposition to demonstrate unity.

In order to come to an interpretation of more complicated dreams, the general knowledge of the circumstances of life is very often not sufficient. We have to get the associations of the patient. It is technically important that one asks for the patient's associations, not to the dream as a whole, but one has to proceed by asking associations to every single part of the dream. This procedure, found by Freud empirically, is not only justified but also of great theoretical importance. I have shown previously that our psychic life consists of constructive efforts. In these constructive efforts we take parts of our experience and put them together till they fit into the situation. Whenever a psychic effort is made, we put wholes together, not merely by evolving a pattern by some kind of mysterious force, but we put the wholes together like a mosaic or a jigsaw puzzle. Of course, in order to do so we must have a plan, a tendency, or a goal. The dream is pieced together in a similar way according to a plan, a drive, which is very often counteracted by other drives. The associations to the above dream are as follows: He is very much impressed by Anthony Eden, whom he envies for his self-assurance. Pitt was prime minister when he was twenty-one or twenty-four. Gentiles have bigger penises. He is more interested in gentile girls, whom he considers better-looking. He had masturbated vividly between twelve and fourteen. At this time he wanted to be a journalist and felt that he would have been a great leader of the Jewish people if he did not masturbate. He speaks now about his early literary activities and continues to talk about his unwillingness to fight. He hit back only at smaller boys. His father had always taught him that Jews do not fight. The hour ended with various remarks of the patient concerning the father, whom he admired very much and who had given him much attention when he was young.

Some important points in the analysis pertaining to the dream may here be mentioned. His relation to his father became hostile after his tenth year. The patient has a double attitude towards his superiors. He tries very hard at first to win them and to make them love him. Very soon he feels disappointed, feels that they do not like him, and answers with hostility. He is afraid of them. His fear is increased at the present time because of literary activities which might be disapproved and punished by his superiors. We point at first to his identification with Eden and Pitt, which serves the fulfillment of his wish for greatness. Feeling inferior as a Jew, he does not transform himself into a Jewish prime minister (although England had a Jewish prime minister in Disraeli). It is also obvious that his identification with gentiles serves him further in overcoming the smallness of his penis, which is, according to his opinion, due to masturbation. One may also be sure that the prime minister is the picture of his father, whom he admired so much. His father had a big penis, too.

One sees how many trends are condensed into his being a prime minister. The father—prime minister—shows a peaceful attitude towards the man in opposition. He was in opposition to his father, too. Material which had come out in the previous analysis revealed infantile jealousy of the father in the sense of the Oedipus complex.

Now the father is peaceful towards him, and he may also reckon that his superiors will treat him as well and love him in spite of his opposition. One sees that such a dream serves a great number of various tendencies. It is also a condensation, in so far as many trends and complicated experiences are united in a short scene which can be expressed in a few sentences. The dream puts emphasis on the appearance of unity. We have reason to believe that the patient wants his superiority and that the unity is a less important feature. The dream furthermore eliminates all fears and is in this respect a wish fulfillment.

Freud would formulate it in the following way: Tendencies were present to assure the patient of sexual and professional success. We shall consider these tendencies later on in detail. These wishes are the latent meaning of the dream. They are transformed into the manifest content of the dream by the dream work. One cannot deny that Freud's description is accurate. We deal, indeed, with a process of reconstruction. This reconstruction leads, as Freud has also emphasized, to pictures. Therefore, the categories of language cannot be applied. There is no grammar, and as in a picture riddle, logical and grammatical connections can be merely expressed by the arrangement of the picture. Freud says succinctly: "All the verbal apparatus by means of which the more subtle thought relations are expressed, the conjunctions and prepositions, the variations of declension and conjugation, are lacking, because the means of portraying them are absent: just as in primitive, grammarless speech, only the raw material of thought can be expressed, and the abstract is merged again in the concrete from which it sprang." If words and sentences are present in the dream they are mostly taken from actual conversations of the preceding days. Logical relations between sentences are also merely expressed by juxtaposition of parts of the dream or by two dreams in one night.

The following is an instance coming from the same patient. We may make the preliminary remark that the patient once attempted intercourse with a sister, seven years younger, and saw the other sister, who is thirteen years younger than himself, naked, with strong feelings of guilt. He had frequent dreams concerning intercourse with her. In this dream he is in a theater. On the stage is an actress whose name is practically identical with the name of the younger sister. An actor, famous for his big nose, is there too. The actress is very high up. A stage elevator is rising. Another dream follows: he has to be in the analyst's office. Some other people are there. The analyst says, "There is no next week; you are through." The patient thinks he does not need any more analysis.

This actress, not very young, is supposed to have an affair with a playwright whose plays were successfully produced by a company which had not yet accepted the patient's play. The big nose of the actor (the father had a big nose, too) and the rising elevator hint to the big penis he would like to have in order to satisfy his mother and sister. To be a successful playwright will do, too, but still he is not sure of his independence. One could express that in the following way: Since my penis is not big enough and my play is not accepted, I would like to have at least the continuous care of the father-analyst. The last part of the dream seemingly means the opposite of what it says. Such use of opposites can be found in dreams as well as in other forms of primitive thinking.

Psychoanalysis speaks about the latent dream thought, but one has to be careful not to fall into the error of believing that at first a primitive wish is formulated in the unconscious, and later on is translated. What is present is a directional attitude on the basis of past material. Furthermore, I do not think that the so-called unconscious is outside the field of awareness. It is merely a different type of awareness and is endowed with the particular characteristics of thinking as shown above. It is further understood, and is obvious in these two dreams, that the material is utilized freely even if it belongs to the past. Freud speaks correctly about the timelessness of the system of the unconscious, but it should be added that no experience disappears from the horizon of psychic experience. The time relations in the conscious material are merely better co-ordinated.

The first dream is decidedly better co-ordinated than the second and third dreams just mentioned. Psychoanalysis uses for the processes of this co-ordination the term "secondary elaboration." The content of the first dream thus comes nearer to the ways of conscious thinking. A process which brings primitive material into the form of logical thinking and motivation is also called rationalization. Secondary elaboration and rationalization both serve the repressive tendencies directed against the unconscious material. These repressive tendencies in the dream are also called the *censor*.

It is obvious that symbols play a large part in this process. We have previously formulated that symbols express two conflicting tendencies. They appear on the crossroads of two drives. Since the dream nowhere comes to definite decisions, symbols are bound to be frequent.

One may generally say that the sign function in the dream is not verbal and that many characteristics of the dream can be understood in this way.

Freud has justly pointed to the important fact that the dream has no outlet into action and that the hallucinated world of the dream is not so far distant from an imagined world. In a world without action the difference between reality and imagination, between perception and representation, is likely to disappear. The dream represents, therefore, a mental preparation without real responsibility, as the dreams which have been analyzed show.

There are the unsolved problems of the day, the reminiscences of the day. These are thoughts which are not clearly in the mind of the person. They are half forgotten, but of the type of everyday thinking. They are called the preconscious. According to Freud, they are reinforced and get their driving power from the unfulfilled wishes of early childhood, which wait for an opportunity for satisfaction. They are hindered in appearing in the unchanged form by the censorship which tries to block their way from the unconscious to the preconscious and from the preconscious into the conscious. They undergo a secondary elaboration, and even then may be finally forgotten. They preserve the sleep by assuring the sleeper that the desires and wishes are fulfilled anyhow.

Even when the manifest content of the dream is anxiety or punishment, the latent thought of the dream is wish fulfillment. It fits completely into the general attitude of Freud when he states that the dreaming individual is merely directed towards the past and towards satisfaction. He has overlooked, therefore, also concerning the dream, that every psychic attitude points also to the future. Adler sees the dream from another side. He writes in his book, *What Life Should Mean to You,* as follows:

" 'My most frequent dream,' she related, 'is very queer. I am usually walking along the streets where there is a hole that I do not see. Walking along, I fall into the hole. It is filled with water, and as I touch the water I wake with a jump, with my heart beating terribly fast.' We shall not find the dream as strange as she finds it herself;

but if she is to continue to alarm herself with it, she must think it mysterious and fail to understand it. The dream says to her: 'Be cautious. There are dangers about that you know nothing of.' It tells us more than this, however. You cannot fall if you are down. If she is in danger of falling, she must imagine that she is above the others. As in the last example, she is saying: 'I am superior, but I must always take care not to fall.'"

Jung stresses the fact also that the dream has a creative function which points to the future task based upon the creative process of the unconscious.

We may stress, from our point of view, the following points, which may facilitate the interpretation of dreams: 1. Every dream has a relation to the present situation. To the present situation belongs the outward world and the state of the body of the dreamer which, as is well known, may express itself in the dream. In dreams of children and in dreams in connection with an urgent problem of the body, the actual situation may be the only one of importance, although, as our example has shown, the present situation is always in some way connected with the past. The present situation has social as well as sexual elements. They may appear in varying proportion in the dream.

2. We have to ask further, what does the dream mean from the point of view of the infantile situation? The infantile problems also are partially social, partially sexual. Although symbolizations will very often pertain to the sexual sphere, that they may also pertain to the social sphere of wish formulation only those will disapprove who extend the connotation of sexuality very far. Animals may, for instance, substitute for parents. We may further expect that in symbols the relation to the infantile sphere of experience will be more outspoken.

3. We have to ask, what does the dream mean from the point of view of the past, what does the dream mean from the point of view of the future? It does not serve merely the satisfaction of infantile wishes; it brings the infantile problem in connection with the present problem and its solution. Adler is right in this respect. He sees merely the individual problem in all too schematic a way. In order to come to a dream interpretation, we have to get associations to every part of the dream.

4. We have further to ask, what does a dream mean from the point of view of the body and the body image? It is obvious that sexual

material, for instance, will have relation to the body image of the dreamer.

The body image is the picture of our own body as we perceive it and as we imagine it.[5] It does not merely consist of perception in the ordinary sense but it comprises elements of representations and thoughts. It is an immediate experience like the experience of any other object. However, it is the experience of a specific object with which one is acquainted from earliest childhood. It has a particular importance and vividness and carries with it a very great number of memories of specific life situations. As an object experience it has a greater variety than any other object experience. It is inexhaustible in details and parts. It undergoes continuous changes. It is the object experience most persistent in time with which we are acquainted. It has, furthermore, parts which are not accessible to the perception of other individuals and some parts of the optic experience of this object are not accessible to the individual himself, at least not without a particular or artificial effort (mirrors). This object body is furthermore characterized by the fact that for its recognition, perception of the bodies around it is almost indispensable.

It is astonishing how little attention the psychological literature gives to this object in general. The tendency prevails of taking it for granted that we have a body and that we know about it. The knowledge of one's own body and the perception of it have appeared to psychologists and philosophers alike as a simple and reliable datum. Psychologists and philosophers have even very often attempted to deduce from this supposedly immediate and simple experience all the other experiences of human beings. One has overlooked that this experience of one's own body has to be built up in a constructive process. The experience of one's own body is perhaps in many respects more impressive than experiences of other objects. However, this experience is at the same time almost spiritual in character since it sums up and integrates vast parts of the individual's life. It is partially for this reason that I have chosen the term *body image*. This terminology indicates also that the problem reaches further than that of the postural model of the body (cf. Henry Head). Head has stressed the system of references to which we refer single postures. The postural model of the body has as its basis not merely postural sensations but also

[5] Reprinted in part from "The Body Image in Dreams," *Psychoanalytic Review* 29:113–26, 1942.

optic impressions—in short, sensations from the whole realm of the senses. At the same time every single experience is meaningless unless in relation to the body image. Scherner had a clear insight since he says that every nerve excitation takes place on the body which is its general basis. According to him, phantasy will erect a basic symbolic picture for the body. The gĕneral phantasy picture for the human body is a building with its walls, bricks, and beams—the house. Scherner was merely interested in this problem from the point of view of the dream. He speaks correctly about phantasy pictures in general of which the dream pictures are merely one, although a very important, instance.

Freud in his book on *Dream Interpretation* has taken up the ideas of Scherner, and he stresses the fact that the symbolism of the body and its organs plays an overwhelming part. Freud is only rarely interested in the symbolism of the body as a whole. However, he has a great interest in the symbolic representations of parts, especially sex parts. He writes, for instance (page 371 of the Modern Library Edition): "All elongated objects, sticks, tree trunks, umbrellas (on account of the opening which might be likened to an erection), all sharp and elongated weapons, knives, daggers and pikes, represent the male member. A frequent but not very intelligible symbol for the same is a nail file. Small boxes, chests, cupboards, and ovens correspond to the female organ; also cavities, ships, and all kinds of vessels. A room in a dream generally represents a woman; the description of its various entrances and exits is scarcely calculated to make us doubt this interpretation. The interest as to whether the room is 'open' or 'locked' will be readily understood in this connection." Freud relates, furthermore, the symbolizations of bladder, anus, urine, birthwater, feces, uterus, in symbolism in dreams. The sexual act may be represented by all kinds of activities. "Smooth walls over which one climbs, façades of houses across which one lets oneself down often with a sense of great anxiety correspond to erect human bodies and probably repeat in our dreams childish memories of climbing up parents or nurses." "Wood, generally speaking, seems in accordance with its linguistic relations to represent feminine matter." "Baldness, haircutting, the loss of teeth and beheading may represent castration." "Breasts are symbolized as sisters, the buttocks may be symbolized as brothers." According to Stekel, symbols for genitals mean the female as well as the male genitals. However, Freud doubts that this bisexuality of symbols is a general trend. Freud, furthermore, refers to the frequent displacement from below to above, and the genitals are displaced to the face, the buttocks to the cheeks. The labia minora are displaced to the lips. Furthermore, the eye may stand for the sex parts. Freud also reports that clothes and especially hats may represent the sex parts. It is worth while to know that according to the remarks in dream interpretation, what is symbolized belongs almost exclusively to the sexual sphere, mostly to the genitals themselves or to the anus, whereas Freud says very little about the symbolization of other parts of the body.

Scherner, on the other hand, writes: "Since the body is erect and goes high up and strives high up the phantasy chooses accordingly the high house consisting of several stories as a symbol; the one story is above the other and stretches high up. The picture of a single room of a floor of a house or of an attic may also express the height and roominess of the body. Sometimes even a bridge becomes the symbol of the body; however, mostly human habitations and dwellings are pictured nearby. Sometimes the whole house becomes the symbol of a single organ of the body and still more often a multiplicity of houses. If the phantasy wants to express the organ of the stomach it chooses frequently a village or city square surrounding the houses. Following the outline of the stomach the square has very often an oblong shape. A dream of sexual excitation may symbolize the narrow touch of the thighs by an oblong narrow space. The length of the intestine is symbolized by long streets, and the symbolization of the large intestines is given by broad and long streets. The stomach may be symbolized by a completely empty room, the mouth by walled and arched rooms of the house, for instance, an attic. The adjoining staircase symbolizes a descending œsophagus. The process of breathing is symbolized by burning in the upper stories. The ceiling very often symbolizes the head."

The difference between Scherner's and Freud's symbolism is therefore more incisive than Staercke has realized. It might be mentioned here that neither Freud nor Scherner seem to be of the opinion that every dream is concerned with problems of the human body. The general psychoanalytic literature is, of course, full of discussions on symbolizations and of instances of symbolizations. However, the general importance of the body image in symbolizations has not been studied specifically, especially not concerning dream interpretation.

This is somewhat understandable when one considers that psychoanalysis clings to the opinion that the knowledge of one's own body does not need any particular consideration since it is given to the child rather completely from the moment of birth. The problem of the building up of the body image of oneself and that of others does not exist for psychoanalysis.

The problem has also not found any specific formulation in the newer comprehensive literature on dreams (Binswanger and Sharpe). The scanty remarks of Adler's concerning dream interpretation and the discussion of the Jungian school (Koenig-Fachsenfeld) do not give any specific attention to the problem. Only Gutheil devotes some remarks to the body image in dreams.

Federn has repeatedly pointed to the changes in body image occurring when we fall asleep and has described that we lose parts of the body image, especially those which are not particularly interesting from a libidinous point of view. However, we lack a description of body-image changes in dreams and a discussion of the relation of the symbolizations to the problem of body image in dreams.

The problems can be classified as follows: Which are the changes in one's own body image in the manifest contents of the dream? In which way is the body image of other persons changed in the dream? Which parts in the manifest contents of the dream are symbolic expressions of problems of the body image? Which are the relations of the body image to the latent contents of the dream? What is the general significance of body-image problems for dream interpretation and for the understanding of the essence of dreams?

It is, of course, to be expected that most dreams will, even in their manifest contents, deal explicitly or at least implicitly with human bodies. Always the dreamer himself is present even if one should merely dream of a landscape. Every human experience is, of course, connected with the experience of one's own body and also of bodies of others. This is not more than a commonplace, and even in the manifest contents of the dream we must be interested in a great deal more than the mere fact that human beings endowed with bodies appear in it.

The following dreams, taken from a twenty-one-year-old young man S., may elucidate the problem.

DREAM 1: *"There is a field of horses in Kentucky. It is a wedding procession. My horse did not jump. Later we jumped the fence again.*

A piebald small horse chases and bites my horse and me. I slapped it with a rope."

The associations of the patient are as follows: The horse is one which he really likes; he is afraid of horses and never feels quite safe when riding. He has read about a wedding procession in Italy on bicycles. He himself is an expert bicycle rider and is very daring at it. The patient had very severe difficulties with his potency before he came to treatment. He has two younger stepbrothers of whom he is extremely jealous and who are also better horseback riders than himself.

In the manifest content of the dream there is merely the dreamer in his natural appearance and horses in their natural appearance. There is furthermore the act of biting. The difficulty the horse has in jumping is probably closely related to his potency problem. However, he himself refuses very often to show his capacities also in other respects. The horse represents partially a spiritual aspect of himself. It represents also his body and his penis. The jumping means the act of intercourse. However it means also his general difficulties in action and achievement. The dream expresses the hope of final achievement which seems to be more probable since his potency difficulties lately have cleared up. The piebald small horse represents the horses of his brothers and the brothers themselves. The biting of the horse represents the aggression of the younger brothers.

During the same night a second dream occurred.

Dream 2: *"I wanted to take a shower. A naked girl came in. She made the remark that she had young and undeveloped breasts. The room had an oriental bead screen. I started to comb my hair, and teeth came out of the comb. I started to dance. I had pimples on my face, and I wanted to fix the pimples. I started to squeeze them at the dance."*

In this dream the manifest dream content contains the naked body of the girl and an allusion to the virtues of this body. In contrast, the dream contains a reference to one of the most painful experiences of the patient, his deep dissatisfaction with his complexion. He has had acne since puberty. Although this acne has almost disappeared the patient still feels deeply humiliated by it. This is closely related to the general idea of the inferiority of his body, which he refers chiefly to bad posture and bad odor. He actually takes great pleasure in squeezing out pimples and blackheads. He likes to exhibit the blemishes of his body and his inferiorities in general and so tries to gain a greater amount of attention, especially from his mother. The inferiority of his body is connected with earlier experiences when at the age of about five he asked the fat cook to roll over him. She refused by saying that he was not strong enough for that; one could do that with his father. He is also dissatisfied with his hair and thinks that he has too much dandruff. One sees that the objective fact which is alluded to in the dream has very deep emotional connections with childhood problems. One may suppose that "teeth breaking out of the comb" symbolizes the danger which he might incur when concerned with his own body. He masturbates indeed rather often. However, there are no specific associations in this direction.

One sees that the differentiation between the manifest and the latent contents of the dream is not always easy. It can be surmised that in this particular dream "the squeezing of the pimples" has still deeper roots. There was a whole series of dreams in which the squeezing out plays a very important part. Great masses may come out either from his skin or from his penis. In some dreams the anal connections of these motives are rather obvious. In a second series of dreams wild animals appear, especially tigers with protrusions coming from their cheek bones. These protrusions are sometimes like horns, sometimes like bronze, and serve a particular expression of ferocity. They are connected with associations concerning moles on the neck of the mother or on the face of a beloved physician who treated him during childhood and finally also with the one or the other excrescence of his brothers. They represent lastly a threat connected with protrusions of the body in general. There is also fear of what might come out of the body of others and the pride in what he might squeeze out of his body. He has, however, at the same time a terrific fear that something of his body might be taken away.

The following dream comes from a female patient with an anxiety neurosis who is in her early thirties. *The patient dreams of an enormously wide telescope. A Jewish lady falls down, floor after floor—J's wife is standing near by.*

The dreamer primarily had no associations to the dream besides the superficial ones that the telescope reminds her of a skyscraper and that the dreamer is afraid of high places since she might jump down. She was given now the interpretation that the falling of the lady represents a birth phantasy. The patient remembers now that she had the evening before—it was Christmas Eve—discussed with G. and A., a childless married couple, the problem of children. They do not want to have children since they do not know what will happen to their children. In addition, there is mental disease in his family. The patient herself would like to have children but is afraid to stay with a child, even when there is another person present. The other person would then be for the child, and she would need a third person for her protection. Christmas is the time for children. She likes to give gifts to children, and she feels deprived because her Jewish parents didn't have a Christmas tree. The telescope reminds her of the shape of a Christmas tree. J. is probably Jewish. He wrote a book on races and married a Christian wife of good Boston family. The patient is at present interested in a married man who sent her as a Christmas gift a picture of his child.

The dream obviously deals with the birth of a child which in the dream is represented by a Jewish lady. The child is also herself. She is born in this dream; however, the Jewish lady may also represent her child. The birth process is represented as a falling down. The telescope may represent the womb, the Christmas tree, and a penis.

The human problem and the problem of the body are represented as an accelerated movement in space. The dream is highly symbolic, corresponding to the awe with which the patient treated sex problems in her childhood. There is reason to believe there is not only the problem of the present but also the past in this situation. After a discussion with the patient about this dream she remembered another dream: *"We were riding in a crowded automobile—death or injury are threatened. Holds her child."* The patient remembered that she was in a smash-up with her mother. She obviously wants to be kept in safety by her mother.

Whatever the detailed interpretation of the dream may be, there cannot be much doubt that the problems of the dreamer and of others are treated in discreet symbolism. However, it does not hinder the fact that the function of the childbirth is conceived in an infantile way. To be hurled away from the mother is the center of this dream.

It seems to me that part of the difficulties in dream interpretation can be alleviated if one keeps constantly in mind the question of what the relations of the dream are to the body image. The following problems make their appearance: How does the body image appear in the manifest content of the dream? What is the relationship of the latent dream thought to the body image? In what relationship is one's own body image to other bodies appearing in the dream? Is the body image dealing with the body as a whole, or does it deal with parts of the body? In which way are parts of the body image transposed inside and outside of one's own body image? Which parts of the body image are the result of identification and appersonation, and which parts are projected into animate or inanimate objects? Does the dream deal with the body image of the past or of the present?

If one studies problems of this kind carefully enough, one will find that in a great number of dreams the body image appears in an infantile form and symbolically disguised, even when the body image appears also in the manifest content of the dream.

It is in no way a simple task to interpret dreams, and a good dream interpretation amounts almost to a life history of the patient. In practical psychotherapy we have to ask the patient to report dreams. Sometimes we have to repeat this order. Sometimes the patient will bring so many dreams that it is impossible to come to a human understanding of them, and arbitrary interpretation of symbols is useless. In analytic treatment as well as in any other treatment which uses dream interpretation, it depends, therefore, on the insight and attitude of the physician whether he wants to use a specific dream in the psychotherapeutic procedure or not. Whether he wants to or not, he has to be active in this respect. He has also to decide whether a dream interpretation started in one hour should be continued in the next hour. It is generally considered unwise to insist on the continuation of the interpretation of the dream unless the patient comes back to it himself or shows a definite intention to evade the issue.

It is possible to conduct a successful analysis in patients who do not bring dreams. It very often happens that a dream interpretation which is convincing for the patient is an important step forward. It has to be kept in mind that an interpretation which is given to the patient has to carry with it the force of conviction for him; and it is useless to communicate to the patient merely one's own knowledge, unless the interpretation provokes new associations and with this the possibility of an increased insight of the patient. This is true for every interpretation. A further activity is, therefore, necessary in choosing the interpretations which are available to the insight of the patient.

It is not necessary to interpret a dream immediately. A dream may be interpreted months after the patient has reported it. Dreams which have taken place before the analysis are as important as dreams which take place in analysis. Dreams of simple contents and archaic type to which no further material is brought forward are often considered as the return of the primal scene. One has a right to be skeptical about such an interpretation.

Freud finds his repetition compulsion also in dreams. Since I am skeptical about the repetition compulsion in general, I do not acknowledge it in the dreams, either. Even if one chooses classical analysis as the method of procedure, this problem has no practical importance. One has justly attributed a great importance to the first dream brought to the physician. It very often sums up important problems of the life of the dreamer.

Interpreting dreams cannot be the ultimate goal of a psychotherapeutic relation. It has to be subordinated to the total situation. It has a value only when it sooner or later increases the insight of the patient into his present and past situation. One may ask the patient to write down his dreams. Psychoanalysts usually advise against it. It has disadvantages. Dreams appear in the course of any psychic treatment according to the psychotherapeutic situation. If the patient is resistant, he very often does not bring any dreams. If we force him to get up during the night and to write down his dreams then, his association to the dreams will be useless. In general, I would advise not asking the patient to write down dreams during the night, but he may write them down during the day, if he wants to. If one sees disadvantages in the procedure, one may give it up. One should consider dream interpretation merely as one of the tools of psychotherapy, and not have the ambition to make a complete analysis of a dream unless it is important from the point of view of the therapeutic situation.

INTERPRETATION OF DAYDREAMS

The principles which are valid in the interpretation of dreams are also valid for the interpretation of daydreams. These are particularly common at puberty. The boy may dream of himself as a successful businessman, a general, a hero, a Napoleon, etc. Erotic phantasies belong in the same category. One of my patients told long stories to another girl during mutual masturbation. The secondary elaboration in these daydreams is very often more outspoken than in dreams. They need, at any rate, an interpretation and one may treat any daydream in the same way as any other dream. The same principle should be applied to masturbation phantasies and to the pictures which come into one's mind before falling asleep—the so-called hypnagogic hallucinations, the knowledge of which has been increased by Silberer, who pointed to their symbolic character. Bergler has shown that they may have a rather complicated psychological structure.

INTERPRETATION OF EVERYDAY MISTAKES

Freud has shown that the mistakes committed in everyday life point to deeper-lying motives. Slips of the tongue, for instance, may be connected with streams of thought which were suppressed although in the consciousness of the individual. A person kept away from his farm in Connecticut, for instance, says, when coming from another place, that it was very nice in Connecticut. He is fully aware of his wish to be there. A patient who has at a particular time aggressive impulsion against the analyst smashes a window by accident. She had violent outbursts of rage and hate against her mother in childhood. One has, therefore, to consider the sign function of mistakes, misfortunes, and accidents. Even accidents, which at first sight are seemingly not due to the attitude of an individual, reveal themselves very often as caused by tendencies of the individual hidden to himself.

INTERPRETATION OF FIRST MEMORIES

The interpretation of first memories of an individual has gained a rather important part in psychotherapy. An individual chooses his first memory from among many available early memories. It is, therefore, indicative of early tendencies. Freud has pointed to the fact that these early memories are often symbolic in character and have to be read like a dream. He has analyzed in detail an early memory of Leonardo da Vinci's of a vulture pushing its tail several times into the mouth of the child. He interpreted this memory as an expression of tendencies directed towards the mother with a penis (nipple). Early remembrances may, therefore, cover important material. Such memories are called screen remembrances. I merely give three short instances from my own material. The patient Sch., suffering from a severe anxiety neurosis, remembers her father leaving for Europe when she was four years old. Her second memory is that she asked her stepfather for bread and he gave the bread first to the others and only then to her. The patient does not want to be alone. She demands continually the love and consideration of the analyst and continually feels rejected. The patient Tr., also a case of anxiety neurosis, who, as the analysis showed, is particularly afraid that something may stick in her and explode her from the inside, has a vague early remembrance that she had a splinter in her vagina and asked her mother to take it out. The patient H., suffering from impotency and the inability to adapt to his professional tasks, has been told that after the circumcision he was dropped by carelessness, had a severe hemorrhage, and was in great danger. Masochistic trends are outspoken with him. He harps on this report of others because it expresses important tendencies of his own. His first memory is that his mother gave him bread through the door when he was standing in the street. He was always very dependent upon his mother, felt very sure of her love, and is convinced that she nursed him although he does not know anything about it. He has the confidence that life will finally give him all that he wants, without his doing much about it. Adler reports, "'I remember falling out of a baby carriage when I was three years old.' With this first memory went a recurrent dream: 'The world is coming to an end and I wake up in the middle of the night to find the sky bright red with fire. The stars all fall and we collide into another planet. But just before the crash, I wake up.' This student, when asked if he was afraid of anything, answered: 'I am afraid that I won't make a success of life,' and it is clear that his first memory and his recurrent dream act as discouragements and confirm him in fearing failure and catastrophe."

We are merely interested here in the fact that early remembrances have a sign function similar to the sign function of a dream.

THE ANALYSIS OF IDEOLOGIES

In order to come to an understanding of any individual we have to know his system of ideas and opinions, his ideologies. I repeat the passage characterizing this problem from a previous paper.

Ideologies are systems of ideas which human beings build up in order to have a better orientation for their actions. These systems are more or less conscious thoughts which mostly carry with them large amounts of emotion. Individuals usually believe that their ideologies are the result of pure reasoning, but astonishingly often do not care to find out why these ideologies are so convincing to themselves. Their belief in their ideologies is usually very firm and the ideologies are often not so very different from religious beliefs, with which they share a high degree of inner evidence, very often in contrast to the scarcity of empirical proof.

Ideologies are not only a theoretical belief but they have a profound influence upon our actions and often are the deciding factor in the organization of our lives. It is easy to see that many of these ideologies are based upon traditions. We inherit them from our fathers and teachers and accept them without any attempt at analyzing their contents. It cannot be denied that ideologies are also different according to the social standing of an individual. Every caste carries with it its own ideology. Since ideologies are handed down by tradition and, once accepted, are retained throughout life, we do not wonder that the ruling classes and ruling systems are interested that children should be fitted with their ideologies as soon and as thoroughly as possible.

Every family has, besides its national and class ideologies, its private ideology, too. It is characteristic that an individual may carry ideologies very different in their structure without being aware of the contradictions in the various ideologies in which he firmly believes. Conflicts arise between the various ideologies in one individual and from the insufficiency of ideologies in given situations of life in connection with the fact that ideologies by their inner nature are inflexible, rigid, and unadaptable. It is also characteristic that the individual does not know the true nature of ideologies. They are often expressed in words, and the individual does not care to know their genesis and implications. They cover the whole range of human life. Since the basis of ideologies is mostly not empirical and their formulation not logical, individuals are often embarrassed when ideologies are brought into the field of rational discussion. Ideologies pretend to have their basis in reason and experience. Very often they do not stand either of these tests, and an individual retains them merely because strong emotional forces protect the ideologies from any attempt to analyze them.

Psychoanalysis has shown the way in which ideologies are built up. They arise from the libidinous situation in early childhood and are, therefore, in close relation to the emotional attitudes of the child towards his parents and the other persons around him. Some of these ideologies are built up by identification, and others by imitation. They are very often reactions to the parental ideologies when there is an open conflict between the parents and the child. Frequently they have a complicated genesis of a neurotic symptom, and represent in a symbolic way the libidinous forces as well as the repressing ones.

When we analyze the ideologies we have to force the individual to bring them clearly into consciousness. We have further to insist relentlessly that the ideology is discussed in all of its logical aspects. One will generally be able to bring the patient to a logical insight into the flaws in his system of ideas. A deeper analysis may start at this very point.

It is clear that concrete thinking and interest in a specific situation give very little opportunity for the formation of ideologies. The patient therefore has to be forced to go back again and again to his concrete experiences. Furthermore, if his own experiences are not sufficient, one may help him to supplement his knowledge. He has to be taught the dangers of abstract thinking which, although it seems to be logical, is usually the expression of complexes which the patient wants to hide from himself. The patient has to ask himself why he favors the acceptance of a specific system of ideas, and he will soon come to the insight that he has accepted them, not on their logical value, but by his personal attitudes.

Logical thinking always has two sides. There is the question whether a thought is correct or not, but there is also the problem why it was possible for one individual to find the correct answer, and why it was not possible for another individual equally gifted to find this answer. Ideologies are formulated in words, or at least can be formulated in words, although the individual very often refrains from a clear formulation in order to protect his specific ideology from his own logic. The analysis of words is, therefore, an indispensable part of the analysis of ideologies. Abstract words of general character, loaded with poorly understood emotions, are often the pillars upon which ideologies are erected. They no longer mean anything specific. Sometimes it is difficult, for instance, to decide what the term "my own country" or the term "patriotism" may mean. Children say, for instance, "One has to defend the flag," but they do not know why one should defend the flag.

Our whole social life is based upon ideologies which have become rigid, unadaptable, and do not fit the individual any longer. Very often generalizations play an important part in ideologies. It belongs, for instance, to the European ideology to think that every American is rich; other ideologies insist on the inferiority of one or the other race. General connotations are, of course, necessary, but they must be checked continually by going back to the basic experiences. Problems of this sort are met in every psychotherapy. The analysis of ideologies is a necessary part of every psychotherapy.

Also, in psychoanalysis the individual has to know many things. The defects of his knowledge and the flaws in his logic indicate his emotional attitudes. An individual should be capable of gaining intellectual insight. I have repeated here remarks from a previous book and from a previous paper, because the importance of the analysis of ideologies for psychotherapeutic purposes has so far not been acknowledged. Modern psychology and especially psychoanalysis have erected an artificial barrier between the so-called intellectual and the so-called emotional sides of life. The power of ideas has been underrated. Human beings have opinions. These opinions have been created in a constructive effort to get in touch with reality, but there is the tendency to use patterns from childhood and patterns taken over from those with whom one has been in relation in childhood. It is very difficult for the individual to change such a pattern, and it is furthermore very difficult for an individual without help to analyze the intellectual value of patterns, words, and phrases.

The difficulties in the analysis of ideologies lie partially in the fact that the physician has his own ideologies, too, and in addition the ideologies very often pertain to problems which according to their very nature do not permit a definite solution. The physician has, therefore, to check himself continually as to whether indisputable facts exist which prove his convictions. Furthermore, he should know where mere opinion starts. He will then not make the mistake of imposing his opinions upon the patient; thus he is continually faced with the necessity of making the patient conscious of the facts. It will thus be necessary to give attention to where verbal formulation has retained the relation to objects and where words have become independent of facts. The analysis of ideologies in this respect is indispensable. One has to keep in mind that we do not have to demand of the patient an understanding of all his ideologies, but only of those which are important from the point of view of his specific situation. In concrete psychotherapy and in deeper analysis there will be not only free association in the sense described above, but also an increase in knowledge concerning vital problems.

I have pointed out on other occasions that there are many things which one should know about sex problems. In psychoanalysis the analyst often gives such discussions and imparts knowledge without being conscious of his procedure. There are also many problems of physiology which the patient has to know—for instance, about diet or sleep. I will not go into a detailed discussion of this problem here, since the chapter on group psychotherapy will give the material on the basis of which a practical approach to this problem in psychotherapy can be reached. As mentioned above, in the treatment of children it is obvious that the opinions of children have to be taken into consideration. One should transfer this principle from the treatment of children to the treatment of adults.

THE ANALYSIS OF SOCIAL ADAPTATION

We come to the general principle that psychic experiences, whatever they may be, have a double aspect. They are themselves, but they also point to something else, quite in the same way as every event in the outward world is not an isolated event but an event in a context which has to be considered from the point of view of a regular sequence. Psychic experiences lie in a context and occur in regular sequences. They are signs of something else. The sign function is general, and whatever we may do or whatever we experience has a sign function, too. We are therefore justified in taking every experience in human life to be a sign of other psychic processes and events. When we work, for instance, this work has an obvious purpose in the community. At the same time it satisfies our own tendencies and is thus a sign of tendencies in ourselves and can be analyzed like a piece of a dream or like a symptom. The term "sublimation" in psychoanalysis means that energies which belong to the sexual sphere are used in such a way that they serve purposes which are socially acknowledged, and, therefore, are also approved by the individual's conscience, the superego. The real drive comes, therefore, from forbidden sources, and the achievement is based upon overcoming and utilizing sexual energies. One might thus show to the patient that his interest in painting is merely an expression of his anal tendencies.

From a practical point of view as well as from the point of understanding psychology, it is important to keep in mind that we have not only to study and understand psychic structures which are socially useless or dangerous, but we have to understand also psychic structures which are useful, socially acknowledged, and a source of enjoyment. A logically correct thought and the successful action have a psychogenesis which has to be understood in the course of psychotherapy. One sees immediately that the scope of psychotherapy extends over the whole life of the individual, and cannot be bound to the attempt of understanding symptoms. The underlying theories of Freud, that the structures of the world and the successful action offer satisfaction only in so far as they serve repressed infantile tendencies, have to be rejected. When we try to interpret so-called sublimated experiences, that does not mean denying the genuine interests in reality and its structures. In actual psychotherapy the patient will very often protest against an interpretation of what he considers the positive side of life. He complies with an analysis of his mistakes. He has to be made to understand that even when we do the right thing, we do it in connection with the deeper problems of our lives.

No experience is for itself, and one may always try to show that an experience means something else. One might even seek to show that intercourse means something else: for instance, gaining superiority over one's partner. Psychoanalysts have interpreted the satisfaction of intercourse as derived from the experience of birth. This is, of course, senseless. One has to stop somewhere and ask, where are the basic experiences? There is a sexual satisfaction, there is an immediate satisfaction by food, and studying the structures of organization we must try to find out what the basic situations are. For instance, the attitude of love remains the attitude of love even if we show that it has occurred in relation to early sex experiences with the father or mother. Interpretation generally cannot mean devaluation. The value of the things cannot be decided upon psychogenetic principles but is dependent upon one's final relation to the reality and to the world.

If psychoanalysis shows the importance of pregenital and genital sexuality in child and adult, and has traced it into manifestations which do not seem sexual, we should be aware that the value of cultural and social phenomena does not depend upon the value given to the infantile drive which it "sublimated." If cleanliness and hygiene are sublimations of anal tendencies, their value is still greater than the value of the pleasurable actions of a child with its feces, since the primitive experience is now in the service of an adaptation to reality. Society and social structures are more than sublimated homosexuality since they point to a reality between human beings. Adler and Jung have seen this part of the problem more clearly.

Jung especially stresses the creative forces of the unconscious. He overrates art and the artist and does not see that our whole life is a constructive effort directed towards creation and action in the world. One may ask what considerations like this have to do with practical psychotherapy, but it is of the utmost importance to interpret to the patient every one of his activities in a spirit which does not try to show to patient and physician only a side which is considered as valueless. The infantile sexuality has to be measured by its own standards and not with the measurement of adult ethics. The patient has to be continually aware that infantile homosexuality and infantile aggressiveness have a meaning different from homosexual and aggressive actions of the adult, and he should appreciate their relation to the present situation. The patient has to understand not only the drives but also the relation of the drives to the situation.

ACTIVITY

Interpretation as described in the preceding remarks is an active process. To be silent is activity, too. The physician is constantly choosing what he has to say, what he has to interpret. He directs the patient and he should be aware of it. The so-called passive analysis—

relying on interpretation as its only tool—is merely one form of activity. Passive analysis has proved insufficient. One cannot treat an anxiety neurotic patient or a drug addiction by merely interpreting. The anxiety neurosis case has to be forced to actions which his neurosis tries to hinder. The patient has to be ordered to go into a situation which provokes anxiety. The drug addict has to stand the withdrawal of the drug. We may formulate in a general way that in the so-called active therapy we force the patient to act against his symptom. According to the psychoanalytic theory such an action will bring forward material which otherwise remains hidden, and the interpretation will progress. The activity would be merely a subsidiary tool to interpretation. Ferenczi has taken over this device from other forms of psychotherapy. In other forms of psychotherapy one supposes that the patient, forced into the situation which he fears, will become accustomed to it and will overcome his fear. Activity is merely used as a form of breaking a neurotic habit. The patient learns, by and by, to overcome the difficulties by forced practice. I believe that this factor plays an important part indeed in the beneficial effect of activity, even when occurring in psychoanalysis. By the repetition of the act which the patient fears, he gains a better insight into a situation which, until then, he considered dangerous.

It was shown in the previous chapter that neurotic symptoms very often serve the tendency of escaping a situation which is considered unbearable or dangerous. The patient is taught by his forced actions that there are no insurmountable difficulties in the situation. It is very often important to find out which actions we may demand from a patient. If it is simply an anxiety neurosis, like that of a patient who does not dare to be far away from his home, he is ordered, at first, to walk two or three blocks. When this performance has taken place three or four times and his assurance has increased, he is ordered to walk four blocks. It is important that one should not ask too much from the patient. He should never be thrown into a panic. We can only demand actions from the patient. We should not demand, as mentioned above, that the patient exert will power. We should not demand from the patient that he suppress thoughts. Such demands are useless and increase the sense of failure in the patient. If we deal with a hysterical patient who has difficulties in walking, we may give him tasks of increasing difficulty. We may occasionally order an impotent person to attempt intercourse. Very often it is indeed very difficult to find actions which are appropriate to the symptoms of the patient.

Ferenczi has been rather ingenious in this respect. He ordered, in the treatment for impotency, for instance, that patients keep back their urine and feces as long as they could. He furthermore ordered patients to act out situations in the direction of repressed drives—for instance, obscene dancing. Such methods will rarely be justified. They bear the stamp of artificiality and are too arbitrary.

It is to the credit of psychoanalysis to have shown that mere exercise does not lead very far unless it increases the insight. However, the exercise has a value in itself. It is very difficult to treat such problems with isolated technical advice. They are in very close relation to the situation between patient and physician. You cannot demand anything from the patient unless you enjoy the confidence (transference) of the patient. In psychoanalysis, active methods generally are not employed in the first few weeks of analysis. The understanding and the tact of the physician are necessary to employ the principle of activity and exercise correctly. It always has to lead to a better insight into the situation. It should not be used to browbeat the patient. One may characterize the principle by saying that the patient has to be led into the danger situation. He has to get acquainted with the danger situation. Necessarily, past material pertaining to the danger situation will come up. The patient will gain better insight merely by the fact that he is confronted with the situation.

This principle is probably also valid when thoughts which seem to be unacceptable to the patient are formulated again and again. The mere formulation in words has such an effect. The word "homosexuality," for instance, very often seems to be loaded with dangerous implications. When it is repeated over and over again, when its true meaning is revealed in relation to a concrete situation, the fears disappear and the patient becomes well acquainted with and therefore free in the situation. A horse may get shy when it comes to a strange object. When it has the opportunity of becoming acquainted with the dangerous-looking object, it will go on quietly. This is the principle of active psychotherapy as well as of verbal formulations which are given to the patient. I have mentioned before that we may, in hypnosis, revive a traumatic scene again and again till it loses its emotional value. Activity of this type will be necessary in almost every treatment.

THE USE OF BENZEDRINE [6]

Benzedrine (amphetamine sulphate) is a sympathicomimetic compound structurally related to ephedrine and epinephrine. Prinzmetal and Bloomberg used benzedrine sulphate for the treatment of narcolepsy. It relieved the catalepsy as well as the attacks of sleep.

According to the report of the pharmacological firm which produces the drug and which based its report on the writings of Myerson, Prinzmetal, and Solomon, it was stated that the drug has a good effect upon the mood if administered in small doses. The effect was said not to be accompanied by any change in personality or clouding of the mentality; it also tended to banish fatigue. Myerson also reported good results in depressive states.

Investigations at Bellevue also confirmed the gratifying effects on narcoleptic attacks and catalepsy. It seemed advisable to try to come to a deeper insight into the psychological effects of using the drugs on patients who were in analysis. Drugs which have psychological effects tend to change the deep libidinal attitudes. Pharmaco-psychoanalysis tries to determine the changes in the libidinous and ego attitudes which occur under the influence of drugs (cf. my *Introduction to Psychoanalytic Psychiatry* and "Psychotherapy in Psychosis"). Important material on this subject can be found in the papers by Lindemann and Malamud. Such studies are not merely concerned with the description of the psychological effects but attempt to go beyond the surface phenomena into the dynamics in relation to the psychoanalytic structure of the personality. Here I wish to report on psychoanalyzed cases in which benzedrine was used.

A thirty-seven-year-old sociologist had been analyzed for about sixteen months by other analysts and was in the seventh month of analysis by me. In the foreground of the picture was anxiety when he was alone. In addition there were states of depression when he was unable to work and felt inhibited. During such a period he took two tablets (12 mgms.) of benzedrine at ten o'clock in the morning. He was seen in the afternoon. He had worked with great energy. He wrote a long article and felt very elated. He stated that his ideas came

[6] Reprinted from "The Psychological Effects of Benzedrine Sulphate," *Journal of Nervous and Mental Disease* 87:584–87, 1938.

very fast and he felt that they were better than usual. He got an idea to write an article on the history of ceremonies. He felt tolerant and friendly towards everyone. He gave a dollar to the elevator boy. He talked to his house maid and felt rather affectionate towards her. He even included his sister in this general idea of friendliness. He was not bothered with sex at all. He said, "I had these moods before. I changed my whole mental attitude." When he worked he had the feeling that he was working well, so he reported the next day. His general sexuality, which was otherwise very lively, did not come into appearance at all at this time. He had the feeling of great energy and strength. He had great difficulty in sleeping the following night, but the sleeplessness was not disagreeable. He had the feeling of being wound up and tense. The next day he felt increasingly depressed, apathetic, and without energy, similar to having a hangover after drinking alcohol. This patient had a similar reaction, but much milder, after taking sodium amytal or alcohol. Seemingly the benzedrine gave him the assurance of being loved, similar to alcohol. It was a diffuse object relationship which excludes genitality. Analytic material showed that in this way he regained the love of the mother and father which he had missed in childhood.

He had been brought up by a tyrannical older sister who, as analytic material showed, was for him a female bully with a penis. The parents, although kind, were not affectionate, and he felt deprived of affection, which he tried to get from a combined father and mother imago endowed with a penis. It is remarkable that he once got an effect similar to that given to him by the benzedrine in connection with a dream in which a cosmic ray gave him the assurance of being loved and being safe. He is an amiable person and wants to be loved by everybody. He is afraid of direct sexual gratification, which might impair the love of others for him. The benzedrine gave him a satisfaction at a level which was not completely genitalized and in which a diffuse object relationship existed without differentiation concerning sexuality. As is well known in other patients, benzedrine suppressed the appetite in this person also. The results of the drug are seemingly due not alone to the structure of the drug but also to the structure of the personality.

In spite of the beneficial effects, this patient did not feel like repeating the experience, since he feared the aftereffects. He took the drug only once more (10 mgms.) when he was especially anxious to be freed from his inhibition for work. The results were qualitatively identical but quantitatively less outspoken.

Also, in another case the bezedrine intensified the relationship towards other human beings but not at the genital level. It helped to overcome the social isolation which was based upon masochistic tendencies. The increase in self-love was still more obvious than in the first case. Benzedrine also produced in this case a reaction similar to that seen in the course of psychological development. It served to overcome a fatigue which was determined by deep masochistic trends. It substituted object relationship at a nongenital level and increased the narcissistic pleasures in the patient's own body and his own energy. Under these circumstances the patient could feel loved by himself and by others.

If one understands the pharmacologic action of benzedrine from a psychoanalytic point of view, one will probably be able to use benzedrine in the treatment of neurosis. It will certainly not cure a neurosis, but it will be helpful from the symptomatological point of view and may help to bring forward important material in the course of the analytic treatment. Peoples and Guttmann describe similar psychological effects from the drug.[7]

If the drug is taken without due consideration of the psychological state of the patient, sleepiness, fatigue, and inhibitions will disappear, but the patient will feel a painful restlessness that is more disagreeable than the original symptom.

HYPNOTIC SUGGESTION

We come now to the tools of psychotherapy, which are based upon the relation between physician and patient and which utilize this relation. We start with the discussion of hypnosis. The technique of hypnosis used in psychotherapy is as follows. The patient is ordered to lie down on the couch. He is told that he will come into a state of relaxation and maybe sleep, which will make him amenable to the therapeutic suggestions of the physician. Before one starts the hypno-

[7] Following this work, Lauretta Bender and Frances Cottington used benzedrine with children for neurotic overactivity, anxiety, blocking, inhibition, restlessness, and precocious sexual drives and preoccupations. [L.B., Ed.]

sis one should make up one's mind whether one needs a deep hypnosis or whether a superficial one will be sufficient. A deep hypnosis is advisable if one wants to clear up amnesias. In the treatment of the abstinence phenomena of drug addiction, the treatment of drug addiction in general, and also for the treatment of organ neuroses and tics, deep hypnosis is needed. In the treatment of neuroses, superficial hypnosis will most often be sufficient. If we need a deep hypnosis, we tell the patient that we expect him to go into a deep sleep. If we do not need a deep hypnosis we tell the patient that he will at any rate achieve a state of relaxation and rest, that he may fall asleep but that this is of no importance. We also tell him that he may very well remember whatever has been said. We tell him further that the state of rest and relaxation is sufficient to make him more receptive to the suggestion.

We then hold a key before the eyes of the patient and order him to look at it. We tell him that he will get tired and sleepy. We start to stroke lightly the forehead of the patient, and talk about as follows: "You are in a state of rest and relaxation. Your arms and legs become more and more heavy. You feel like closing your eyes. You get more and more tired and sleepy. You feel like falling asleep. You breathe calmly and deeply. You have an agreeable feeling all over your body." This suggestion has to be repeated again and again till the patient closes his eyes. If the patient does not close his eyes himself, we order him to close his eyes.

The procedure is continued for from five to ten minutes, and the suggestion is given. In a therapeutic hypnosis it is advisable not to make any experiments with the patient. The suggestions should be merely therapeutic. Occasionally one may stroke the patient's arm slightly, saying, "You have an agreeable feeling of warmth in the arm which I touch." The therapeutic suggestion should be repeated several times. We shall hear later that the formulation of the therapeutic suggestion is of paramount importance. It should sum up the important problems of the patient and should show him the way to understand and to overcome his difficulties. If a suggestion is directed against the symptom without taking into consideration its psychological origin, the suggestion should be as detailed as possible. When we give suggestions against constipation, for instance, we may tell the patient, "When you awake in the morning you will feel the urge to go to the toilet. When you are there, you will start with your bowel movement without much pressing." When we suggest to the patient that he should sleep well, we shall not merely tell him so but tell him that when he goes to bed he will experience an agreeable relaxation, all tensions will disappear, he will sooner or later become more and more sleepy and fall asleep, he will have a restful sleep and awake the next morning fully refreshed and active.

It is not advisable to ask any questions pertaining to the depths of hypnosis after the patient has awakened. One may try to raise the arm of the patient during the hypnosis and see whether catalepsy or complete flaccidity are present. One may say aloud two or three numbers, without asking anything. One awakens the patient by touching his forehead and announcing, "I shall awaken you soon. When I count to five, you will open your eyes, you will not experience any headache and dizziness, you will feel completely refreshed." If one awakens patients too suddenly, especially those who are in deeper hypnosis, they will very often react with headaches and dizziness. If the patient does awaken with a headache, a few strokes on the forehead, with the suggestion that the headache will disappear, are very often helpful.

After the patient has awakened, one may ask him what he has experienced. Most patients will report that they were tired, that they felt heavy, and a great many will have experienced the suggested warmth in their arm. One then says to the patient, "There has been an influence and that is all that is necessary." When the hypnosis has been deeper, the patient may not remember the numbers. Patients who have been in deeper hypnosis very often doubt that they have been hypnotized, and it is good to prove to them in this way that they have forgotten their experiences. Many patients are disappointed when they are not in a deep hypnosis, and say, "Doctor, I have heard everything which you have said." One may assure them that a deep hypnosis is not intended, or promise them that the next hypnosis will be deeper. Patients who assure you, after the first session, that they have been wide awake are not very good subjects for hypnotic treatment.

It is generally advisable not to prolong the first session for too long a time. This is especially important when the patient obviously goes into a deep hypnosis, behaves like a sleeping person, shows flaccidity and catalepsy. Patients of this type may go into a dreamy state of their own which might be difficult to handle. One should, therefore, not prolong a deep hypnosis and should interrupt it as soon as the patient shows signs that he does not obey the hypnotizer any more. The depth of hypnosis generally increases at the second or third session, and one may tell this to the patient. One may then extend the duration of a single session up to one hour if one can stand it oneself. Magic gestures and magic implements are not advisable in a therapeutic hypnosis. The room should not be too light and not too noisy. If the patient complains too much about little disturbances, one may justly tell him that the important thing is not the outward situation, but his attitude. It is indeed possible to hypnotize in very noisy and fully lighted rooms.

If the hypnosis is not sufficiently deep after five or six sessions, one may use drugs in order to facilitate the hypnosis. I have mostly used medinal in doses of ten to twenty grains. One may use any other barbiturate in appropriate doses. Sodium amytal can be used in doses of three to six grains. Barbiturates have to be given from one to two hours before the hypnosis starts. It is important that the physician remain in contact with the patient during the hypnosis. It should not be merely a sleep. Although it is possible to awaken the patient after the hypnosis, it is generally advisable to let the patient sleep. However, he may go home and go to bed until the effect of the sedative has disappeared. One may also use paraldehyde in a dosage of one or two drams. The hypnosis can start immediately after the paraldehyde has been taken.

We have described the method of hypnosis used as direct suggestion. The suggestion can be directed against the symptom as such. In some cases it cannot be avoided; for instance, in tics and in organ neuroses, where the genesis of the symptom is not ascertained. Direct suggestion can also be used in clearly formulating the problems to the patient and suggesting to him that, on the basis of the insight, symptoms will disappear. This method is preferable; and it is, of course, necessary in order to formulate the suggestion properly that one know something about the genesis of the symptoms. Preliminary work in this respect will be necessary. One should be careful in suggesting problems and their solutions, unless one has a sufficient insight oneself. The usefulness of hypnosis for increasing the insight by catharsis is limited, as mentioned above. The full implications of hypnosis can only be understood in connection with the general conduct of a psychotherapy. The relation of the patient to the physician has to be fully understood if one wants to make the correct use of hypnosis as a therapeutic method. In the limits discussed above, hypnosis can be of help in short psychotherapy.[8]

SUGGESTION

It is, of course, not necessary to use the full armamentarium of hypnosis in order to suggest. One may rely upon one's authority as a physician, make one's voice sound convincing, give orders to the patient; and one may tell the patient something about his problems based upon the insight one has gained. The value of such a procedure depends not upon the strength of the suggestion and the influence of authority, but upon the amount of insight upon which the suggestion is based and upon the amount of insight which it imparts to the patient. We have discussed this problem when talking about persuasion. Persuasion undoubtedly contains a considerable amount of suggestion.

One may resort to masked suggestion by treating the patient with medicines, which according to the physician's opinion are of no use. One may give physiotherapy, electric treatments, and massage. According to our general principles, we are strongly opposed to such methods, as far as they are used not as physical agents but as methods of suggestion. They obliterate, instead of increasing, the insight. They can be excused only when the state of the patient is such that he cannot avail himself of any insight. The electric current may be used not so much as a suggestion as a threat with pain. With hysterics one may apply faradic currents to a paralyzed limb, and tell them that the faradic current will have a curative effect. The patient gives up his symptoms when the pain inflicted by the faradic current is less bearable than the situation which provoked the paralysis. One may use the pain directly or as a threat. The method may cure hysterical symptoms in the motor sphere and mutism as quickly as anesthesias. It is a cruel method and should be used only when extraordinary circumstances make it very important that the symptoms should disappear immediately. Whenever such a thing is done, psychotherapy should try to proceed to the real problem. There are many more methods

[8] Recent reviews on hypnotherapy include those by Lewis R. Wolberg and M. Brenman and M. M. Gill. [L. B., Ed.]

which combine suggestion with threats and actual discomfort. These are at best very crude methods.

Autosuggestion has been employed by Coué. The patient is at first shown by simple methods the influence of autosuggestion on the body. He is taught to stand erect, his feet close, telling himself that he will fall forwards or backwards. Very soon he will sway in this direction. He is also taught to hold in his outstretched hand a thread on which a ring or any heavy object is suspended and to tell himself persistently that it moves in the one or the other direction. Very soon the pendulum will start to swing in the direction indicated. He is ordered to intertwine his fingers and to say to himself that he cannot loosen the fingers; he will not be able to do so unless the contrary autosuggestion follows. Experiments like this might occasionally, indeed, be usefully employed in bringing the patient to an insight into psychophysiological correlations. But this will be only an exception. The experiment is rather primitive.

Subsequently, Coué orders his patients to repeat to themselves mechanically, over and over again, a formula that they will become better and better from day to day. The formula has to be repeated twenty to thirty times, several times a day. There is a spark of psychological truth in the method, in so far as Coué does not demand any emotional effort from his patient and relies merely on the fact that thoughts and words spoken to oneself will have an influence.

We have seen that in every active psychotherapy one should not demand anything from the patient which the patient cannot fulfill. One can always say something to oneself, but one generally cannot command one's emotions. Since autosuggestion in the sense of Coué is general, it is bound to be ineffective. It has no deeper relation to the real life of the patient. And since the autosuggestion is ordered by the authority of the practitioner, it is not autosuggestion but merely a special type of suggestion. The method as it stands is ineffective and is no real addition to psychotherapy. Although it may seem rational, it belongs in the category of healing by faith.

The curative factor lies in the symbolism of the procedure. In the case of Coué it is self-assurance by an introjected father. The electrical apparatus symbolizes something: mysterious forces of nature. Behind the results of the great shrines like Lourdes stands the symbolic power of the Catholic Church. Behind Christian Science stands the strong wish for the integrity of the body which is elevated to a preposterous doctrine but still has retained relations to a deep instinctual wish. In psychotherapy we avoid symbolic treatments even if we should be able to employ them. The mainspring of modern psychotherapy lies in the desire to help the patient to a better emotional and intellectual adaptation on the basis of insight. Symbolic methods give either no insight at all, or a very incomplete one. Pfister is, therefore, not right when he praises the symbolic insight displayed in the ceremonies of the Navaho Indians as psychotherapeutic procedure.

RELAXATION AND CONCENTRATION

Jacobson has worked out a method of progressive relaxation by which the patient is taught to relax his muscles. The relaxation as such is considered as a therapeutic factor. Relaxation is, according to my opinion, merely a suggestive method. Tension is not the cause of neurosis but a symptom of neurosis. Relaxation may also be used as the basis on which suggestions may become more efficient. I. H. Schultz has worked out a method of self-concentration in which exercises in concentration of increasing complication are demanded. It is the method of the Yogis. Jacobson and Schultz's methods are akin to suggestive methods in which the influence on the body and especially on the muscles is stressed. The state reached in this way may increase the plasticity of interhuman relations, and a better insight might be reached on the basis of this plasticity. Interesting as special methods, they are hardly usable in the everyday approach of the patient. It seems, furthermore, that the technique has a large mixture of symbolic elements and serves only very incompletely our general aim of a dependable insight into an individual's life history.

CHANGING THE SURROUNDINGS

The methods described are so far more or less direct methods of psychotherapy, but one may try to gain influence on the attitudes of the patient by changing his way of living. One may send a patient away to Florida, or send him to a hospital for rest, or put him to bed. There is no curative effect in any of the measures of this type.

However, the change in the surroundings and the other practices mentioned may have a symbolic value and help so that the patient has symbolic satisfactions. To be away from one's family or business situation may be of value. It is difficult to employ these indirect methods. They are useless when not based upon deep psychological insight into the individual problems of the patient. The patient himself should be aware of the situation. If we can make him aware of the situation, then all the procedures mentioned will become unnecessary. If the patient then wants to get away from his family or his business, he will do so on his own initiative, which is better. The physician may try to change the outward situation for the patient; he may change his type of work or may feel as though he were the master of his patient's destiny. Such a procedure is dangerous for the physician and for the patient. The physician grossly overrates his own possibilities, and the patient will at best remain dependent and without insight and capacity for determining his own goals.

THE HOSPITAL AND OCCUPATIONAL THERAPY

A patient who needs psychic help may enter a hospital. The modern psychiatric hospital provides a well-regulated routine of social life and work. It takes care of the occupation of the patient. Occupations are of two types. They can be useful, or they may be merely artificial efforts. Weaving, making straw baskets and metal ash trays can hardly be considered as useful efforts. Carpentry certainly leads one step further. Work in the house, garden, and field are useful occupations. It is obvious that the type of occupation employed should be decided on the basis of an intimate knowledge of the patient's problems. Whenever possible, the patient should make his decision himself. There is a natural tendency to form social groups; as far as the patient is not able to fall into one of the natural groups, the physician should help him in such an endeavor. Such group formations will take place in connection with physical exercises, physical culture, and sport. It is obvious that the patient, in the course of such activities, meets not only the physician but also many other persons who are ready to help him, especially the nurses, and as a second line, the instructors.

The hosptial is, therefore, a rather complicated community which seemingly serves two purposes. It simplifies the outward situation and the problems of the patient. It takes him out of the world of conflicts and puts him into a world which is simple, socially accepted, and moderately useful. In addition, he has the help of a group: the physician, the nurse, and the other patients. The function of this group is twofold. It offers a varied chance for forming human contacts (transference), each of which might offer successful possibilities for the patient to find a leader. Every member of the group might help the patient increase his insight into his situation and his problems. The importance of the nursing personnel in this respect can hardly be overestimated. It is obvious that such a situation is ideal for the psychotic. We shall hear later that the psychotic suffers from difficulties in finding a suitable love object. He is also more threatened by the world than the nonpsychotic individual and is unable to cope with these dangers. The well-directed hospital is, therefore, the ideal place for the psychotic patient who needs psychotherapy. The hospital routine will blend easily with any type of rational psychotherapy given to the patient. The situation of the neurotic and psychopathic patient is fundamentally different. We may expect more from him. The hospital situation makes the adaptation too simple for him. His need for insight is not stimulated by the situation. There is no urgent need to offer him a simplified world. It is, furthermore, comparatively simple to make the right choice in the outward surroundings for a psychotic patient. It is difficult to gain enough insight to find the right world for the neurotic or psychopathic individual. If the neurotic goes to the hospital, he urgently needs, besides the hospital routine, a psychotherapy which gives him deep individual insight.

THE ORGANIZATION OF A CHILDREN'S WARD

The remarks made will also help us in the understanding of the way in which a ward for problem children should be conducted. The routine of a children's ward will include classes in which the child should have a possibility of expressing himself freely, although he should be given definite tasks. There should be occupational activities. The children's ward of Bellevue Psychiatric Hospital organized by L. Bender,[9] on whose work and experience the remarks on psychotherapy in children are largely based, has classes in art, classes in clay modeling, classes in music, and, finally, the puppet shows about which Bender and Woltmann have already reported. There is, further, care taken that the children have sufficient opportunity for play. There are regular school classes in which teaching is adapted to the general plan of the institution. All these activities not only provide a routine in groups, but the expression of the child in any of his activities becomes the basis for a further therapeutic approach. One may compare also the report of Potter on the organization of the children's service in the New York Psychiatric Institute. One should not forget about the aspect of routine, the aspect of an increase in insight, and the possibility for human contacts with the adults who conduct and direct the activities, the nurses and the physicians. There is also the continuous contact with other children, providing the possibility of seeing one's own problem reflected in the others, the possibility of getting help from the stronger, and giving help to the weaker one.

If a successful treatment for the criminal could be attempted, it should be modeled after the pattern which has proved to be successful in the treatment of psychiatric cases and of children in institutions. It is obvious that a new principle makes its appearance here. The individual is not isolated with the physician in the psychotherapeutic contact, but lives in a group, and one member of the group may identify himself with other members of the group. Hospital treatment, in addition, substitutes for the limited transference situation of the individual treatment the offer of a greater number of love objects.

Group activities are a successful way of communing with children, of getting them to express their emotional problems, of giving them full play for their impulses for aggression or love, and of relieving them of anxiety and apprehension.[10] Group therapy, moreover, has a definite socializing effect, in aiding the child in becoming a more successful social personality.

---

[9] The techniques used on the children's ward of the psychiatric division of Bellevue Hospital have been described in Lauretta Bender's *Child Psychiatric Techniques.* (See Footnote 4.) A very brief account is given here. [L.B., Ed.]

[10] From Frank J. Curran and Paul Schilder, "A Constructive Approach to the Problems of Childhood and Adolescence," *Journal of Clinical Psychopathology* 2:125–42, 1940; 2:305–20, 1941.

The essential needs of any normal child are food, clothing, warmth, support from falling until he has learned to walk, protection from an aggressive world, and demonstrations of love from the persons who give him these things. Upon the satisfaction of these needs is built the personality. The essential drives of the child are for a free expression of his own impulses to be aggressive and to love and for the chance to exercise the growing functions of his physical, intellectual, emotional, and social personality. A deprivation of the satisfaction of the needs of the child or a deprivation of the demonstration of love, which should accompany it, results in developmental retardation, in apprehension and fear, in prolonged infantile behavior, and in attention-getting mechanisms. A repression of the drives results in feelings of inferiority, anxiety, and guilt.

Behavior problems, psychopathic reactions, neurotic reactions, and conduct disorders arise from deprivations in the satisfaction of these needs and drives, owing to a failure on the part of the parents or parent substitutes, or to constitutional weakness or organic disease in the child. Behavior problems may be associated with mental deficiency, epilepsy, organic brain disorders or somatic diseases.

The ward activities should be based upon the natural rhythms of sleeping, eating, resting, and physical, intellectual, and emotional activity. This rhythm should be emphasized in contrast to allowing the child to follow his own undirected impulses. The rhythm must adapt itself to the age level, to the intellectual maturation, to the motility problem, and to the attention span.

In order to relieve anxiety and guilt and to provide free expression for aggression and affection, many group projects are utilized. Active sports, shopwork, schoolwork, the use of puppet, art, music, and dramatic projects are provided.

The music project utilizes group singing and rhythm band activities. These music activities have definite value in training the hyperkinetic children whose main problems are of direction and attention, concentration, motivation, goal attainments, and patterning of impulses. The singing classes have definite socializing value.

The schoolroom activities consist of regular Board of Education classrooms and classes conducted by remedial-reading and arithmetic teachers. In the latter group, special tutoring is arranged for those children suffering from scholastic retardation.

Group discussions are frequently utilized. Children with similar problems are interviewed in groups of six to ten; they speak very freely about their sex problems, about aggressive conduct, etc., talking much more expansively than in the individual interviews with the physician.

The most important aspect of the ward is that the patient should be individually understood and cared for as an individual. The individual interview remains, therefore, the most important part of the treatment on the ward. Whatever has happened in the various group activities is summarized and explained in its deeper aspects in the individual interviews with the patient. It is also possible in this way to exemplify his own problems in the problems he sees in others and which he can recognize more readily in other patients than in himself. The problems of leadership, organization, and adaptation appear in varied aspects and help the patient more freely to associate his own experiences in relation to what he has observed on the ward. He learns, also, that his aggressiveness and destructiveness are closely connected with specific difficulties in adaptation, and as a result, his behavior becomes more socialized.

He learns, furthermore, that when the ward discipline forces him into restrictions, these restrictions are socially necessary. In addition, he learns tolerance towards the problems and difficulties of others and understands that many of his aggressive, antisocial impulses are merely a screen behind which he tries to hide his social and sexual shortcomings from himself and others.

The organization of group activities is not merely for solving educational problems and for occupying patients to keep them out of mischief. The real purpose is an attempt to give each child a better understanding of his own problems and, finally, to produce a therapy which reveals to the child his individual difficulties, and finally to make possible for him some form of social adaptation. In the long run the child will become more tolerant towards his own weakness and shortcomings and will give up the asocial behavior, which so often is merely an attempt to escape deep feelings of insecurity and guilt. The problems revealed (and, in some cases, solved) in this way include not only the spheres of activity, passivity, aggression, and submission, but also the sphere of sex. The problems of masculinity and femininity are of fundamental importance to all these children. The whole structure of ideas and ideologies has to be investigated, and the deeper roots of these systems of wrong adaptations have to be eradicated so that a new social orientation of the individual becomes possible.

GROUP TREATMENT [11]

Group treatment plays an important part in religious movements as far as they give relief to the psychological phenomenon of suffering. The members of a church identify themselves with each other. They are also united by a common goal and by a common belief, of which the priest or minister is the exponent. The Oxford movement (Buchmanism) puts particular emphasis on the public confession. It is not our task to discuss the ideology of the Oxford movement. I merely want to emphasize the importance of the public confession. It remains rather impersonal. The principle of guidance and guided experience, although containing a symbolic nucleus, is further psychologically valid. The emphasis on discipline and destiny turns the attention to important parts of the social reality. One may object that the vagueness of the general principle does not increase insight sufficiently.

In the narrower sphere of medical therapy, group treatments have been used repeatedly. Wetterstrand was able to produce a deep hypnosis in an unusually high percentage of patients by hypnotizing them in groups. I have used this principle repeatedly with great success. Wetterstrand used his method merely in connection with the direct suggestion concerning the symptom. There is no reason why one could not use this kind of hypnotic state for a more individual type of psychotherapy. Cody Marsh gives systematic lectures, to groups of selected hospital patients, in which the fundamental problems of human life are discussed. The method may be useful if followed by a free discussion and "confession" of the participants. Otherwise, its results are liable to remain on the surface. Greene has worked out a method for the treatment of stammerers in which the stammerer is performing before a group, so that everybody participates in the fate of others.

[11] The following are pertinent references from the large amount of literature on group therapy for the past few years: Giles W. Thomas, "Group Psychotherapy; A Review of Recent Literature," *Psychosomatic Medicine* 5:166, 1943; S. R. Slavson, *The Practice of Group Therapy* (The International Universities Press, Inc., 1950); S. H. Foulkes, *Introduction to Group Analytic Psychotherapy* (Grune and Stratton, 1949). [L.B., Ed.]

Trigant Burrow seemingly has done group psychoanalysis; the patient and the analyst live in one community and analyze each other. It seems almost impossible that a reliable technique could be worked out in this way. At any rate, it is not published. L. Wender has used group treatment based upon analytic principles. I have followed a similar technique, which will be described in detail in a later chapter of this book. Simon has induced the patients of a state hospital in Germany to do work in groups. Almost all chronic cases could be made to participate in the group work, which partly served the hospital and partly was work in the field and garden. The result was beneficial even for the deteriorated patient, who was taken out of his isolation with its asocial consequences. Even some of the acute cases can benefit by this work therapy. This is a more methodic use of principles which had been utilized in progressive state hospital systems before (cf. Wertham).

One sees that modern psychotherapy has a great number of technical tools at hand. But one should not forget that no technical tool is of any use unless one knows what to use it for. If one does psychotherapy, one needs more than technical tools. The man who does psychotherapy must have a plan and a system of co-ordinates with which he brings the experiences of himself and of his patients into relation. Furthermore, the discussion so far has not touched the fundamental problem of psychotherapy, the relation between physician and patient. This is a definite variety of human and social relations. It has to be studied in detail.

Chapter 7

THE RELATION BETWEEN PHYSICIAN AND PATIENT

THE DISCOVERY of transference is one of the most consequential made in the history of psychotherapy. Freud found in 1901, when analyzing Dora, that the patient had transferred her attitudes towards her infantile love objects to the physician. The physician had taken the place of father and mother and also the place of the actual love object. The emotions had been transferred to him. These emotions were the emotions of love, in its full sense, and of hate. We speak of positive and negative transference. He discovered further that the transference develops in psychoanalysis without any display on the part of the physician. The emotions liberated by the psychoanalytic process of free association have to find an object and take the object at hand, the analyst. If the analyst remains passive, does not display his own opinions and personality, the more apt he will be to receive transference.

It is obvious that the transference cannot be merely a positive transference. Most of the patients have been afraid to acknowledge the hostile tendencies towards those whom they love. They have been repressed and have not lost anything of their infantile energy. A psychotherapy in which these negative transferences do not make their appearance is superficial, and analysis in which negative transference does not appear is a failure.

The symptomatology of transference has to be studied. It is obvious that the patient has some choice concerning his physician. He has heard about him. He may have had a friend or relative who has been successfully treated. He comes to the treatment with the definite expectation that something will be done for him. He expects help and relief from his suffering. The situation is only different in children, psychotics, criminals, and psychopaths, i. e., in all those who come to the physician not so much because they suffer themselves, but because they make others suffer. When the patient pays, he obviously sacrifices something for the physician and for the help he expects to receive from him. Material of this kind is, of course, not fully conscious to the patient.

The patient also has from the very beginning a distrust of the physician. He may doubt his professional qualification. He is furthermore afraid that the physician may not have any real interest (love) for him, may have problems of his own, and finally may be more interested in the money he receives than in the patient and his cure. If the patient does not pay, he is still more suspicious. The physician, not compensated, may not make any real effort. The patient also resents it when he suspects that the physician is scientifically interested in him. The ideology of the patient, hidden from himself, is that the physician should not have any other interest than helping him. He demands the unconditional love which the child expects from its parents.

It is obvious that the mere fact that the patient talks to the physician and that the physician does not criticize him has to increase the positive transference. The physician participates now in all the experiences of the patient. When the patient confides, he gives confidence. One may therefore reckon with an increase in the positive transference in the analytic procedure. This will appear in little remarks of the patient. He will come a few minutes before the time he is expected, and finally there will be either associations or dreams in which there is a partial identity or similarity between the analyst and the one or the other of the important love objects of the present situation or of the childhood. The patient may remark that the voice of the analyst reminds him of the voice of the father or of the mother or that the picture in his room is similar to a picture which was owned by the family and which the patient likes.

At this time the associations very often start to flow freer; there will be dreams which disclose important elements of the childhood. The patient will acquiesce with any interpretation given by the analyst. He will praise the skill and the qualities of the analyst to his friends, and there will be a relief or maybe even a disappearance of the symptoms. Very often dreams occur in which the analyst visits the house of the patient as his guest, and the associations of the patient center around the idea of how nice it would be to have personal contact with the analyst.

Sexual phantasies follow. They may occur more easily when the analyst and the patient belong to different sexes. The patient very often keeps these sexual phantasies to himself. Occupied with them and keeping them back, the flow of associations may stop or the associations may become superficial, as mentioned above. Pretty soon the patient will suffer by the positive transference, he will feel again that the physician has no personal interest in him, remains cool and impersonal, is interested merely in the money, and the way is paved for negative transference.

The interpretation of the positive transference situation should not be given too early. The patient will very soon find out about it himself. It is also important that the interpretation of any transference situation should not be given merely as a hint to the relation between physician and patient and that the patient should be made to understand the transference situation in relation to the context of his life and to his attitudes concerning other love objects. It is obvious that the physician very often takes the place of homosexual as well as heterosexual love objects. He substitutes for father and mother. He substitutes, further, for persons important to the patient in his present situation. It is a general rule of interpretation that one should not discuss infantile material with the patient before he has come very close to this discovery himself. In the first stage of psychoanalysis, material of the present will generally prevail, unless the patient has knowledge of psychoanalytic principles, which he uses then very often as a resistance and as a protection against any real free associations.

When the negative transference appears, the patient hides it still more carefully. His associations may become tardy, his dreams scarce, he may come late to the analytic hour, may complain about the office of the physician, about the noise or the ventilation. The symptoms may reappear. He may not accept the interpretations of the physician, may discover logical flaws; thoughts that he has chosen the wrong physician may pop up. Finally, there will be the one or the other distinctly hostile dream or association, either expressed openly or veiled.

It is advisable not to wait too long with the interpretation of negative transference; this is quite in contrast to what has been discussed concerning the positive transference. Even when the interpretation of the negative transference has been given, the outbreaks of hostility do not stop. It will very soon be possible to find out towards whom the hostility is directed. It may be an object either of the present or of the childhood. The hostility will be the stronger the more the infantile material comes into appearance. The hostility will extend from the analyst to his office and the persons who help him in the office or the persons whom the patient suspects of being the relatives of the analyst. One of my patients, for instance, meeting the mother of the analyst on the staircase and recognizing her by her similarity, remarked that the analyst and his mother have the same vulture-like faces. He may develop phantasies of seducing the analyst's wife or, more modestly, the analyst's servant or secretary, or he may wonder that the analyst is not afraid that the patient might hurt or kill him. If the negative transference is properly recognized and interpreted, the patient continues with the analysis and the negative transference is very soon followed by a positive phase again. Positive and negative transference may follow each other repeatedly in the course of an analysis. We expect that the analyst in turn will play the part of any important love object in the patient's life, in the positive aspect as well as in the negative aspect. Furthermore, the analysis repeats and exhausts all the stages of development which the patient went through. At one stage of the analysis the analyst may play the part of the father when the patient was five, and at a subsequent stage the part of the father when the patient was three or four. He plays, furthermore, the parts of the mother, sisters, brothers, nurses, etc.

The negative transference may come out in the beginning of analysis very strongly. I have seen this especially in obsession neurotic cases. In one case the patient, who came in for treatment because of severe inhibitions, had had a very unsuccessful love affair with an analyst and her hatred repressed in this relation poured out in the very beginning of the transference situation.

Progress with the analysis goes hand in hand with a deeper understanding of the changing transference situation. It seems that the infantile situation remains pale unless it drinks some blood in the present situation, and only in the transference situation does the past come fully into life. We may justly speak about two stages in the analytic situation: the winning of the transference and the working through of the transference. I venture to say that positive transference remains the basic note in analysis, even when the negative transference seems to be most violent. Towards the end of the analysis the problem arises how to finish the relation and to break the transference. The patient has to understand that he cannot keep the analyst forever and that the analyst must be finally substituted for by love objects in real life, who are able to give full satisfaction. He has to understand that the analyst is a symbol not merely for the past but also for the future.

The analyst is not allowed to try to keep the transference of the patient for himself. He has to point, by interpretation, to the necessity of finding new love objects. Very often the patient projects, towards the end of the analysis, his problem onto the analyst and uses the analyst as a pattern of how to overcome one's own difficulties. Associations very often liken the process of ending the analysis with the process of leaving the maternal womb. Rank has especially emphasized the maternal role of the analyst towards the end of the analysis and has, furthermore, stressed that symbols of rebirth come into the foreground at the end of the analysis. He has also tried to shorten the process of analysis by giving to the patient a term of about six weeks, after which the analysis would come to an end. This method, sometimes helpful, is in a great number of cases unsuccessful and one has to continue the analysis after the term set for its end, which is not very desirable.

The difficulties in finishing the analysis are sometimes very great. Towards the end of the analysis patients very often produce all the symptoms of their neurosis again, in order to force the analyst to continue the analysis. Even when the analysis is finished blandly and the patient has been discharged as completely analyzed, the patient may soon react with an outburst of rage against the analyst who has deserted him, may have a recurrence of his symptoms, and demand a continuation. I have seen this in a patient who had been discharged after the analysis had lasted for three years.

This is a fairly accurate description of Freud's view of the transference situation. One should not forget that the analyst is not only a representative of the infantile love objects in sexual respects. He represents them in their social aspects. Furthermore, in his supposed adaptation to reality he represents society in general. He thus becomes the mediator between the demands of the reality and the libidinous demands of the patient. He takes the place of a more appropriate and adaptable superego and ego.

It is not to be doubted that this description is fundamentally correct. During the process of working through the transference situation the individual comes to an increased insight into his own problems and, in connection with it, to a better insight into the structure of human situations.

The process of transference is not confined to the analytic situation; it is characteristic of the relation between patient and physician. Every psychotherapeutic approach has, accordingly, three stages: (1) winning the transference; (2) working through and using the transference; and (3) breaking the transference. The transference can be used to educate the patient or to make him accessible for direct therapeutic suggestion. We insist at the present time, especially, that the transference should be used to help the patient to a better insight by the various methods discussed above. The patient should be enabled in this way to give up his symptoms. Breaking of the transference should enable the patient to approach the problems of real life in an independent manner.

A psychotherapy in which the transference keeps too much of the energies of the patient bound to the physician cannot be considered as completely successful, even when the patient is free from other symptoms. One will generally be able to break off the transference unless one deals with patients who are not capable of full adaptation, and it is better to keep those emotionally bound to the physician. This is particularly true about schizophrenic patients, who may be protected against the recurrence of symptoms merely by the love which binds them to the physician.

By hypnosis we very quickly get a very deep transference based upon the boundless admiration of the child which ascribes magic powers to its parents. One should be aware that the physician has to use this transference for a better adaptation of the patient, preferably on the basis of an increased insight in the middle period, and must carefully assure the patient that his dependence on the physician can only be temporary. The breaking of the transference does not then offer any serious difficulties. On the average, it is easier to end a hypnotic treatment than a psychoanalytic treatment.

In short, in psychotherapy of any kind the same problems arise. If the brief psychotherapy is not merely of a suggestive or advisory type, material will be worked through which gives the patient a greater insight, but it will mostly be impossible to come to an understanding of the transference situation as such. Psychoanalysis is the only method which analyzes the transference situation as such.

When a physician treats a patient for a somatic disease, the three stages discussed will also make their appearance. The physician is only able to approach the patient when the patient has given him a sufficient amount of confidence. The middle period is substituted by the physical procedures the physician employs, which have the purpose of adapting the patient's body to regular functioning. Towards the end of the treatment the patient gives up the physician, sometimes rather incompletely; sometimes there are even strong reminders of negative transference for which the actual behavior of the physician may not offer sufficient explanation.

It is not the choice of the physician whether he wants the transference or not. The transference comes regardless. He has merely the choice whether he wants to understand and analyze the transference situation or not. The whole problem of transference is still, in spite of the pioneer work of psychoanalysis, incompletely understood. We do not know in which way the individuality of the physician influences the transference situation, even if he is as passive as classical analysis demands him to be. The sex of the analyst plays a more important part than one would suspect when one studies psychoanalytic literature. The transference demands and the transference resistances of the patient are more urgent and more openly genital when the analyst is of a different sex than the patient, at least in heterosexuals. It is well to be aware of this fact and to take it into consideration in the interpretation and in the handling of the transference.

In the psychoanalytic situation the analyst has to show the attitude of the passionless observer. He is not allowed to show more than a moderate degree of interest. He is not supposed to display any deeper interest, and he should not be moved by either positive or negative transference. If he has feelings and emotions of his own concerning the patient, he should keep them to himself. There is no question that this dispassionate attitude of the analyst puts the patient in an inferior position, which he naturally resents. He blames the analyst, not quite without reason, as being inhuman and ruthless. The weapons of the analyst are silence and interpretation. The weapons of the patient are revolt, hate, reproaches against the inefficiency of the analyst and the incorrectness of his interpretations, and, finally, the persistence or reappearance of the symptom. The situation of the analyst can only be understood after we have discussed the counter-transference. At any rate, the relation between analyst and patient is full of human dangers, even for the analyst who maintains the correct analytic attitude throughout the whole course of treatment.

Individual psychology ascribes to the physician another role. The physician helps the patient to understand his attitude towards the problem of the outside world. He is merely an older and wiser brother who knows more about the goals and aims which are worth while and how to reach them. The physician thus becomes a guide and mentor who stresses the necessity of seeing the useful side of life. He explains to the patient that he has to fulfill his duties towards the community, towards his friends, and towards his love objects, and he shows the patient how and why he has shunned his responsibilities and gone to the useless side of life. It ends in some way in common sense. It is difficult for the physician using this method not to become too didactic. It is more a process of education. American psychotherapy, and especially the psychobiologic approach of Adolf Meyer, has a very close inner relation to the approach of Adler, without acknowledging it fully. It seems that Adler's approach, in comparison with Meyer's, is more ruthless towards the patient and forces him more to confess his mistakes. But the older-brother attitude, the common sense, the stress of the necessity of social action, and the direction are common to both, although more precisely formulated in Adler's approach.

In Jung's approach the therapist becomes a half-mystical leader to the secrets of the archetypes and to the hidden creative forces of the collective unconscious and mankind. He is really a psychagogue. It is not by chance that one of the pupils of Jung gives one of her books the title *The Secrets of Women.* It must be hard for the physician to keep up such a role, and Jung justly warns against the inflation of the ego of the analyst. From personal reports I get the impression that the community spirit carefully cultivated plays an important part in the circle of Jung. In the older methods of psychotherapy the physician took the role of the father who makes demands or punishes.

One cannot deny that every one of these attitudes has in itself great difficulties, and the man who does psychotherapy may come into serious danger in any one of these roles. He may overrate his power to help, and the power of kindness; he may overrate the validity of his advice and his intellectual insight; he may assume a too superior role, by which the analyst is particularly threatened since he provokes the deepest reaction in his patients. The problem of countertransference arises. It is a general principle of social psychology that an emotion of a person with whom we are in contact must necessarily provoke an emotion in the other person fitting the situation. We may suspect, for instance, that the passivity, the helplessness, the masochistic attitude of the patient who is hypnotized provoke aggressive attitudes mixed with sexuality in the hypnotizer. He may easily also feel in possession of magic power. If he feels so, he will not be able to keep a full grasp of the situation and will not see the limits of his powers. The positive transference of the analytic patient is liable to provoke an erotic countertransference which will not help the physician in the handling of the situation. He may answer the hostility of the patient with counteraggression, which will come out in the way he interprets. Overrating the patient's need for his help and wanting to keep the patient dependent upon him, he will prolong the analysis unnecessarily. Accustomed to play the superior role, he may overrate himself considerably. He is, furthermore, under particular stress, in so far as he refrains from expressing any of his emotions to the patient. The analytic situation thus becomes fraught with ambiguities, and the openness of the patient is not answered by the physician. To be conscious of these dangers diminishes them but does not eliminate them completely. The psychotherapeutic situation, especially in analysis, is not fully satisfactory from a human point of view.

The physician who by the particular method he chooses is able to express himself more freely is psychologically in a better situation. But he is in some danger of overrating his ideologies, of coming forward too much with his own opinions, and of impressing on the patient a style of life for which the patient is not fit. It is the important task of the physician to develop the patient's personality according to the capacities, endowments, and characteristics of the patient. He will be better able to do so if he has the conviction that the other human being is an entity of its own and is valuable in so far as it is a definite person. Every psychotherapist is in danger of forgetting this and of making out of the patient a mirror image of himself.

Very often perfectionistic ideals will make the physician demand tasks from the patient which he is not able to perform. Human beings have different degrees of adaptability. Not every individual is capable of reaching an adaptation on a high level. We should be modest in our demands of the patient. The analyst, although supposedly passive, is continuously exerting pressure in a specific direction and very often makes remarks which are only justifiable from his personal point of view. I quote here the remarks of an analyst concerning friendship as they were understood by the patient, who was a long time in analysis with him. It may be that the remarks were not made in this way, but they were understood in this way.

"The concept of friendship is exaggerated in our society. It is romantic but it often leads to trouble. You have seen it; two men are friends then the one gets married, the other one is unhappy, he hates the wife. The wife sees it and makes it tough for him. Friendship! Bah! When I was ill my nonanalytic friends sent me candies, called every day in great anxiety, etc. My analytic friends phoned once a week to see how I was and that was all." The suggestion was very definite that their interest in him was not very great. It is at least questionable whether this particular view concerning friendship should have a general application.

The psychotherapeutic relation is, therefore, not only difficult for the patient, whatever method the physician may choose. When the physician keeps the principle in mind that he has to respect the personality of his patient, he will not err too much. He has, furthermore, to keep in mind the specific social reality in which his patient lives. He should be further aware of the necessary limitation in his own point of view and should have, at the same time, a concept of his goals in life and the concept of the goals in life of the patient. The basic attitude in psychotherapy is that there is one human being who needs help and another human being who wants to give help. The attitude of the physician is the attitude of helpfulness and understanding. His aim is to relieve the patient from his suffering, and his conviction is that this aim can be reached by a better adaptation to the inward and outward reality, preferably by an increase in insight.

It is necessary that the physician experience many other strivings and tendencies closely following the primitive strivings and tendencies displayed by his patient. He lives his own social life. He has to have an interest in his professional skill, in increasing his knowledge, and in making a living by what he is doing. He cannot remain unmoved by the erotic tendencies the patient displays towards him. He may answer to the sexual wishes of the patient with infantile attitudes—for instance, the wish for absolute authority concerning his patient. He may indeed want to play the role of the father and mother assigned to him by the patient. He may feel inclined to answer the aggression of the patient by counteraggression. He may further want to experience, by identification, gratifications which the patient may get. He may further be narcissistic in relation to the patient and overrate his capacities in comparison with him. No therapeutic system protects completely against this danger.

Psychoanalysis has preached for a long time that the physician should be indifferent to his patient and display this indifference to the patient. However, I have heard analysts justly say that there are occasions in which the analyst has to show compassion and sympathy. This has found a rather exaggerated expression in the last attempts of Ferenczi, who postulated that one should give love to the patient and even not refrain from moderate caresses. This opinion has been rejected by Freud, but we may formulate the principle by saying: Be human and respect the personality of the patient as much as possible.

It is, furthermore, an important question, what to do with the religious, moral, and social convictions of a patient who is in psychotherapy. It is obvious that some of these convictions are more or less closely connected with his suffering. What we can do is to bring the patient merely to an insight into this connection and let him decide what he wants to do about it. There will also be in the analyzed person the possibility of adhering to religious and moral standards in which the analyst does not believe. The great religious systems as well as even strict moral systems, if rightly understood, leave room for an adaptation to reality which should be sufficient for everyone. I have professed my skepticism concerning advice given to the patient without having sufficient insight into the problems of the patient. If the patient gains sufficient insight he will mostly find his way himself.

The advice to marry, to divorce, or to have extramarital relations has to be considered from this point of view. In cases of impotency we very often have to insist upon an attempt at sex relations even with "love objects" for whom the patient does not and cannot care, but such advice or order can be given only if the style of life of the patient goes in this direction. The advice becomes, then, an immediate therapeutic measure. Whenever any advice is given or whenever the patient comes on the basis of his experiences to a decision, he should know all the facts. He should know, for instance, the dangers of extramarital relations. He should also know that marriage is a task which can only be undertaken on the basis of the full appreciation of the other person.

Psychoanalysis demands that the analyst should be analyzed himself. This is a comparatively easy way to become informed about the psychoanalytic technique and to receive insight into one's own problems. It cannot substitute for clinical experience, study, and respect for other human beings. Since Freud himself has not been analyzed and since many of his followers who have contributed largely to the progress of analysis, and as I have convinced myself are competent analysts, have not been analyzed, I cannot consider his own analysis as an indispensable requisite for the psychotherapist or even for the analyst. I have not myself been analyzed. The danger of the analysis of the therapist lies in the possibility that he may become too much imbued with the principles and the technique of the man who analyzes him. An all too rigid technique may be handed down from one analyst to the next generation, and a standardization of the technique may result which may be good neither for the physician nor for the progress of psychotherapy. At the present time the average duration of a so-called didactic analysis is between one and two years. The pupil is expected to gain, besides the knowledge of his own complexes, a deep conviction in the correctness of the analytic doctrines. Such a procedure, serving the preservation of the tradition, may serve as well the preservation of errors if not handled with inner freedom by the man who does the didactic analysis. At any rate, a didactic analysis does not protect the therapist from being led astray by his own emotional needs and prejudices. For one "blind spot" in human problems it may substitute other ones.

The problem of countertransference is one of the basic problems of psychotherapy. The psychoanalytic literature is not rich in investigations devoted to this point. It is more often considered in private discussions.

The therapeutic situation necessarily gives the physician the position of superiority. He may be clad with the attitude of the magic father, the father, the older brother, or mother, or sister. One should keep in mind that this superiority pertains only to the specific situation. If the therapist considers the patient as a fellow human being equal to himself he will be able to avoid many mistakes. Human relations are based upon the principle of mutual help. In our innermost feelings we are convinced that we have a deep interest that the other human being should exist and should exist free from suffering. The true relation between patient and physician rests upon this principle. If the patient stays with the physician and if, as I have stated, the positive transference is prevalent throughout the course of a psychotherapy, it is due to unconscious insight of the patient into this fundamental human relation.

In the analytic and psychotherapeutic situation, the patient sees in the physician all the persons who have been of importance in the psychosexual and social development of the child.[1] All these emotional attitudes are transferred to the physician. The social process, more or less crystallized before, becomes more fluid, loses its rigidity, and reveals its meaning in a clearer way. However, the psychoanalytical situation is a more or less artificial one. Two individuals are closeted with each other, and the analyst by the mere fact of his silence becomes more or less a mythical factor. However in the psychoanalytical situation we observe a real group foundation. It is a complicated social and psychosexual situation between two human beings. The objective situation puts the analyst into the situation of authority and gives him an enormous social preponderance. He furthermore demands financial sacrifices from the individual. Predominantly the patient feels that his life is at the mercy of the analyst. The analytic situation, therefore, will in its immediate functioning show the forces of authority and dependence at work. It is true, a rivalry will make its appearance too, although in a more shadowy way.

From a purely theoretical point of view it would seem advisable to change the set-up in order to see the problems appearing in the psychoanalytic situation from a new angle. It would be, at any rate, interesting to see a group which is less restricted than the psychoanalytic unit in its making. Groups are, of course, fundamental in education. Group leadership is in many situations delegated from the teacher or leader of the group to individual members of the group. The value of such groups and of group education has been stressed

[1] From Paul Schilder, "Introductory Remarks on the Group," *Journal of Social Psychology* 12:83–100, 1940.

by S. R. Slavson. However, it is difficult to come to a deeper insight into the psychological structure of such a group. The spontaneous remarks during the process of group activity may be enlightening. This is a hit-and-miss procedure from the point of view of deeper insight into the structure of the group, even when the group is not organized for the specific purpose of occupation, information, and amusement. It may be valuable to observe groups in action as Tarde, Le Bon, and Trotter have done. One would like better to hear from an individual who participates in the group what he experiences while he is in the group and would prefer the insight into such an immediate reaction to an analysis of his experiences after he had left the group. In this relation our interest in group activities as such is limited. We are chiefly interested in group activities which not only liberate the social forces in connection with group life but bring them also to clearer expression. One might gain considerable insight from studying mass movements, like the movement of Father Divine, especially when one analyzes the individual follower.[2] However, it would be more interesting if one could study the group in formation and action. Spontaneous social groupings do not give this opportunity. Such an opportunity is only given if one does psychotherapy for groups of neurotic and psychopathic patients. One could proceed in such a way in the wards of psychopathic hospitals where the patients are placed more or less against their will.

The hospital and its representative, the physician, not only are authorities but impose their will on the reluctant individual. In such a situation, authority becomes hostile authority, and the preliminary process of getting the interest and attention of the patient will be necessary. I do think that this winning-over process on such wards takes place more easily when the individual patient is seen not only in an individual interview but as a member of the group which has been collected by chance and force. The fear of the hostility of authority will be of paramount importance in such a situation. It will be lessened when the other members of the group are present. At the same time, the other members of the group might realize that there is no hostility directed against the other members of the group, and they might finally be reassured concerning themselves. The physician

[2] See L. Bender and Z. Yarrell, "Psychoses among Followers of Father Divine," *Journal of Nervous & Mental Disease* 27:418–49, 1938. [L.B., Ed.]

and his staff and the patients might finally become a rather closely knit group after the hostility is allayed. Individuals are afraid of the hostility of others and do not dare to show their sympathy before they have given up their apprehensions. In hospital groups, group activities of all kinds may help in answering the fear of the group concerning the physician and also concerning the other members of the group. This will be particularly important for schizophrenic patients in whom distrust and fear play such an outstanding part.

One should never forget that the winning-over process and the socialization in the group are only a small part of the psychotherapeutic task. The psychotherapeutic task demands that the individual should gain insight into his social and psychosexual adaptation and into the premature solutions which he built up in his childhood. These premature crystallizations are obstacles to an adaptation which considers not only the early situation but also the situation and the social reality of the present. Only when the individual dives down into his personal experiences or brings them forward in the group does the crystallized individual development come into a flux again which allows a new adaptation to the situation. In other words, during the process of group treatment the individual should bring forward his individual experiences for the group and so help everybody else to bring forward similar experiences. This process is the more important since human experiences in their deeper layers are very similar to each other. The fundamental pattern of human experience is determined by the psychophysiological structures and the social conditions of a given society. To understand another individual completely means also to have a deep insight into one's own problems, although there are many psychological obstacles which hinder the transfer of insight from another individual to oneself. However, the probability of such a transfer is increased when there is a group situation which tends to lower the barriers between single individuals. Group activities which allow a free expression of one's individual problems and which make it possible for the individual to elaborate later on the expression of the problems which have been mobilized in the group are therefore of particular value. Such a procedure is, for instance, followed by L. Bender and A. G. Woltmann in their use of puppet shows, which allow emotional expression during the puppet show, which is continued in a group discussion following the presentation of the show.

The individual interview may be necessary in order to bring other material, since groups and societies contain small units and the connection between two individuals is one of the fundamental experiences of social life. Such a one-and-one connection may be a connection of a quality of superiority and inferiority in its varied aspects from a social point of view, or it may be a more or less outspoken relation in which problems of equality and inequality are again of paramount importance. Similar expression has been sought in the dramatic activities of the adolescent ward as worked out by F. J. Curran. Moreno advocates the impromptu theater as a method of expression. Whatever the specific mode of expression may be, the final value of a group psychotherapeutic method is dependent upon the degree of sociological and psychological insight upon which it is based. It will increase this insight when it is used not as a rigid scheme but as a social experiment which by trial and error leads to better adaptation. There are countless possibilities of variations. Under specific circumstances, as in Trigant Burrow's group, the role of the leader may not be fixed. The analyst of the one situation may become psychoanalyzed in the next situation. The group connection might not be a passing one as in most of the psychotherapeutic situations but a lifetime association. This is obviously one extreme form of the principles discussed here, and it will have to face the test of its social usefulness outside of very special circumstances.

Group psychotherapy in this sense does not intend to give an insight which is of symbolic character. It appreciates that the symbolic confessions in the group provided by the Oxford Group may be of importance. However, a symbolic confession which does not go back to concrete situations of one's individual life has only a preliminary value. It will not always be possible to give the final solution to a symbol; however, this should be the intention. Public religious confession is inclined to take the symbol as a final solution. As stated, group psychotherapeutic methods can be used on psychopathic wards. Their use is not confined to them. Individuals suffering from somatic ailments which force them into a hospital for a short or long time are under very similar conditions. Attempts at group psychotherapy of cases with somatic ailments have been made. Irrespective of the questions of how far psychological methods can influence organic processes and which the curative effect of group psychotherapy may be, hospital groups as groups need psychotherapeutic assistance. Such an assistance should be organized. Human beings thrown together by the chance factors of medical classification form a group just as well as children thrown together by the chance factor of age and vicinity. Moreno has given a preliminary scheme for the dynamic forces of the attraction between the single members of the group, which should be supplemented by a deeper analysis of the relation of individuals to each other on the basis of a deep knowledge of their individual history. Moreno has called his approach sociometry.

In out-patient departments groups can be formed of those who seek psychotherapeutic help. I have conducted such group psychotherapy for several years. In such a group, the physician necessarily plays the part of the leader. He conducts the group and assumes a role of superiority. However, his purpose is obviously not to be superior to his patients, but he strives towards the aim of giving to the patients a sufficient insight into their history so that they should be able to give up the wrong adaptations they have built up in their individual development. He assumes the superiority merely in order to help. However, besides this conscious motivation, he is obviously bound to the aims of his social setting. He gains satisfaction by increasing his scientific insight. He is curious about the lives of his patients as everybody else. He wants to participate in other human lives. He wants to enjoy his superiority. Furthermore, he continually measures his own life by the lives of his patients. As a human being, his interest cannot merely be a social one. He has to live out his homosexual and heterosexual desires on his patients although he lives also in a well-defined social reality with aims, purposes, and gratifications. He lives in different psychosexual and social levels and has to change continually from one level to the other. He expects and receives the gratification, admiration, and sexual desire from his patients, but he is also the target of their hatred and criticism, to which he is only allowed to answer in his own mind and which he has to recognize as symbolic expressions of experiences in early childhood which have to be integrated into the total social situation, which is dependent upon the social structure. His success in conducting this psychotherapy will be largely dependent upon his ability to understand his own tendency to incomplete experiences in infantile symbolizations. In his relation to patients he will play the role of the father, mother, and sibling, but he will also play the role of the teacher, spiritual guide, and social leader. The complexity of social realities will appear in his situation. He will finally be not merely the leader of the group but also a member of the group and will also be the connecting link between this group and established social groups.

It is easier to describe what is going on in the members of the group since they have the right and duty to free expression, which is denied by this particular situation to the analyst. I do think that he should express himself as freely as possible, but the social situation makes it inadvisable to reveal his complete individual history. A patient coming into the group will experience reticence at sharing his experiences with others. However, he is deeply interested in the fate of others as far as it seems to give him a clue to the understanding of his own experiences. At the same time he experiences a keen rivalry when the other takes too much of the time and seemingly of the interest of the analyst, whose undivided attention and love he craves. The other individual's experience is primarily a help for his own purpose. Later an interest in the other person as a person may develop. The seriousness of difficulties of others is almost continually underrated. His own difficulty looms as all-important. Only occasionally a human interest develops which leads to more or less loose contacts outside of the hospital. It is astonishing that most of the patients overcome an initial hesitation of talking in the presence of others very easily. Outbursts of open hostilities in the group against other participants are rare. Occasionally one patient demands that the analyst should be less patient with other patients. On the whole, the attitude of the single patient in the group is definite. He has come with the special purpose of being cured. His interest is chiefly directed towards the leader of the group, who is expected to help him. As far as the others try to gain the attention of the analyst they are his rivals. As far as he sees his own experiences in them they help him in the understanding of his own problems and relieve especially his guilt feelings. He follows the progress of their cure with interest, and if a patient is a long time in treatment he uses this fact as a method of expressing his doubts concerning the analyst and the treatment. Only with the deeper progress of the treatment does the patient gain a deeper understanding of the similarity of his problems and the problems of the other patients. Generally the other patient is considered merely as a colorless exponent of society whose tolerance is appreciated and returned.

There is no question that the relation of the patient towards the analyst who conducts the group is a much more intensive one. The analyst takes all the roles he plays in the individual analysis, and in successive order he plays the role of the father, the mother, the brothers and sisters, and of all the persons who were of any importance in the childhood development. The physician appears as the love object, and the positive transference finds almost always an open expression, and it is particularly astonishing how open the expression of hate can be. The complaint that the analyst does not give enough attention, that he is heartless and experiments, comes in a great number of instances. It can be easily shown that these complaints are dependent upon the parental situation in childhood. Often the attitude of hate expressed by one patient finds a sympathetic response from other patients. Very often there is also a defense of the physician by other patients. Often the patients project their own problems into the physician and have the feeling that he must have gone through them, and finally identify themselves with the physician as the man who has solved problems identical to theirs. At the same time, the physician is the link to social reality. He is supposed to know, to advise. In the specific situation tested, the analyst is also considered as a member of a higher economic stratum.

However, this latter point comes only rarely to discussion. The patients are more concerned with the human side of the problem and the human side of social problems than with the economic and political side. Only rarely does the one or the other patient use the group for expounding political and economic views, especially communistic ones. It is obvious that any intellectual and crystallized pattern does not fit into the specific purpose of the group. The specific situation makes it often necessary that the physician help the patients in the social problem of employment and public aid. However, the problems of work and adaptation primarily appear from the point of view of the adaptation of the individual. Occasionally the analyst has been helped in the group by other physicians present although their activity consisted chiefly in helping to protocol. The patients considered them mostly as friendly helpers, and did not resent it when occasionally other physicians took an active part in the analysis.

It would be easy to express the problems involved from the point of view of psychosexual development. The problem between the patients and the problem between patient and physician are, of course, psychosexual problems. It is possible to trace them back to definite situations in early childhood. The attitudes in the group reflect the attitudes of individual life history. One can also study in such a group the social factors which go into the formation of a group. Not only has one the chance to see how the group is built up, but owing to the analytic process, one can see the social forces at work.

One has to recognize that there is a definite purpose which binds the group together. This is a purpose in which the analyst plays the leading part. Furthermore, because of the specific circumstances, the connection between the leader of the group and single members of the group is particularly strong, whereas the bond between the members of the group is otherwise comparatively weak. The analyst represents father and mother, and the importance of the family tie, the relation to both parents, becomes apparent. The group, furthermore, allows a free expression without the fear of dangerous hostility of any participant of the group. It becomes again apparent that it is one of the definite functions of the group to neutralize hostilities and so give opportunity to the possibility of a human contact of curiosity. The rivalries are put into a definite form which is not dangerous any more. Furthermore, it does not appear that any individual is merely fulfilling a cultural pattern. He is nowhere a slave of the collective or objective spirit. Guilt, anxiety, despondency, and helplessness remain individual problems which can be brought nearer to an individual solution when they are freely discussed in the group.

It seems advisable to study groups in formation, and group psychotherapy makes such a study possible. In such a group all the forces will appear which are important in the structure of society.

[Dr. Pauline Rosenthal participated in the group psychotherapy sessions conducted by Dr. Schilder for many consecutive sessions before his death. It thus devolved upon her to adjust these abandoned patients to the death of the father figure, "a task beyond the means at her disposal." The productions of twenty-seven patients under her care, including dreams and associative material, were recorded by her for the light they might throw on the role of the leader in the group.—L.B., Ed.]

Recent experimentation with group therapies has brought into the foreground the pioneer work of Dr. Paul Schilder.[3] For a number of years, up to his death in December 1940, Dr. Schilder treated groups of psychoneurotics, many of borderline or outspoken psychoses, by group psycho-

[3] From Pauline Rosenthal, "The Death of the Leader in Group Psychotherapy," *American Journal of Orthopsychiatry* 17:266–77, 1947.

therapy, in the out-patient department of Bellevue Psychiatric Hospital. Schilder has fully described his own methods, and has explicitly stated his point of view regarding the role of the leader.

Schilder set a higher value upon the "different" and the variants than is usually the case. It was his conviction that one could best gain insight into the forces which determine group living and underlie social movements of all kinds by studying the psychoneurotic in the process of acting out his individual and social conflicts in immediate and direct relation to the group under observation. He believed that neither hereditary, constitutional, nor familial factors comprise the whole story of human development, but that social-environmental factors play an equally determinant role. Therefore, since social factors play a role in the genesis of the psychoneuroses, they could also play a determinant role in their correction. Furthermore, social and sexual adaptation being understood as equivalents, access to the problem of psychosexual development would also open the door to the problem of social development. The group situation, he considered, is a step nearer to reality as opposed to the classical analytical twosome. In the latter, the analyst and the patient are bringing into artificial play the opposing forces of authority and dependence, repeating earlier relationships of the parent-child pattern. In the group, the analyst is much more directly the representative of group (social) authorities. It is not intended to pose the controversial aspects of these points of view; they are included because they bear upon the psychodynamics of how the conscious purposes of the leader can deal with the unconscious strivings of the group. After Schilder's death, less than half of the patients returned for treatment. They were seen individually at first, and later in the group.

A representative case was George, aged thirty-one years. His father, who had always been inadequate and dominated by the mother who is still living, had died of cancer when the patient was twenty-seven. The patient felt that his own failure in life had contributed to the father's death. The mother looked upon him as a "mental cripple"; his four sisters called him "Gyp the Blood." Patient regarded his wife as his humble disciple, servant, and slave, whom he had molded to his purposes, although he admitted that she was demanding more practical proof of his greatness than he could deliver. He was schizophrenic; a psychiatric description emphasizes that he was "manneristic, loquacious, boastful, vain, opinionated, hypercritical, grandiose, pedantic, and exhibitionistic."

Following Dr. Schilder's death the patient came to the clinic. He told an admitting officer that he had spoken of hundreds of dreams, and that he wanted another analyst. He began his first interview with the writer by speaking of his many recent nightmares and went on spontaneously to speak of his father's death. "I couldn't summon any tears." He had not been on speaking terms with his father, he said; they had practically been strangers all their lives. He had a mental image of his father sitting in the kitchen, suffering, dying from cancer, and he remembered a dream in which "Dr. Schilder is reading from a platform that the patient was kind to his father, and that he doubted this sentiment." He said that he had an active resentment against Dr. Schilder and was going to tell him his students were a lot of half-baked neurotics, and that's why they were in psychiatry.

Two days later, the patient's free associations ran as follows: "I'm not superstitious [it was Friday, the thirteenth, exactly a week after Schilder's death]. I said, let the dead bury the dead. You looked at me askance. I had a dream: the analyst was a one-eyed ogre . . . you had looked at me out of one eye. A WPA superman . . . I hated him . . . he had one arm crippled . . . Schilder had two fingers missing . . . Ulysses and his travels . . . it was the one-eyed ogre who captured Ulysses . . . I was going to tell you the last time, I felt partially responsible for his death. There seemed to be a titanic struggle raging between us, it tends to break down something . . . he felt attacked by working class . . . he stepped often from psychiatry to economics . . . I'm a terrific Communist, I have grandiose illusions about myself, a sort of twentieth-century-Christ concept, a Savior who wants to get disciples around him, to preach, to steal. Of course it would have been important to get one of the world's leading psychiatrists as a disciple, then through him to get to the section of the ruling class—Marx said, 'A section of the ruling class will cut itself adrift.' He rejected the class struggle, said proletarians were contemptible fools. I felt a definite antagonism to him. When I spoke of the analyst's impassive screen, his face became like a death mask, as if he were saying he'd rather die than agree with me. Rather than recognize me, he chose Death. I wonder he never regained consciousness. If he had, I think he would have mentioned my name, I think he would have acknowledged me with his dying breath."

In this schizophrenic patient, the sense of guilt is expressed in the form of grandiose delusional ideas which derive their content from the ideology of Communism, and from the feeling of being persecuted, expressed in the idea—"rather than acknowledge me, he chose Death." The homosexual bond which is concealed behind the castration wish is revealed in the patient's association that the one-eyed ogre is the analyst, and that it was the one-eyed ogre who captured Ulysses. In this connection, the patient, now identifying himself with the analyst, spoke of a young Negro of his acquaintance, one of his own little band of disciples, whom he proposed to break in to become a leader. Here the patient admitted the overt homosexual bond, adding that his purpose was "to break down in him that something which creates a wall between white and Negro." In subsequent interviews, the patient "recognized" the analyst. He brought an article by him on group therapy, which he praised, and quoted him as saying that the content of his dreams was changing; for two weeks there had been no nightmares. He was contemplating an article on "Buttocks I Have Seen and Known." The "recognition" is on the oral-anal level, colored by aggression, and represents the wish to bring back the father.

Later, George told the group that he had organized a group of his own, calling himself a psychiatrist without a license. "But," he added, "they resent me, they don't think me a Savior." The patient's need for punishment, expressed also on the oral-anal level, is represented in such fantasies as these: The analyst is sitting up in bed, laughing at him. In another fantasy, in which he projects his self-destructive impulses upon the analyst, the latter is seen as having "joined a soul-mate in another world." A dream of this period: "I'm speaking to my supervisor, there are walls between us . . . words not making an impression . . . he is setting up a mental resistance against my words . . . suddenly, it's dark, I'm standing on the street-corner . . . realize there are walls between everybody. I start yelling. I wake up shrieking . . . walls close in . . . I'm alone in the world."

When this patient returned to the group after his individual interviews with the writer, he immediately took on the role of the analyst, identifying himself completely with Dr. Schilder, asking questions, making interpretations, and so on. His associations during this period throw considerable light on the transference to the woman psychiatrist. He said that he was thinking kindly of his father. He thought of the trunk his father used to have in which he kept his belongings. After his death, "I got into the trunk," he said. "I sold some of the articles." He felt that he missed him. Thinking of him in this kindly way, he fell asleep and had a nightmare in which he is pursued by the woman. He runs away, only to land in the arms of the father.

In all of the 27 patients who came under the care of the writer, the reaction to the death of the leader was clinically manifested at the emotional level of development reached in each patient, in terms of the peculiar and habitual response to conflict, either frankly neurotic or psychotic, or characterological. The gamut of affective response ranged all the way from apparent indifference to fear of annihilation. The death of the father was experienced as guilt and/or need for punishment, and was followed by an attempt (also at level of emotional development reached) at "subsequent obedience." The reaction to the death of the father would seem to be the expression of castration wishes superimposed upon the more immediate homosexual, or (it might be) incestuous strivings (perhaps more accurately described as bisexual).

Schematized, the sequence would be: (1) Psychic need for the father (homosexual and incestuous impulses). (2) Ambivalence toward the father (identification and castration fantasies). (3) Guilt, need for punishment, "subsequent obedience." (4) Moral reaction, with or without failure.

The questions that arise are: How do the conscious therapeutic purposes of the therapist deal with the unconscious strivings of a group of psychoneurotics? What can the group situation do for them? Are they able to develop group emotion in relation to a leader as do normal individuals? The outstanding characteristic of the psychoneurotic is that he is highly ambivalent, that the balance between aggressive and libidinal components is only precariously maintained, so that he fails repeatedly to achieve a workable mastery over his conflictual impulses. At the same time, he is subjected to too excessive a drain upon his total energy resources to maintain this delicate balance. To protect himself, he is driven to keep his distance from the group, a situation into which he has in any event fallen because of the sense of his personal uniqueness or "difference." On the other hand, he is equally beset with a yearning to be in harmony with it. He fears, yet wishes to belong, since the need for group identification is older than the need to remain apart. In these young men and women, the aggressive components of instinctual drives were almost continuously in process of stimulation not only from within, but also from the life situations to which they had to make some sort of partial adjustment. Their only "object in common," when they came into the group, was, paradoxically, their difference, which each member in the group recognized in the other.

This group may be described as a spontaneous group formation whose difference *brought* them together, and whose common need for the father *held* them together. One is led to conclude from the case material that the release of the libidinal component of the instinctual impulse is attended by the emergence in psychoneurotics of severe anxiety, too severe to be dealt with in the group. It is questionable whether the group situation is able to pull the psychoneurotic out of his private world into an identification with other psychoneurotics in relation to any leader for other than hostile aims. Even in the group he tends to be alone with his object, at his own point of fixation.

Chapter 8

THE PSYCHOTHERAPEUTIC SYSTEMS

WE HAVE considered in the previous chapters the tools and technical possibilities at the disposal of the physician who intends to do psychotherapy, but technical tools and the use of one or the other technical possibility do not constitute psychotherapy. If the psychotherapeutic tools are to be useful, they must be used in a systematic way, and we have, therefore, to ask which are the psychotherapeutic systems and what is their methodology. Systematic psychotherapy offers the following systems: (*a*) Psychoanalysis. (*b*) Adlerian individual psychology. (*c*) Jungian psychology. (*d*) Psychobiology. (*e*) The so-called short psychotherapy.

A. PSYCHOANALYSIS [1]

According to Freud, psychoanalysis is the method which systematically uses the phenomena of transference and resistance. Transference has been discussed in the preceding chapter. Resistance is the

[1] For some recent comprehensive surveys of psychoanalysis, see: Therese Benedek, *Insight and Personality Adjustment* (Ronald Press, 1950); Edmund Bergler, *The Basic Neurosis* (Grune & Stratton, 1949); Felix Deutsch, *Applied Psychoanalysis* (Grune & Stratton, 1949); and Leon J. Saul, *Emotional Maturity* (J. B. Lippincott, 1947). Books which are more specific in regard to psychotherapeutic techniques or procedures are: Maurice Levine, *Psychotherapy in Medical Practice* (The Macmillan Co., 1942) and Sandor Lorand, *The Technique of Psychoanalytic Therapy* (International Universities Press, 1946). [L.B., Ed.]

force which hinders repressed material from coming fully into consciousness. One might also define it as the force of repression which has to be removed or dissolved before the repressed material can appear. It is obvious, therefore, that the resistance can originate from various sources. Libidinous tendencies strongly directed towards heterosexuality may repress homosexual tendencies. In analysis there will be, therefore, a resistance against bringing forward such repressed homosexual material. We may talk about resistances originating in the id. The individual, being highly moral, will not be inclined to bring forward material aiming in the opposite direction. We may talk about resistance originating in the superego. Further resistances may originate from the transference situation. The patient may not be willing to display to the analyst positive and negative transference. Other resistances may originate from feelings of guilt. Individuals who have adapted to their neuroses may also be unwilling to give up the advantages connected with neurosis. We did not discuss resistance in detail prior to this point, since our previous chapters show that there is a continuous activity going on in the mind and that experiences which are excluded must be kept out by some force. The term "resistance" refers this general principle to the analytic situation and makes it clear that there are forces at hand which hinder the appearance of repressed material in the analysis.

When resistances are closely connected with the character pattern of an individual, we speak, with W. Reich, about character resistance. This is the pattern which organizes the repressions and systematizes them. One has spoken about countercathexis in relation to the energy of repression. The term "cathexis" in analysis means the amount of libido invested in a specific experience. If the libidinous cathexis is not counteracted by countercathexis, the repressed material is liable to come into the foreground. But we are here more interested in the practical problems of how resistance appears in analysis. The patient may not talk at all, he may say that he does not want to report a specific problem, he may bring superficial material, or he may use infantile experiences as resistance for bringing forward material of the present, which he wants to keep repressed. The opposite may occur, too. The patient may try to involve the physician in a discussion. He may even use his analytic knowledge.

When Rank tried to show that birth phantasies and the trauma of birth are the basis of every neurosis, analysts agreed that material pointing to the trauma of birth is not uncommon. They interpreted the data as the patient's bringing such material forward in order to protect himself against producing experiences pertaining to the Oedipus complex, which might be more painful. Obviously it might be very difficult to decide whether material brought forward is merely due to resistance, or to true free association. The weapon of the physician against resistance is to remind the patient of the necessity of saying everything, to tell him when, according to the opinion of the physician, resistance is present, and most important to show him the material and the motives of his repressions on the basis of associations. One sees that the analysis of the resistance parallels the whole analytic procedure.

I have mentioned before that resistance may be a sign of negative transference, but otherwise negative transference is a psychic phenomenon different from resistance. Negative transference may even bring forward important repressed material and so remove the resistances. How much the patient will accept of the analyst's interpretations depends upon the state of resistance in which he is; but this also depends on the state of transference.

One may start the analysis by telling the patient, who is lying on the couch, with the analyst sitting behind him, that he should tell the history of his life. The basic rule of free association has, of course, to be told to him at first. Even when the patient tells his life history, we may hear some of his dreams, some of his free associations. One should not start too early with interpretations. The interpretations should be obvious, and should be gained preferably by merely putting the material into a form from which the patient may draw his own conclusions. According to psychoanalytic rules, symbols generally have to be interpreted to the patient even if his association material is not sufficient. In the further development, interpretations can be given in a freer way. There is no necessity to interpret positive transference early; negative transference should be interpreted whenever sufficiently clear.

Active therapy in the sense mentioned above should not start before a sufficiently deep transference is reached. The patient should refrain from making important decisions during the analysis. In acute situations the analyst should refrain as much as possible from giving advice. He should not give too much satisfaction to the patient, should not give encouragement, and should not make promises. Freud says succinctly that the patient should not have satisfaction by the analyst. One will generally let the patient go on with his ordinary social and sexual activities. Prohibitions and admonitions should be given in accordance with the rule of active therapy. Putting a term for the end of the analysis is generally not advisable. Recurrence of the symptoms just before the termination of an analysis may be expected. At the end of the analysis the patient should be capable of forming satisfactory human contacts in a social and sexual sense.

It is not essential that the patient should dream during the analysis. Whether and when to interpret a dream depends on the situation in the analysis. The patient chooses the topic of every analytic hour for himself. One is entitled to break this rule only with old persons or when the patient obviously avoids coming back to his previous hour. Contact with relatives is not advisable, and information from relatives is useless. It is generally advantageous if the patient does not discuss his analysis with other persons. There should be no social contact between the patient and his analyst. Remarks made after the hour are a part of the analysis. The patient should be forced to be punctual. He hires the hour and has to pay whether he comes or not. Punctual payment by those who can pay is considered as essential. The resistance often appears in relation to money. For a while it was considered impossible to conduct an analysis for which the patient did not pay. This point of view was given up when the experiences of psychoanalytic institutes proved the contrary.

This is a description of the analytic procedure. It is often difficult to determine when the analysis is finished. Around 1920 Freud postulated that the period between the third and the fifth years has to be completely elucidated. Most analysts at the present time desire to push the analysis further back. So does Freud. Freedom from symptoms is no criterion, as it may be due to transference. The symptoms are liable to appear again. One might say the patient has to be free of his symptoms. His life history, his resistance, and his transference situation have to be worked through, and he must have shown an adaptation to his life situation.

Special techniques have been recommended in cases in which the patient shows more or less severe character deformation. Reich recommends starting with the analysis of the negative transference and the resistance. His procedure has been called one-sided. In making one's decision, one should be guided by the material as to what to analyze first and what to analyze later. Reich uses the capacity for achieving a successful intercourse as criterion for the cure. He has shown that an individual who is potent in the ordinary sense might orgastically be impotent and not derive the full psychic satisfaction. Freud has declined this criterion. Although there is obviously a correlation between the completeness of orgasm and freedom from neurotic disturbances, this correlation is far from being absolute. I know of cases of neurosis in which the orgasm is perfect, even when one applies the severe criteria of Reich. He demands absence of phantasies during intercourse and a complete relaxation which facilitates sleep. The need for another sex gratification should be absent for a while. There should be a gradual increase of the pleasure, a peak, and a complete and rather sudden decline of the desire after the peak has been reached. In reading Reich's book, one is astonished by the severity with which he insists on what he considers the ideal type of intercourse and orgasm. His "morality" is no less strict than Mid-Victorian prudishness. We need a more liberal attitude concerning sex. There are no strict laws prescribing how intercourse and orgasm should take place, and we should not have perfectionistic ideals concerning intercourse.

This has so far been merely a report; we may now try an evaluation of the procedure. It cannot be denied that it gives the patient deep insight into his psychological problems. The psychoanalytic practice is very often less rigid than the theory, and the patient not only sees his problems merely from the point of view of the satisfaction of his somatic needs but also from the point of view of goals, aims, and purposes. It is a great advantage that, at least in principle, psychoanalysis lets the patient seek his own salvation on the basis of the insight he has gained in the analytic procedure. Psychoanalysis declines to give to the patient any guidance or to direct him anywhere. It has overlooked the fact that insight as such gives us specific orders about what to do and what not to do. The difficulties of psychoanalysis lie in the psychoanalytic situation. We may characterize them as follows: (*a*) It is a secret relation between two persons closeted from other human beings. (*b*) It is a relation in which money plays a very important part. (*c*) In stressing the constitutional and instinctual side of human problems, psychoanalysis is in danger of stressing the individual too much rather than his relationship to society. (*d*) The prevalence of sexuality in psychoanalysis looks like a reversal of the

Mid-victorian repression of sexuality; at least the terminology of psychoanalysis stresses the sexual side of human experience. (*e*) Since the analyst does not have the right to speak about his counter-transference there is an artificial stress in the analytic situation. (*f*) Since the theory of free association is stressed, there is considerable danger that the conscious adaptation of the patient, his actions, opinions, and ideologies, are not sufficiently elucidated.[2]

The therapeutic efficiency of the method is beyond question. There are severe neuroses which cannot be cured in any other way. In neuroses of medium degree it is often the surest way. Character deficiencies very often react favorably. Efficiency and the capacity for happiness are increased after almost every analysis which has been carefully conducted for a sufficient amount of time. The advantage of psychoanalysis lies in the fact that it has for a long time directed its attention, not to the symptom, but to the person. Whereas previous attempts attacked the symptom, the analytic procedure does not take the symptom into consideration. It is, therefore, by principle, a character analysis.

The duration of an analytic treatment is long. Eight or nine months is considered at the present time as a very short analysis. Two, three, four, and even five years of analysis are not uncommon. Sessions of one hour take place six times a week.

The statistics so far available show that the method is not always successful. We have the statistics of the Berlin Psychoanalytic Institute and the reports of Hyman and Kessel. It is astonishing that the statistics of state hospitals show almost the same percentage of cures and improvements of their cases of neuroses as Carney Landis reported in L. E. Hinsie's *Concepts and Problems of Psychotherapy*. Hinsie also pointed to the social inefficiency of the method, since only a very limited number of patients have so far been treated, and the number of persons who can be benefited by an even larger number of analysts is very small. I am inclined to believe, considering my own experiences with hospital patients, that the cure of the patient by psychoanalysis is not the same as the so-called cure by a state hospital.

---

[2] Many of these criticisms have been met in the work of Erich Fromm, Karen Horney, Abram Kardiner, and Harry S. Sullivan, who have emphasized interpersonal relationship and cultural factors. Cf. Clara Thompson, *Psychoanalysis, Evolution and Development: A Review of Theory and Therapy* (New York, Hermitage House, Inc., 1950). [L.B., Ed.]

The psychoanalytic cure comes much nearer to the ideal cure.[3]

The value of psychoanalysis in the treatment of psychosis in its present form is debatable. Alexander is obviously much too optimistic. There are some cases of schizophrenia which profit by analysis. Zilboorg reports such a case. In manic-depressive psychoses successful treatments have been reported by Freud and others. Many cases do not react sufficiently. In others it is difficult to ascertain whether the disease is self-terminating or whether it was cured by the treatment. We may state that psychoanalysis is not the method of choice in psychotic cases. Selected cases may profit.

The neuroses of medium and severe degree and especially perversions and character deviations are the field for psychoanalysis. In appreciating psychoanalysis one has to keep in mind the fact that the method has still not been tried on a sufficiently large number of cases. The present technique is cumbersome, expensive, and is very often handled with an unnecessary rigidity. However, the method is indispensable, and Freud's work is the basis for every psychotherapeutic approach. Much of what is valid in modern psychotherapy goes back to him and his co-workers. There is invaluable advantage in a definite technique. Persons specializing in psychotherapeutics should have full insight and knowledge of this method and should be able to handle it. Further development of psychotherapy which does not utilize Freud's work is unthinkable.

B. ADLERIAN INDIVIDUAL PSYCHOLOGY [4]

Many of the principles of individual psychology have been discussed in the previous chapter. It stresses the goals and aims of the individual and his life plan. It tries to find out the individual's style

[3] See C. Oberndorf, P. Greenacre, and L. Kubie, "Symposium on the Evaluation of Therapeutic Results," *International Journal of Psychoanalysis* 29:1–27, 1948, and Paul Hoch (ed.), *Failures in Psychiatric Treatment* (Grune & Stratton, 1948). [L.B., Ed.]

[4] For recent reviews on Adlerian individual psychology, see: Alexandra Adler, *Guiding Human Misfits, Practical Application of Individual Psychology* (New York, Philosophical Library Inc., 2nd ed., 1948) and Rudolf Dreikurs, *Introduction to Individual Psychology* (London, Kegan Paul, Trench & Trubner & Co., 1935). Adlerian group therapy is reported by Joshua Bierer in *Therapeutic Social Clubs* (London, H. K. Lewis & Co., 1948). [L.B., Ed.]

of life. It asks whether the attitudes and the actions of the individual are on the useful or the useless side of life. The individual's tasks are defined as tasks pertaining to profession, social life (friends), and sex. The neurotic individuals and the psychopaths have chosen the wrong style of life. They suffer from feelings of inferiority, they are not up to the task to which they are put, they have to overcompensate by feelings of superiority and refrain from serious attempts. The wrong style of life has been acquired in early childhood. Under ordinary circumstances one's style of life becomes crystallized at the age of five. One might expect that when an individual has been pampered in childhood he will expect to get everything without effort, and will devise various devious methods in order to get what he wants. When an individual has inferior organs he will not be sufficiently appreciated by his surroundings or he may be pampered too much and will develop a wrong style of life. The organ inferiority does not act as a biological factor but merely as the basis on which wrong attitudes of the others are developed, making it impossible for the child to acquire the right style of life. The parents and the persons who nurse the child are of particular importance in this respect. The actions and dreams and early memories indicate the wrong side of life as well as the neurotic symptoms. The task of psychotherapy is to show the individual his wrong style of life, to have him give up his feelings of inferiority and superiority and subordinate his will for power to the community spirit. The regard for other human beings should be paramount also in sex relations. The only really valuable form of sex relations is marriage.

It is difficult to get clear insight into the technique of psychotherapy in individual psychology. Although Adler does not use the term "unconscious," it is a matter of course that the individual does not understand himself in choosing the wrong style of life. He also does not understand his symptoms. A process of interpretation is therefore also necessary for the individual psychologist. I have quoted, above, two instances from Adler's writings. In his first independent book, *The Nervous Character,* Adler's interpretations, although stressing the aims and goals, are much more closely related to the analytic way of interpreting. His method of interpretation has become more and more simple. For him, symbols at the present time are merely exaggerated expressions of one part of the situation which hide other important sides of reality. They have the purpose of directing the aims and goals into another direction which is not always useful. Whereas in his first books sexual interpretations were not uncommon, they do not play any important part in his later writings. A period of preparation is seemingly necessary in order to make the patient ready to accept the interpretation and change to a better style of life. There is a growing tendency to rely upon common sense, and oversimplification follows.

My own experiences are limited in respect to this method. I do not doubt that it may be efficient in one or the other case. It is doubtful whether more complicated cases will react at all. Successes are reported in children. I would recommend a method of this type only for comparatively uncomplicated cases.

It is unjust when Freud says that Adler stresses merely the inferiority of an organ and that his inferiority complex is but a variant of the castration complex. The important part in Adler's system is his interest in reality and especially in social reality. It is further valuable that he stresses the community spirit, the style of life, and the various techniques of the affected individual in compensation and overcompensation. Psychoanalysts mostly do not reproach Adler as being incorrect in what he says, but they justly say that it is incomplete.

It is indeed to be regretted that Adler does not have more to say about the structure of the social problems and the outward world. It must also be acknowledged that his opinion that human beings are fundamentally equal has a very important insight as its basis. His attitude towards the problems of masculine and feminine is clear and decisive, since he does not acknowledge fundamental differences and points to the different social standards concerning masculine and feminine. The severe disadvantages of the method lie in its meagerness. It is also not possible to maintain the attitude of the wiser, older brother for a very long time. The patients very soon feel that the physician has given to them all that he is able to give and feel compelled to seek the help of others. From a scientific point of view there is no deeper relation to biology. The difference between the thinking of the child and that of the adult is not sufficiently acknowledged. I may reproduce a discussion which I once had with Adler, which I think makes his position pretty clear. The talk was on anal erotism:

I: "We have experiences in relation to the body which cannot be analyzed further."

A: "Behind it is the defiance."

I: "There must be final constants. One of them is the body. There is not much sense in going beyond this point on which one can rest."

A: "There is no rest."

I: "But rest is the background without which movement is not possible."

A: "Individual psychology can see nothing in isolation."

If individual psychology reminds us again and again to look also for the structure in the outward world and especially to the social structures that surround us it has done a valuable service. Indeed, human beings have goals, and Adler is right when he says that the meaning and the goal are very closely related to each other.

C. JUNGIAN PSYCHOLOGY [5]

It is difficult to characterize Jung's approach. He has simplified the libido problem by calling everything libido. He has succeeded in desexualizing libido by this simple method. Freud also later came to the point of view that the clamor of life is merely due to libido, whereas the death instincts are silent. Freud, however, really sexualizes the world by making the counterpart of libido imperceptible. I do not see that there is a great advantage in stressing the common basis of life experiences, although it has to be conceded that human beings strive as unified personalities. There is no denying that there are well-characterized differences in attitudes and goals. There are sex instincts and there are other instincts in connection with other life functions. Why deny this and stress merely the unity and neglect diversity?

Jung's doctrine of extroversion and introversion has, according to the preceding remarks, a rather limited value. It has no immediate bearing on psychotherapeutic procedures. Since Jung acknowledges an unconscious he needs also a method of interpretation. Whereas psychoanalysis uses for interpretation the individual experiences, especially those of childhood, Jung tries to find out the meaning of the

[5] See Jolan Jacobi, *The Psychology of Jung,* translated by K. Bash (New Haven, Yale University Press, 1943), in addition to Jung's own writings. [L.B., Ed.]

manifestations in dreams and symptoms by comparing them with folklore and myths. Since folklore and myths offer an almost unlimited number of pictures, it is almost arbitrary which one is chosen for the interpretation of the individual psychic experience in question. As far as I know, Jung has never given a classification of his archetypes. It is true he has pointed to many important symbolizations in his book, *Variations and Symbols in the Manifestation of Libido.* I doubt whether such a procedure ever can reveal very much of the individual life of the patient. His increase in insight remains limited. One may suppose that the prevalence of animal figures in the associations and drawings of the patient, and the appearance of symbols for the magic healer and fertilization, have partially something to do with the special method employed and the community spirit developed in his circle.

The concept of collective unconscious is, as pointed to previously, exposed to serious doubts. It is only justified in so far as the fundamental reactions of human beings are common to all of us and comparatively limited in number. Even the last part of the statement has to be specified. Human situations show an unlimited variety, and only by abstraction do we come to a comparatively limited number of basic situations. Jung and his followers stress the creative force of the unconscious. They are right in this respect, and I have often objected to the formulation of Freud that all drives are regressive in their final tendencies.

But the creative character is a characteristic of human existence and not only of the so-called unconscious. I would also prefer not to use the term "creative," which is loaded with more or less mystical tendencies and stresses too much the artistic creation. It is conceded that artistic capacities are present in everybody, as testified by the art of children, primitives, and psychotics, but the artistic creation is merely a step towards the conquest of the world which has not been completed and therefore retains the charm of varied possibilities. Stressing the artistic side of life, we are not likely to lead the individual to a full reality and the real problems of life, which lie in the moral problems in relation to other human beings and go beyond the artistic problem. It is in close relation to the emphasis on art that mystical tendencies play a very great part in Jung's theoretical and, as far as one can see, practical approach. It does not increase confidence in the reliability of such methods when Jung, on the basis of them, discovers the difference between Jewish and Aryan psychotherapy. One feels so much in the vicinity of a type of thinking which praises intuition in order to further one's own prejudices and ideologies. A thinking which remains in the symbolic sphere sooner or later ends in premature crystallizations. Jung's theory and, as far as one can see, also his practice remain, in spite of very valuable and interesting findings in detail, in a sphere of mental and emotional ambiguity which is far from being a synthesis. Jung has created the valuable connotation of the "persona," which means the social mask everyone is wearing, but the term is merely a transcription of psychoanalytic findings. He thinks that every human being has to repress the tendencies belonging to the opposite sex, and these repressed feminine tendencies in the man ("anima") and masculine in the woman ("animus") are likely to provoke disturbances. This view of masculinity and femininity seems rather narrow and does not exhaust the real problems.

I do not know, therefore, especially after the perusal of his pupil Heyer's books, whether Jungian psychotherapy deserves the name of a psychotherapeutic system and has any place in the treatment of specific cases. Many of his insights may be usefully subordinated to other types of psychotherapy.

Jung used the word-association test in order to find out "complexes" of the individual. The individual has to answer to a word given to him with the next word coming into his mind. When complexes are present, the reaction time is increased and unusual words may be chosen. If a series of words is prepared, one may come to an insight into the situation. The test itself, although in no way testing associations, offers some theoretical interest. It is useless in the course of psychotherapy. It is also useless to order the patient, as Stekel does, to say a series of words in reaction to a chosen stimulus. Answering in mere words is an artificial effort which does not promote the bringing forward of repressed material. In this respect a note of Milton E. Erickson's is interesting. The word-association test contained hints that the patient had gone through an abortion (unrecognized by the physician), but the patient did not report this to the physician. She confessed spontaneously, later on. The word-association test got its meaning merely by the spontaneous "confession."

D. PSYCHOBIOLOGY [6]

This is the term used by Adolf Meyer for a rather eclectic system of psychotherapy, based upon the acknowledgment that humans are physical beings as well as personalities. The importance of the present situation is stressed in this approach. Infantile experiences are not systematically taken into consideration although accepted when offered by the patient. The patient has, in this approach, more freedom than in any of the psychotherapeutic approaches mentioned above. Strong emotional reactions of the patient are avoided; his social duties and obediences to the ruling social code of morals are stressed. The patient is taken as much as possible out of the atmosphere of conflicts, and his reality is simplified as much as possible. Common sense is stressed. The complaint is taken as a starting point. Diethelm speaks about synthetic and distributive analysis. Neither goes very deep into the analysis of the problems of the patient. The same attitude is prevalent in the child psychiatry of Kanner. Although some of the analytic knowledge is taken over, it is not fully utilized.

Sexual interpretations are used with all too great precaution. It is characteristic that great stress is laid on panics, especially in connection with the sex problem. The patient is supposed to get help in being led out of the panic. He should not be excited any further. According to my experience panics are rather rare. It is true that they occur under the influence of earthquakes and similar catastrophes which provoke fright, as described by Stierlin and Kleist. Otherwise, the panic is on the side of the physician who is overwhelmed by the strength of the drives of the patient which he considers as inopportune.

One may summarize this therapeutic approach by saying that it puts the patient into a simplified situation of which the physician, slightly soothing and slightly helping to understand, is a part. But

[6] Adolf Meyer's teachings on the subject of psychobiology are now available in Alfred Lief (ed.), *The Commonsense Psychiatry of Dr. Adolf Meyer, Fifty-two Selected Papers with a Biographical Narrative* (New York, McGraw-Hill Book Co., 1948); Oskar Diethelm, *Treatment in Psychiatry* (Charles C. Thomas, 1950); and Edward G. Billings, *A Handbook of Elementary Psychobiology and Psychiatry* (New York, The Macmillan Co., 1943). [L.B., Ed.]

every deeper analysis, whether it stresses the goals and the approach to the outward world or whether it stresses the psychosexual and somatic problems—and they should both be stressed—is bound to upset and disturb the patient. This is the price he has to pay preliminary to his better adaptation. The adaptation reached by psychobiology will therefore be of a more or less superficial character. However, Meyer's method is invaluable for those human beings from whom we do not demand a full adaptation—the psychotics. The Phipps Psychiatric Clinic is indeed an admirable institution which provides for a simple routine in occupation and social life, and takes the patient out of the atmosphere of conflicts into a well-regulated atmosphere of moderate social usefulness. The effect of this institution on psychiatric development in this country has been very great, and leading University institutions are modeled after it. In psychoses this psychotherapeutic approach, using to a great extent indirect methods, has proved to be successful. Its usefulness, in my opinion, is limited by the fact that the so-called functional psychoses, such as schizophrenia and manic-depressive psychosis, are largely based upon organic factors. They are helped by preparing the ground and aiding organic recovery. We may not expect that such an approach will be particularly successful in the treatment of neurotic persons, from whom we may demand more and whom we should force to a deeper insight into their problems.

E. THE SO-CALLED SHORT PSYCHOTHERAPY [7]

The problem of short psychotherapy is urgent. The costs of psychoanalysis are large for the patient as well as for the hospital. The amount of time necessary for such a treatment is great. We do not have exact figures as to how long the average treatment by individual psychology, or by Jung, takes. In the remarks on the technical tools I have emphasized that every method which increases the insight of the patient can be of use, if applied with the correct attitude of the physician. The result of a shorter treatment will depend on the depth

[7] See *Conferences on Short Psychotherapy of the Institute of Psychoanalysis,* Chicago, 1944, 1946. Also Franz Alexander and Thomas M. French, *Psychoanalytic Therapy* (New York, The Ronald Press, 1946). [L.B., Ed.]

of the neurosis in relation to the depth of the psychotherapy. One has to take into account that many of the more searching methods are partially dependent on the faculty of the patient to verbalize. This faculty has some relation to his degree of education. Beyond that there exists another factor which is difficult to appreciate. Some patients are able to bring forward an astonishing amount of material. Their experiences and memories are wide open to them. Others, though intelligent and educated, are hardly able to formulate anything about their memories and experiences. This difference is generally independent of the clinical type of neurosis under which the patient suffers. I once tried psychoanalysis on a well-educated and efficient physician who was interested in the subject, but did not bring forward any memory pertaining to events before his twelfth year. He did not dream and what material he brought forward was merely a report of his everyday experiences. He was well adapted and reasonably happy. I gave up after six weeks of futile effort. It is doubtful whether such an individual, when inflicted with a neurosis, can be treated by searching methods.

Whereas psychoanalysis neglects the symptom, shorter psychotherapy will very often have to start with the symptom. It has, accordingly, to use the method of discussion; but it will be advisable, even in a shorter therapy, to use the method of free association and dream interpretation. It will very soon turn out that from the analysis of the present situation one has to proceed to earlier and even infantile situations. Even in short therapeutic procedures, the use of first memories will very often be advantageous. Even in such shorter treatments it is indispensable that one give the patient a synthesis of his conflict and reconstruct the life history from the specific angle of the understanding of his conflict. The interpretations given under such circumstances cannot, of course, have the relative reliability obtained by methods such as psychoanalysis for instance, which allows for checking the validity of interpretations again and again and does not interpret before the patient has brought forward convincing material. The knowledge and skill of the physician will, therefore, be particularly necessary in short treatments. He will generally not have them unless he has analyzed a number of cases before.

It is very important that one should keep in mind even during short psychotherapy that the same fundamental relation exists between patient and physician as in the forms of treatment which take a longer time. The treatment consists of winning the transference, working through and using the transference, and breaking the transference. The attempt to adapt the patient in the middle period to the reality has to be more energetic and more direct, and the breaking of the transference may also be difficult in such a treatment. But I do not see any particular difficulty in helping the patient in difficult situations even after the main treatment is finished. Very often it will not be possible to bring the patient to a full insight into the structure of the transference, and especially of the negative transference which necessarily is present in this form of treatment, although mostly repressed. Even the so-called short therapy takes some amount of time. One may reckon with about thirty hours. Very often the relief of the symptoms starts early. The symptoms may disappear after the first ten or fifteen sessions. It is advisable not to stop the treatment after success is reached. A relapse is common. If one is able to explain some of the motives of this relapse, the patient very often reaches a lasting degree of adaptation. I have followed cases treated in such a way for years after the treatment was finished and the good results were permanent.

It is very often advantageous to combine hypnosis with short psychotherapy. I proceed generally in such a way that in the first few sessions a preliminary insight into the problems of the patient is attempted. A hypnotic session follows, in which the insight gained in this way is used for the formulation of the therapeutic suggestion. In the therapeutic suggestion the patient receives a succinct interpretation of his symptoms and at the same time is shown that his symptoms will disappear when he has fully acquired this insight. No session is entirely devoted to hypnosis. The patient brings his associations and dream material in the first part of the session, and the last quarter of an hour is used for the hypnotic session in which no emphasis is put on the depth of the hypnosis. The period of the working through of the life history of the patient after the transference is accomplished has also to stress that the patient is only at the present time dependent on the physician. However, such a dependence is but transitory and cannot last. The emphasis has to be put on the preliminary character of the situation of dependence and upon the efforts of the patient to progress to formulations of his life plans for himself. It is furthermore necessary that the patient should gain at least some understanding of the transference situation in general and the hypnotic transference. If one does so one will hardly be troubled by a too great attachment of the patient to the physician.

It is obvious that we use in such a treatment, besides the discussion, also free association and dream interpretation. It is true that without any particular effort of the physician, the patient may fall into deep hypnosis in such a treatment. I may repeat then what I have said about the difficulties of deep hypnosis. It is particularly important that no experiments should be made with the patient. Hypnotizers were particularly proud, previously, to have good "mediums." They kept the patient in dependence and thus sinned against the cardinal principle of every psychotherapy, namely, to respect the patient as an independent human being. They pushed the patients into passive infantile situations and not only prolonged their neurosis but even deepened it. I have seen such artifacts in the beginning of my psychiatric work, residuals of the wave of hypnotism which swept the Continent about 1890. This was not therapeusis but showmanship, to the detriment of the patient. However, this has nothing to do with the technique of hypnosis as such.

One may get similar artifacts by any other psychotherapeutic approach if this approach does not take place in the right spirit. The attachment of the psychoanalytic patient to the physician can be deeper than the attachment of hypnotic patients and may lead to the same undesirable effects to which hypnosis leads if the transference situation is not properly handled. Even in the face of such difficulties, one should not forget that there are neurotic cases which are not fully curable and in which lasting dependence on the physician, whatever method he uses, is the lesser evil, as long as the physician is conscious of his ambiguous position. It is not always the physician's fault when a treatment, even one which was intended to be a short one, cannot be brought to an end.

Let us return to our topic of short psychotherapy. The proper field for short psychotherapy is a neurosis in which a deformation of the character has not taken place yet and where one deals chiefly with symptoms. It should be kept in mind, however, that it is very difficult to separate the character from the symptoms, and very often so-called monosymptomatic neuroses reveal themselves at closer inspection as very deeply rooted in the life plan of the patient or, in psychoanalytic language, in infantile genital or pregenital fixations. This is particularly true of difficulties in potency and orgasm.

It is generally true that patients who once have reached a sexual adaptation show neuroses of a less severe degree. Furthermore, patients whose difficulties lie in the Oedipus situation are generally easier to treat than those in whom pregenital fixations are prevalent, as in obsession neurosis. (Cf. also the remarks about the Oedipus complex and the infantile sexual organization in the chapter on the Oedipus complex.) The nucleus of a psychopathy or perversion usually cannot be reached in short psychotherapy; however, psychopathic individuals often develop symptoms, and those symptoms very often do not need more than a short psychotherapeutic effort.

In psychotherapy we should, anyhow, be aware of the fact that we are not always able to change our patient into the ideal human being, and the psychotherapist should ask himself from the beginning how far he may be able to change the basic attitudes of the patient. Therapy which changes the character of the patient and gives him a reasonable security against the recurrence of the symptoms is not always easy to perform. Relapses after a seemingly successful psychoanalysis are not uncommon. Witness, for instance, the case of Freud's "History of an Infantile Neurosis" who, after three and a half years of analysis which was considered successfully concluded, showed relapses almost every year and finally had to be reanalyzed by Ruth Mack Brunswick. He was apparently cured after this analysis. One may doubt whether this result will be final, and I have heard rumors that the patient has since been cured again by another analyst. It is true that the psychiatrist will suspect that this case is not a neurosis but an atypical manic-depressive psychosis, which diagnosis has been made by one of the psychiatrists who saw the patient.

My own results in short psychotherapy with and without hypnosis, extended over many years, are on the whole satisfactory. I prefer to discuss the situation with the patient. I prefer not to promise the patient too much unless I am myself convinced that the chances are very favorable. On the other hand, if such short psychotherapy should be unsuccessful, the possibility for a psychoanalysis or another type of deeper treatment is still open, and the difficulties of starting an analysis after a short psychotherapy are in no way greater than in starting an analysis after another analysis has been unsuccessful for one reason or another.

Psychoanalytic literature has been rather reticent about the treatment of the type of neurosis which Freud called actual neurosis, and which he considered as the result of the toxic influence originating from incomplete sex satisfaction by masturbation, coitus interruptus, coitus condomatus, or continence. Freud has adhered to this conception. I have never seen such a case. The cases to which Freud alludes are very often those in which the conflict lies chiefly in the present situation. These are, therefore, particularly favorable objects for short psychotherapy. The mere regulation of the sexual diet of a patient is useless. Although the satisfactions mentioned above may be insufficient, there remains the chief problem of why the patient had refrained from getting fuller satisfaction. Freud's statements, never retracted, also imply a vast overevaluation of the technical side of intercourse. A sex relation with condom or with interruption, with a person for whom one cares, is decidedly more advantageous for the psychic health of a person than very complete sex relations with a person for whom one does not care. As to continence, one will always have to raise the question, why is the person continent, and what for? Continence in itself is neither a neurosis nor the symptom of a neurosis. It can be, of course, the symptom of a neurosis, and may mean an unwarranted attempt to escape sex.

In the evaluation of masturbation many factors have to be considered. As we shall discuss later, we have primarily to ask what it stands for. It is, of course, at best an inferior substitute, an expression of an incomplete adaptation to sex which in the one or the other case might be the result of a particularly difficult reality. These problems have been mentioned in connection with short psychotherapy, since the patient has a right to be informed about the fundamental sex problems (birth control included). I do not see any virtue in sexual ignorance, which is very often one of the starting points of neurotic symptomatology. In every type of psychotherapy obvious lack of knowledge concerning vital problems, and misinformation, have to be corrected. The further question has to be considered, where the lack of knowledge and the misinformation originated from.

Various attempts have been made to shorten the course of analysis. Stekel has propounded a particularly active type of psychoanalysis in which interpretations are forced upon the patient, and are very often shocking to him. Owing to insufficient information of the physician and of the patient, such attempts are more or less arbitrary and therefore dangerous. I have occasionally seen therapeutic results which were achieved by a rather passive psychoanalytical approach which was extended over only two or three months. This is in no way an ideal procedure and is only justified by urgent outward circumstances.

It might properly be debated at this point whether we have the right to shock the patient in the course of any psychotherapeutic procedure. This is debatable even in forms of treatment like psychoanalysis where we have the patient under perpetual control. It depends very much on the formulations. Some analysts prefer the occasional use of vulgar words for sexual parts and for sexual functions, but it will also make a great difference whether we tell the patient, "You have the wish of having intercourse with your mother," or whether we tell the patient, "This points to an infantile wish for sex relations with your mother. This wish is not the same as when an adult person wants to have intercourse with a love object." The same problems arise when so-called unconscious homosexual tendencies are discussed. My general advice is that the physician has not the right to shock a patient unless it is necessary, and he is not allowed to choose the formulation which might seem more striking to the patient if he has not the conviction that the striking formulation is the correct expression of the situation. This warning has to be still more emphasized in short psychotherapy, where we have the patient less in control than in the extended form of treatment.

It is advisable, even in short psychotherapy, to see the patient at least four or five times a week in the first two or three weeks of the treatment. One may then gradually decrease the number of hours per week and may finally see the patient once a week or once in a fortnight before one finishes the treatment. If the necessity arises, one may increase the number of hours again. An average duration of an hour for a session will be preferable for most of the cases. I have never seen anything good come from lengthening a single session over an hour. (Concerning the prognosis of neuroses treated with similar methods, cf. book by T. A. Ross.)

Chapter 9

GROUP PSYCHOTHERAPY

THE WORK done so far in group psychotherapy and its literature have been discussed in Chapter 6, and the problem of the relationship of the physician, as the leader, to the group has been discussed in Chapter 7. I shall try here to give a detailed description of a method of group psychotherapy which I employed in rather large measure in the out-patient department of the Psychiatric Division of Bellevue Hospital.

After the first interview, the patients were seen individually by the physician. They reported their life history, as in analysis. The principles of free association and dream interpretation were taught to them. When, after several sessions, a preliminary insight was reached, the patient was asked to write down his biography in detail. The following advice was given:

"When you write down the history of your life, you must not keep back anything. There may be situations and experiences which you would prefer not to write about. Still you have to write them down. Do not attempt to make a masterpiece out of your biography. Write it down as it comes into your mind and do not polish it. Contradictions and repetitions may finally help us to an important insight. It is of great importance that you write down every remembrance pertaining to your early childhood up to the age of five. Give particular attention to your first memories. It will help if you keep in mind that the relation to father, mother, siblings, and nursing personnel are of particular importance. Write down, therefore, whatever you can remember about them.

"You certainly have not always experienced love only. There must also have been some experiences of hate. In the world of the child there is a great interest in food, in urination and defecation. Write down whatever you can remember about this. Sexual experiences are not uncommon, even in early childhood; try at any rate to give an accurate description of the development of your sexual attitudes and also do not forget that your opinions about sex problems are of importance.

"Follow these fundamental relations through the school age to puberty, and describe the relation to all the persons who played an important part in your later life. These relations are relations to friends and to love objects. Also give consideration to your professional achievements and to the persons you have met in your professional career.

"Give an idea of your aims, goals, and interests and how they have developed. In every person's sex life are facts and experiences which they feel do not conform to the professed moral standards. Do not hesitate to write these experiences down. The human life is not merely filled with experiences and memories. Everyone has phantasies, wishes, dreams. Write them down as far as you can remember them. There is no necessity that you give this report quickly. Take your time. No detail is unimportant which comes into your mind. Give us also a general idea of your surroundings in childhood and in later life."

This is merely a general outline; one may vary the instructions according to the education of the patient and according to the material which the patient has brought forward in the preliminary session. At any time one may ask the patient to add to the one or the other part of his life history.

It depends on the course of the psychotherapy how much one uses this report of the patient. The patient is very often helped already by the necessity of letting his whole life pass before his eyes. However, almost any part of the life history will need an interpretation in the course of the treatment.

After the patient has reached the preliminary orientation, he is seen together with a group of other patients who are in various stages of the treatment. The session begins with the report of any one of these patients, and is conducted in a way similar to individual psychoanalysis. An interpretation is given to the patient if the situation warrants it. If there are patients in the group who are far enough progressed, any one of the other patients can give his interpretation or may add associations and experiences of his own. Demands to associate may be directed towards any one member of the group. The physician gives an interpretation when he sees fit to do so. Whenever the material brought forward by one or the other patient is sufficiently clear, a general remark about the mechanism involved may be added. If one or the other patient tries to monopolize the situation, one has to turn to other patients. If the material brought forward by a patient is very archaic and shocking in character, one must give immediately an interpretation which may reduce the shock by showing the relation of this material to infantile situations and by explaining the dynamic significance of infantile material.

The groups I have seen so far did not number more than six or seven. The patient is not seen more than once a week in such a large group. Occasionally, I take two or three patients in one group in which the preliminary investigation has shown a similarity of underlying mechanisms. Release of new material may reasonably be expected in both when the further progressed patient brings forward his associations.

Most of the patients can easily be convinced that such a procedure can be of advantage for them and they show, sooner or later, a great interest in the group. In some cases the resentment of talking before others is not immediately overcome. The patient may then be, for one or two sessions, a silent participant, till he feels like talking. If he does not, no pressure is exerted to continue in the group. When I see a group or six or seven patients, I spend from two to three hours with them. Smaller groups are rarely seen for more than an hour.

Every patient who participates in groups is also seen in individual interviews, on the average of two times a week. If the time of the patient and the time of the physician permit, the patient is seen even more often, especially in the beginning of the treatment. Many of the patients are employed and cannot be seen as often as the physician would like to see them. However, it seems very important that the patient should not be taken out of his professional work unless that is absolutely necessary. I have made myself as accessible as possible for the patients and see those who come in at a time when they are not expected, if I can so arrange.

The interpretations given during the session depend upon the material and the situation of the patient in question, even if the other patients should not be as far progressed as this particular one. The physician does not refrain from generalizing and expanding on material which has come to the surface. It is obvious that the analysis of ideologies which are a comparatively higher socialized experience will play an important part in the discussion of these groups. The general problems of sex will naturally appear again and again. It is important that the individual genesis of any ideology should be made as clear as possible to the patient himself and to the group. Obviously, the goals and aims of the individual, his attitude towards the future, have to be considered under the same aspect. The situation naturally gives a preponderance to the analyst which the patients may resent. He has to account for it, and there is no objection to his bringing forward the one or the other part of his experiences and his own free associations, if he sees fit. A complete freedom of associations of the analyst is neither expected nor desired. I have not seen any objection in having other physicians participate in the group, and I have repeatedly listened with pleasure when other analysts conducted the group, made their interpretations, or completed my own interpretations.

It is obvious that an individual in such a group sees the fundamental identity of his problems with the problems of others. It takes him out of the isolation into which the neurosis has led him. The members of the group easily identify themselves with each other. The fact that one member of the group brings forward material which another very often tries to hide lessens the resistance and brings forward conscious as well as unconscious material. Frequently it is easier to see one's own problem when it is brought forward by another. Any problem of money, occupation, or sex that may be met has its true meaning only in a social setting of which it is a part, and it cannot even be thought of apart from this. It is to be expected that the meaning of any detail of an individual life history will be better delineated if brought forward in a group and appreciated by a group.

The phenomena of positive and negative transference to the analyst were not less outspoken in the group than in the usual psychoanalytic treatment, and a serious attempt was made to bring the patient to an insight into the transference situation. It expressed itself in generally known terms. The reaction of one patient to the transference situation of another patient was very often remarkable. The patient in positive transference felt the need to defend the analyst against the negative transference of another. In the negative transference the group particularly stressed that the physician was not sufficiently interested in their fate and that as a public employee he must spend his hours regardless, and that he was less interested in the fate of the patients than in the scientific problems they offered. Very often, discussions of problems of this type have an important effect on the fate of the group. The physician should freely state his position. He should confess his human and individual interest in the patients, but he cannot deny his scientific interest, or that work is expected from him. The patients can be shown that nobody has the right to expect the complete emotional surrender of another person, and that the other person has to live his own life even if he should happen to be one's father, mother, sweetheart, wife (husband), or physician. The physician has to emphasize, when the occasion arises, that his natural superiority in the group is merely a result of the particular task and the particular situation. This situation should not be used to push the other into an inferior position. The fundamental equality of the physician with any one member of the group, and equality of members of the group, should be stressed.

I have so far avoided mixing the sexes in the group, for obvious reasons. When the technique is worked out more in detail there should be no serious obstacles to trying to see persons of different sexes in one group. I have occasionally done so in smaller groups, when the female patient had been analyzed for a long time and had a comparatively good insight into the fundamental problems. Social contacts between the members of the group outside of their regular meetings were neither encouraged nor discouraged. They were the exception.

I do not put any limitation in time on the duration of a treatment. The patient comes as long as he feels that he is not completely adapted to his situation. The disappearance of symptoms is never considered as a sufficient reason to give up the treatment, unless the physician feels that the infantile history and the present situation are sufficiently elucidated and that the patient knows what his purpose in life is. On the other hand, no necessity is felt to force the patient to go on with the treatment when a social adaptation and insight have been reached, even when details of the early history remain unsolved. It is felt that only comparatively severe neuroses should be treated in such a group. The results with social neuroses and obsession neuroses have been particularly beneficial. The results in anxiety neurosis cases were very good. The majority of depersonalization cases were benefited, though not sufficiently, but there were some cures. Character problems could be brought to solution. Only some of the cases of hysteria treated, which were very severe, were influenced. No results were obtained in depressions of the manic-depressive group. There was one astonishing result in a case of schizophrenia, concerning the diagnosis of which there were no doubts when the treatment started. Other cases were influenced; many cases could not be influenced at all. This is not a definite recommendation but a hint as to the usefulness of the method.

One may object to the method on the ground that it is too intellectual. I believe in the power of the intellect. I think that patients have to learn many things in every psychotherapeutic procedure. Furthermore, the patients show very deep emotions in no way less powerful than those experienced in individual psychoanalysis. It is unquestionable that in many cases, perhaps even in the majority of cases, individual psychoanalysis may be the more efficient method. However, there are cases in which material comes forward in the group which does not come out in the individual treatment. There is, furthermore, a group of patients who are so strongly repressed and bring forward such scarce material in individual treatment that one has to try to decrease the resistance by their participation in the group. There is the further advantage that a single physician can treat a greater number of patients and fulfill social obligations which he otherwise would have to neglect. I have so far made unsystematic attempts to use this approach on psychiatric wards and to discuss problems of one patient in front of a group. As far as I can ascertain, the results were beneficial and there was progress in the adaptation of the patients to each other on the ward and in their relation to the physician. Most of the individual problems brought out in psychotherapy lose their magnitude when presented before a group and recognized as common to every member of it. It is obvious that the group activities on the wards should be conducted in this spirit of self-expression and of revealing one's hidden problem. The children's ward in Bellevue Psychiatric Hospital is conducted by L. Bender with such an attitude, with excellent results.

I have devised a number of questionnaires which indicate the fundamental problems involved in this procedure. One should keep in mind that these questionnaires, which state the questions with absolute frankness, can be understood only by the experienced and cannot be put in the hands of the patient. They are merely a guide for the physician who has to give them, in the discussion with the patient, in the form which is appropriate to the patient and the degree of his insight. I have added to these questionnaires some general remarks of orientation for the physician which indicate not the solution of the problem but the way in which the problem can be utilized in the group discussion.

The questionnaires are arranged in the following way:

1. *Relation to other persons.*
2. *Relation to one's own body.*
3. *Relation to the functions of one's own body.*
4. *The attitude towards oneself as a psychic personality.*
5. *One's social functions and relations.*
6. *Two special questionnaires on aggressiveness and death.*

One will realize that these questionnaires not only ask for memories, phantasies, and associations; they also ask for opinions and convictions. A questionnaire of course addresses itself, even if orally administered as it should be in this case, to the clear conscious thinking of the individual; but it is obvious that when we do not interrupt but let the individual talk on after the question, we shall soon come to material which the individual generally hides from himself. Clarence Day's *God and Father,* for instance, describes very well the religious ideology of the wealthy middle class. It should be easy, even if one merely uses logical reasoning, to find the flaws of ideologies and so force the individual to the question of how he happened to develop such an ideology. It is, furthermore, obvious that the ideologies lead into the social aspect of the individual's life. They are a part of the social life which has not been less standardized than the products of custom and material culture; instruments, furniture, buildings, churches, art, food habits, clothes, are in some way indicators of ideologies no longer fully alive. The product of an ideology may survive after the ideology as such has changed. It is true, of course, that ideologies may be survivals of attitudes which have long ago lost their adaptation to the situation.

1. *Relation to other persons*

a. Father and mother. It is obvious that the relation to one's father is one of the most important parts of every individual's life. The economic status of the family is usually dependent on him. He and the mother constitute the first social reality for the child. The child sees things not only with his own eyes but also with the eyes of the parents. Every child has two realities before him: the one which he perceives, and the other which is transmitted by the parent. Many persons, in their later lives, do not see anything in the world independently but always in relation to their parents. The parents are important transmitters of reality, especially in its social aspect, even before the child has identified himself with father and mother and has made them a part of himself (superego).

It is obvious that the child does not see the parents as spiritual entities. It has a relation to them as persons with a body. Obviously, the child has to overrate the power and influence of the parents, who have a command over the real things which the child cannot achieve. In the earlier stages of development father and mother are, therefore, endowed with magic powers. They generally remain objects of admiration even when the belief in their magic power has vanished from the foreground of consciousness. The child is naturally interested in the body of the parents, since it needs a somatic gratification by the action of the parents. It needs love by stroking. The parts of the body which have a specific capacity to provoke strong sensations of erotic type (erogenic zones) will naturally be objects of interest on the bodies of others, particularly since the erotic feelings (in the widest sense) are to a large measure provoked by the care and caresses of the parents. The parents in this way become erotic love objects. According to Freud, we have reason to believe that the erotic interest of boy and girl is primarily directed towards the mother, who is in closer contact with the child. At this time, naturally, the importance of the genital organs is not yet fully established. When the sexual organs start to play a more important part, which generally happens around the age of three, the erotic interest may be directed chiefly towards a person as similar as possible to oneself, and we may call this primitive relation homosexual, if we are aware that an infantile act and attitude cannot be identical with the same attitude in the different organization of the adult.

It is furthermore obvious, and proved by experience, that children are insatiable in the demands for love. Correspondingly, they want to have competitors removed. To be away and to be dead mean the same for the child. Since the child does not believe in complete annihilation, it may wish also to destroy the competitor for a while. This is called the homosexual phase of the Oedipus complex. With further development, the interest of the boy in the mother and the girl in the father is increased and the sexual interest is now directed towards the parent of the other sex, the rivalry and the death wish towards the parent of the same sex. The questions concerning father and mother and other persons try to help the patient reach an insight into these important relations which have a social and a sexual side. It is important not to overlook the somatic side. Attitudes in later life are very often closely related to such early attitudes. Every human being has to be in some relation to his parents; every individual has an Oedipus complex. Of course the child shares the general human quality of wanting the love objects (and both parents are love objects) intact. It may also have some insight into the possibility or inappropriateness of its desires. Fears of retaliation which may threaten the child, especially in those parts which are particularly valuable from an erotic point of view, may deter it from sexual wishes concerning the parents.

According to Freud, the Oedipus complex is even destroyed in later development. Its destruction is more complete in the boy. However, it is rather difficult to understand how a psychic structure should be destroyed. I do not believe in a destruction of psychic experiences. We see that attitudes which have lost their inner meaning are reorganized and subordinated to other units. We might also suspect that after a certain degree of maturity is reached, the individual may try to find his own solutions in a larger world. This discussion has chiefly followed Freud's ideas but puts a greater emphasis on the social situation of the child.

Such general remarks, to which instances may be added, may be still more popularized for use in discussions which have the following questions as a basis:

What do you remember about the body of your father?
What do you remember about the sex parts of your father?
What do you remember about the anus of your father?

Were you impressed by another part of your father's body?
Did you ever compare your sex parts with his?
What are your first memories of your father?
Can you remember what he looked like?
Was your father kind or severe?
Did your father hit you?
In what other way have you been punished?
Which acts of kindness do you remember?
Which caresses do you remember?
Did you ever sleep with your father?
Did you admire your father?
Did you see your father sick?
Did you see your father dead?
Did your father ever touch your sex parts?
Did your father ever touch your anus?
Did your father touch your breasts?
Did your father ever touch any other parts of your body?
Did you ever see your father during intercourse?
Did you ever see your father urinate?
Did you ever see your father defecate?
Did you see any other act of your father which impressed you?
Did you think your father was strong?
Did you think your father was good-looking?
Did you think your father was gifted?
Did you and do you love your father? and why?
Did you ever hate your father? and why?
Were you ever afraid of your father?
Were you afraid that he might look at you?
Were you afraid that he might hit you?
Were you afraid that he might hurt you?
Were you afraid that he might hurt your sex parts?
Did your father ever scold you?
Did you ever wish to have sex relations with your father?
Did any sexual scene ever take place between you and your father?
Did you ever wish to kill your father?
Did you ever wish to hit your father?
Did you ever wish to be loved by your father?
Did you ever wish to be seduced by your father?
Did you ever wish to be hurt by your father?

Did you ever wish to be punished by your father?
Did you ever think that your father was not your real father?
Did you ever wish to have another father?
Did you ever want to help your father?
Did you ever give any presents to your father?
Were you interested in the well-being of your father?

You have been asked, so far, concerning actual memories and wishes. Report also about any phantasies you may have had about any one of these points. Report also about any present opinions and wishes concerning your father in any one of these points.

Naturally, the same questions have to be asked about the mother. Special attention should be given to the question of the breasts of the mother and, furthermore, to the question of being within the body of the mother.

b. Siblings. It is furthermore obvious that the same or similar questions may be asked about any person with whom one has been associated. If one investigates the relations to siblings one has to give particular attention to the question of sibling rivalry, and has to take into consideration that the relation concerning the sibling should also be investigated from the point of view of what relations were supposed to exist between the sibling and other persons, especially the patient. There can be no question that sibling rivalry plays a very important part. L. Bender has reported a boy who from the moment of the birth of another child, when he was eighteen months old, showed violent aggression against the other child. He not only tried to kill this other child but from this moment on showed hate against the mother.

Sexual plays between children are natural. Unless prohibited, they start to explore the body of the other sibling. Tendencies of this kind are not only present in earliest childhood but may extend into later periods. In one of the groups this question came up, and among five patients present who had sisters, every one remembered, since the report of one patient relieved the resistances of the other, that there were interests in the bodies of their sisters and they had displayed sexual interests by peeping and acting. In one case, an attempted intercourse at the age of six, about which the mother found out, played a very important part. The mother told the grandmother about this, and the patient felt that she had given him up completely. Whenever this scene was touched upon, the patient showed great emotion. He felt deserted by everybody, which was a psychological factor in the development of the depersonalization picture in the frame of a probable schizophrenic psychosis. One should not forget, however, that the patients have a genuine interest in the well-being even of siblings against whom their rivalry is directed, and that the sexual interest in the sibling is in no way their only interest.

c. Children. As mentioned, it is sometimes difficult to get a deeper insight into the attitude of the parents towards their children. In obsession neurosis cases, the hostile impulses towards the children very often become paramount. This is also true in depressions. The subject of parent-child hostility has been discussed, for example, by Zilboorg. One should not forget to ask how much gratification the parents expect from their children. However, they also have a genuine interest in their existence and well-being as independent entities. The patient L. demands that she should love her children continually. She has symptoms of compulsion concerning the children, and has obsessions and compulsions of killing them. She has a great interest in the body of her daughter, whom she admires inordinately and of whom she is jealous. Unfulfilled homosexual wishes thus find their expression. She dislikes the sex part of her son and also his reddish pubic hair. This is in close relation to attitudes she has concerning the male sex organ.

Did you want a boy or a girl as a child? Why?
What pet names did you give to your children?
When did you first wish to have a child?
Why did you want to have a child?
Why is it good for parents to have children?
What do you expect from your children?
Do you want to help your children or do you want to be helped by them?
Are your children good-looking?
Are your children gifted?
Do you want to have them good-looking or gifted?
Do you want your children to be rich, famous, happy?
Do you worry about the health of your children?
About which part of their bodies are you particularly concerned?
Do you worry about the gifts of your children?

Are you interested in the sex parts of your children?
What do you think about their defecation and urination?
Did you ever check the sex activities of your children?
Did you ever have sexual thoughts about your children?
Did you ever hit your children?
Do you think that one should hit children?
Did you ever want to hurt children?
Did you ever have death wishes against your children?
How should one punish children?
Which is the most enjoyable situation you have had with your children?
Do you want your children to look like your family and you, or like your husband and his family?

d. Animals. There is hardly any psychotherapy in which animals do not make an appearance, as in the case of Gr., for instance. He was bitten by a dog when he was three years old and had wanted to kiss the dog. During his life he has been bitten by animals several times. In his early dreams he was persecuted by men and animals which became larger and larger. The relation to his father is of paramount importance. In one of my obsession neurosis cases the fear of dogs is always in the foreground. In another of my cases, the early family situation is reflected in a dream where he saw three apes. He was probably the third and smallest. He feared the second smallest one, who was obviously an image of the mother. For the child, the animal is probably a magic counterpart of the parent. The probability is that the child also uses it for expressing his ambivalent feelings. The body of the animal is, of course, a source for interesting observations. I reproduce here an autobiographical report I received from a patient whose difficulty, impotency, was obviously coupled with a general lack of interest in sex and early discouragement in sex.

"Surrounded by many domestic birds and animals, as a child, I frequently saw sex activity in animals. Unlike civilized human beings, animals apparently made no attempt at repressing their sex urge.

"Among the first things I recall is the sex activity of the domestic birds: chickens and ducks. The rooster very frequently would chase his beloved object, the hen, who like other females would attempt to run away from the male, but she would not run too far. On catching up with the hen, the rooster would mount her and the entire act of sex would be rapidly performed. I saw two or three body movements and the male would dismount from the conquered female and continue about his business, seeking worms, grain, etc. Not always would the rooster chase after the female (hen) for frequently he would mount when the birds were together at feeding time or while roaming about in groups. I do not recall what my reactions and interpretations of these observations were. I did know that unless the rooster were present in the group of domestic birds, the eggs of the chicken and ducks were not fertile and would not yield chicks or ducks. The sex acts of the cattle, horses and dogs, also were observed. All these animals would begin the so-called sex play with their sense of smell. The male usually smells the tail end, vagina, of the female. Neither the dog nor the bull would usually walk around with his penis visible in an erected state. The male horse, however, frequently did that. I saw these animals in their sex acts, and at an early age. Having been born and lived until the age of twelve on the farm, I cannot date the earliest observations of this sort. However, I think I was aware of these animal activities about the age of seven or eight. I cannot recall, by thinking back, what I may have thought of the sex act of the animals nor do I recall interpreting it in terms of human behavior."

What are your earliest remembrances concerning animals?
Did you play with animals?
Were you ever afraid of animals?
Have you ever had the fear of being eaten by animals?
Were you ever bitten by animals? How many times?
Did you ever torture or tease animals?
Did you ever see others torture or tease animals?
Did you ever see animals urinating?
Did you ever see animals defecating?
What do you think of the udders of a cow?
Did you ever see cows milked?
When did you first hear of the castration of animals?
Did you know the difference between a bull and an ox?
Did you ever compare your sex parts with the sex parts of animals?
Did you ever see the birth of animals?
Did you understand what it meant?
Did you ever see the intercourse of animals?

Did you ever hear that dogs cannot separate in intercourse?
Did you ever see the sex parts of animals?
Did you ever touch them?
Did you ever pet animals?
Did you ever have sex relations with animals?
Did you ever phantasy this?
Did you ever compare animals with human beings?
Did you ever imagine that a person looked like an animal?
Did you ever dream of animals?
Did you ever have phantasies of animals?
How do you feel about touching animals?
Do you feel any disgust for animals—e. g., rats, mice?
How do you feel about insects?
Do you like snakes?
How do you feel about worms?
Did you ever think one ought not to kill animals and eat them?
What do you think of eating animals?
Are there any animals which you particularly dislike eating?
Did you ever wish to slaughter animals?
Is killing a dog or horse more painful than killing insects?
How did you react to the story of Jonah and the whale?
Did you ever think animals had magic powers?

2. *Relation to one's own body*

What do you think about your own strength?
What do you think about your own beauty?
What do you think about your own health?
How strongly are you sexed?
How many characteristics of the other sex do you have?
Are your own sex characteristics outspoken?
What do you think of your future development?
Will you age early?
What does beauty consist of?
Which is the most important part of the body?
What do you think about your head?
What do you think about your eyes?
What do you think about your nose?
What do you think about your mouth and teeth?

What do you think about your chest?
What do you think about your abdomen?
What do you think about your bosom?
What do you think about your buttocks?
What do you think about your sex parts (penis, testicles, vulva, vagina, womb)?
What do you think about your arms and legs?
What do you think about your hands and feet?
What do you think about your skin and complexion?
What do you think about your lungs and your breathing?
What do you think about your digestion, stomach, and anus?
What do you think about your potency and quantity of semen?
What do you think about your menstruation?
What do you think about your faculty of having intercourse and orgasm?
What do you think about your faculty of having children?
What do you think about urination?
What do you think about your sense (seeing, hearing, smelling, tasting) organs?
Which part of your body is most beautiful?
Which part of your body is most ugly?
Which part of your body is best in function?
Which part of your body is worst in function?
What do you think about your mind?
What do you think about your memory?
What do you think about your emotions?

We have furthermore to ask not only what are his opinions, but whether the individual has developed any phantasies about any one of these parts of the body and any one of these functions, and in addition, whether there are any remembrances concerning earlier attitudes in relation to any of these items.

a. Castration complex. Every individual wants to preserve the integrity of his own body. Parts which are particularly valuable are naturally especially cared for. The sex parts belong to them. One generally sees that boys have a very great interest in their penis, in its color and in its size. This becomes particularly obvious when one is confronted with a group of patients. All of them are also inclined to compare the size of their own sex organs with the sex organs of adults, especially with the sex organ of the father. Competitions in urination concerning the stream of urine may follow. For instance, the patients Gr., P., and Sch. saw their father's penis and were appalled by its size. Perl. realized the size of his father's penis, too, but did not give much attention to it. The fact remains remarkable, since children mostly do not wonder at the difference in size concerning other organs. Only P. was also interested in his father's feet, which were large, and hoped he would have the same size feet when he grew older. However, the size of the feet has a symbolic significance of power to P. P. is abnormally small, almost a dwarf, and feels continually attacked by stronger forces. The interest in the size of the penis may be partially due to the fact that these parts are usually hidden and also show more variations than other parts. B. dreamt once of a copper-colored snake and showed in his subsequent associations a great interest in his penis. He would like to have his penis lighter, as he has seen it in his cousin. His whole neurosis, in which shyness and sensitivity prevail, centers around his cousin, by whom he feels continually attacked. There is, after all, no part of the body which may not be compared with the body of others according to the total constellation. We are always aware of our own bodies in relation to those of others. I am inclined to believe that one should speak rather about the tendency of preserving the integrity of the body than about castration complex. Psychoanalysis acknowledges pregenital analogies to the castration complex, the fear of losing the intestines or other valuable parts of the body. It has even gone so far as to consider the loss of the nipple of the mother as a castration of the child when it is weaned.

The attitude of psychoanalysis, mainly a man's psychoanalysis, concerning the female castration complex is hard to defend. The little girl, according to Freud, feels castrated from the beginning, since she has no penis. She experiences merely penis envy, and Rado even speaks about the illusory penis the child (girl) produces when she sees her defect; and neurotic complications are supposed to arise from the awareness of the girl that the real or illusory penis is absent. Better observers, like Karen Horney, justly stress that the girl is very soon aware that she has receptive organs. She fears being hurt in these receptive organs. I may add that the fear of occlusion in the female and the fear of being robbed of the container inside of the body are common and point to early fears in this respect. One will not be wrong if one supposes that children, from the earliest ages, are aware of their sexual organs and sexual abilities and have considerable fears concerning them. This is only a specific expression of the general fear of an impairment of the integrity of the body and should not be seen in isolation. Many symptoms have been considered as a symbol of castration, but very often the so-called castration complex as such is a symbol for other difficulties. In the case of B., for instance, the competition with his cousin has very deep roots which are not merely of sexual character and are in close relation to his attempts to gain an appropriate place in the family and in society.

One should furthermore be on guard and not see these general problems merely from the angle of the man. When the girl actually demands to have a male sex organ and male possibilities, the boy demands female organs and female possibilities as well. One finds, in psychoanalytic literature, many theories concerning the early sexual development in boys and girls, and the particular formation of the theory is dependent on the attitude of the analyst concerning the problems of the so-called castration complex. Freud has always stressed that the mother is the first love object for the boy and for the girl. The girl may even want to have a child by the mother. Since this attachment cannot be completely satisfied, hate may result, and the mother emerges as the persecutor who has withheld milk from the child. The final disappointment of the girl, according to Freud, is due to her discovery that she has no male sex organ. Penis envy thus becomes the cardinal point in the psychology of femininity, according to Freud.

He completely overlooks the genuine pride present even in the little girl in her own possibilities. This has been stressed by Karen Horney and myself. Melanie Klein has developed a rather complicated theory according to which the child acknowledges merely a combined father and mother image. The mother has in herself the penis of the father, which both girls and boys try to get for themselves. The child tries to scoop out the inside of the body of the combined father and mother image, take out the milk, the intestines, and the sex parts and wishes to attack with the poisonous weapon at its disposal in feces and urine and with its sex organ or substitute. On the other hand, it fears that it might be attacked and destroyed and robbed of the inside of its body by the same weapons of the parents. I have quoted this rather exaggerated and one-sided formulation in order to show that the so-called castration complex and the fear of dangers, in general, are very closely related to each other.

In discussions in the group psychotherapy, inferences concerning early situations may very often be drawn in connection with fundamental fears concerning sex. One should refrain from one-sided formulations and should see in the human being's attitude towards his sex organs, whether it appeared in later life or in very early childhood, an indication of tendencies concerning the body as a whole and concerning life situations in general. However, no psychotherapy can overlook what an important part the attitudes towards the sex organs play in the psychology of everybody. In this spirit, the following questions concerning castration can be used:

Do you have fears that something may happen to any part of your body?
Are you afraid of being hurt?
Are you afraid of disease?
Which parts of your body are easiest to hurt?

Questions directed to men:

Are you afraid that your penis may get hurt?
Are you afraid that your testicles may get hurt?
Are you afraid that intercourse might harm your sex parts?
Are you proud of your penis?
Do you think that masturbation has harmed your penis and testicles?
Do you think that masturbation has harmed your health?
Do you think that some part of your body is too big or too small?
Are you afraid of the female sex parts?
Do you have a knowledge of the anatomy of the female sex parts?
Are you afraid of the smell of female sex parts?
Do you think there is something missing in the female organs?
Did you ever think that girls have a penis or testicles, too?
When did you find out that girls have different sex parts?
How did you find out about it?
Are you ashamed when somebody sees your sex parts?
How do you react when seeing the sex parts of other men?

Questions directed to women:

Do you feel ashamed of your sex parts?
How do you react when you see the sex parts of other women?
When did you find out that the male sex parts are different?

Did you wish to have a male sex organ?
Did you feel that something was missing in your sex parts?
When did you first find out about your clitoris?
Are you afraid that your sex parts may get hurt? By masturbation?
Are you afraid of a venereal disease?
Do you think that intercourse harms you?
Are you proud of your sex organs?

In the sense mentioned above, the following questions should be answered concerning the fear relating to the integrity of the body:

Are you afraid of being cut to pieces? Do you wish it?
Are you afraid of being hurt? Or of being deprived of any part of the body?
Do you feel threatened by superior forces of nature? (Storm, hail, snow, earthquake, thunder and lightning, world destruction.)
Are you afraid of machinery? (Autos, fire engines, locomotives.)
Are you afraid of superior man-power? (God, Devil, giant, boxer, father, mother, brother, sister, bully, racketeer, Chinese, Italian, Catholic, Jew.)

3. *Relation to the functions of one's own body*

a. Masturbation. The problems of masturbation are, of course, in very close relation to the problems of the castration complex. It is today generally maintained that masturbation is not harmful in itself, but is merely a symptom; we mostly inform our patients, who very often come loaded with feelings of guilt concerning masturbation, that there is nothing wrong about it and, furthermore, that no harm either to the sex organs or to the health in general can come from it. It is questionable whether this attitude is completely correct. Masturbation is at any rate an escape from the actual problems of sex, and is at least indicative of an undesirable human incompleteness. It is, in addition, questionable whether the continuation of such an attitude may not be an expression of difficulties in further development. Without losing the general attitude of tolerance, the patient should be informed about the physician's attitude to the problem. The first awakening of sex may occur in this primitive form, and masturbation may then indicate progress, but it should never be more than a passing phase in progress. Many patients complain about all kinds of physical discomfort after masturbation and after wet dreams. We have not the right to deny the physiological basis of such complaints, although they are obviously modified by fears in connection with the castration complex and by the feelings of guilt. Undoubtedly, masturbation is an act physiologically different from intercourse, and this should not be denied in a discussion with the patient.

We are, of course, very much interested in what masturbation stands for. Phantasies and drives of various levels may find their expression in it. Masturbation phantasies can be (in the case of a temporary difficulty in getting other gratifications) of the adult type; they may belong to the Oedipus complex; they may also belong to homosexual, oral, anal, and sadistic experiences. They may, further, be of such a primitive type that no formulation in phantasies is possible. It is sometimes very difficult to get a report about these masturbation phantasies. We generally have the opinion that masturbation in puberty and later life originates from the earlier masturbation which is in connection with infantile problems. Freud therefore stresses, justly, that the patients are right when they ascribe importance to their masturbation. Masturbation should, therefore, be treated as a symptom. The way in which a patient masturbates may be indicative of fundamental attitudes concerning sex and masculinity. The masturbator very often plays in his masturbatory action, not only his part, but also the part of the love object. The following questions arise:

When did you masturbate first?
Under what circumstances?
Were you taught to do so or did you find it out for yourself?
How do you masturbate?
Do you use your hands?
Do you press your legs together?
Do you rub against objects?
Do you put your fingers on the clitoris (girl)?
Do you introduce your finger into the vagina (girl)?
Do you touch your penis (boy)?
Do you touch any other part of your body (nipples, anus)?
Do you hurt yourself during masturbation?
Are you afraid to hurt yourself during masturbation?
What phantasies do you have in masturbation?

What psychic process goes on in you before masturbation?
How do you feel after masturbation?

We are of course, as always, interested in the following categories: *a.* present opinion; *b.* memories and past opinions; *c.* present and past phantasies. If mutual masturbation has taken place we shall also be interested in the distribution of action between the two partners and the complications arising from it.

b. Intercourse. Nietzsche once said that the sexuality of human beings expresses their highest and their lowest possibilities. We should say the same about intercourse as such. An intercourse is never an isolated act. It is difficult to separate the physical from the spiritual side. The human attitude one has towards the sex partner is of fundamental importance. Furthermore, the preliminary play, the gaining of the love object, the attitude after the intercourse, can only be artificially separated from intercourse itself. We are here merely interested in gaining insight into what we have to know about the intercourse of a patient in the course of a psychotherapy. We have to keep in mind that intercourse unites the manifold strivings of an individual in one act. It is in some ways the highest expression in the body of which a person is capable. Freud has justly pointed to the fact that the preliminary acts and the preliminary play run through almost all infantile part functions of sexuality. There are no norms about intercourse as far as we can see, if only intercourse ends in the union of genitals which may potentially lead to fertilization. Feelings of guilt connected with techniques which deviate from an artificial but socially approved ideal of normal intercourse are common. If the physician has to discuss these problems with the patient he must be careful that he says what he actually thinks and that he has sufficient knowledge about sex problems not to fall into rigid pseudomoral evaluations.

One should not believe that intercourse as such has a curative function. It depends upon what degree of human adaptation is expressed in intercourse. If the individual has no regard for the function as such, and for the love object, it does not mean very much whether he has intercourse or not. It is obvious that full adaptation includes sexual adaptations and intercourse as its essential parts. There are only very few situations in human life where the outward circumstances make such an adaptation impossible for a long stretch of time. It is the task of psychotherapy to investigate carefully whether the circumstances actually warrant continence. If not, the patient has to find out in the course of the psychotherapy what has driven him away from sex.

Many neurotics are astonished that after having performed intercourse they are still neurotic. One cannot even say that all of them have an incomplete orgasm. Obsession neurotic cases especially, but also even depressions of a severe degree, may have a satisfactory intercourse from a physical point of view and it will not help them at all. One should never consider sex merely as a physical problem but as a psychosexual phenomenon. The problems of intercourse can, therefore, be understood only in connection with the problems of love. On the other hand, the problems of love can only be understood when the sexual and physiological part of the situation is taken fully into consideration. It is obvious that not every love relation will exhaust the ultimate human possibilities of the participants. Dissociations are common, especially in men. They are, under the present conditions, socially fully acknowledged and it would be one-sided to say that sex gratification without deeper attachment is not possible.

This also happens in women, although social convention is less favorable for women to have this kind of sensual satisfaction. It is very often difficult for the analyst not to infuse his own moral standards into the situation. The fanaticism of morality has to be avoided, as well as the fanaticism of immorality. Generally, it will be necessary to let the patient find his own way in a matter which is so complicated that the person has to find his individual law by some kind of experimentation. The ideal of the complete love and sex experience conforms, to all appearances, with the reality, and there is no reason why the patient should not be informed in this respect.

What ideas do you have about intercourse?
What was your reaction to your first intercourse?
How often do you have intercourse now?
With how many persons have you had intercourse so far?
To which sex did they belong?
Where are your strongest sensations localized?
How great is the enjoyment of intercourse in comparison with other enjoyments?
What conditions add to your enjoyment?

What conditions decrease your enjoyment?
What variation from the so-called normal position do you use?
Do you like to spend much time in the preliminary play before intercourse?
What are your thoughts during intercourse?
What are your thoughts after intercourse?
What other sex play do you enjoy?
Do you like to kiss the nipples, mouth, sex parts, anus, or any other parts of your sex partner?
Do you like to be kissed on any of these parts?
Do you like to inflict any kind of pain on your partner?
Do you like to experience any type of pain from your partner?
Do you like to play a more active or passive part?
Do you like your partner to play an active or passive role?
Are you interested in overcoming the resistance of your partner?
Do you appreciate love objects more when the love object has put up a great resistance in either the preliminary phases or immediately before the act?
How often have you been impotent or frigid?
How often did you commit homosexual acts?
How often did you insert your penis into the anus of men?
How often did you insert your penis into the anus of women?

Many questions concerning the different types of perversions could be added. However, it is not necessary to give detailed questions in this respect; they can easily be deducted from the principles evolved here.

c. and *d. Urinary and anal tendencies.* In almost every psychotherapy interests of the patient in urination and defecation become obvious. Children are naturally curious about what comes out of their bodies. The sensations connected with these functions have at least some similarity to sexual function. After all, urination is anatomically very closely related to organs which serve sex, and the defecation uses an opening very near to the sex openings. Most of the parents acknowledge the close relation between sex, urination, and defecation in so far as they display a unified attitude towards all these functions. In repressed families, modesty concerning sex and excretion is preached with the same religious fervor.

B. thought, as a child, that during the sex relations the man had to fill the crack of the woman with urine and to fill the woman's bag (bladder). Another of my patients (around the age of four) thought that sexual relations consisted of urinating at each other's genitals, and she induced a little boy to do so. The first patient is the one interested in the size of his penis and participating in urinary plays of competition. In many individuals, sexual excitement expresses itself in a urinary urge, as for instance in the patient T., who writes as follows in her autobiography: "I don't know how old I was when I learned to masturbate with the girl next door. It seems that I was around twelve. Now it seems to me that it must have been earlier. She had a younger sister whom she would be stationed to take care of. In the evening after supper we would sit on the back porch and start to tell stories. Then when it was dark enough, my friend and I would masturbate each other. I don't remember what the stories were of. I think they were about kings, queens and castles and about King Arthur. I know that my imagination was fertile and that I could go on endlessly, a gift I have since lost completely. I didn't know what masturbation was. The orgasm was associated in my mind with an intense desire to urinate. I think that's what I thought it was: inducing myself to need to urinate. I felt that I was doing something wrong and was petrified that my mother might catch us. . . . Roughly contemporary with the masturbation, this girl and I became interested in exploring each other's bodies, exploring each other's breasts, watching each other going to the toilet to try to discover just where the urine came from."

I could multiply the instances very easily. The question is, what deeper significance do urinary experiences have? A function occurring so often must of course give cause for many observations and speculations. That could be merely an intellectual operation which is fascinating since it is quite difficult to understand urination and its many variations. The urine has, furthermore, qualities of a part of the body and must have, in connection with this, narcissistic and erotic value. Urine is a base and smelly substance, and must provoke accordingly a tendency of rejection whenever any state of cultural adaptation is reached. The disgust concerning excreta is a rather general phenomenon in all cultures. Even if urination and defecation (for which the same considerations are valid) should not have any sexual tinge (which they have), they should be of psychological importance, since cultural and esthetic rejection and infantile evaluation of body products (and curiosity) contradict each other. However, there can be little doubt that there is not only a topographical relation to the sex parts but also a deep similarity between the local sensations of sex, defecation and urination.

In spite of all this, urinary and anal sensations point merely into the past. Sexual sensations point as well from the cultural as from the individual point of view into the future. Furthermore, urination as well as defecation is, basically, an individual business. Sex is a social one. The following questions arise concerning *c. urine:*

What is urine?
In what way are urine and semen different?
Where does it come from in men and in women?
Do you like the smell of it?
What is your first memory concerning urination?
Did you ever compare your urination with that of another boy or girl?
Do you think that urine is dirty?
How often did you wet yourself?
Up to what time?
What do you think of fellows who wet their beds?
When did you find out that the other sex urinates with a different organ?
Did you ever see your father, mother, etc., urinating?
What did you think of it?
Did you try to see others urinate?
Do you urinate more when you are sexually excited?
Did you ever urinate with another boy or girl?
Did you ever try to find out who can urinate farther?
Do you think you have more urine than others?
Did you ever extinguish fire by urinating?
What happens to a person who cannot urinate?
Do you think that urine is poisonous?
What were your phantasies about any of these subjects?

d. Anal problem:

Do you want to be alone on the toilet?
Do you want to have somebody with you?
What are feces?
Are feces poisonous?

Do you like the smell of feces?
Could you eat feces?
Do you look at them?
How often do you think of feces and defecation?
How often should one have bowel movements?
What quantity of feces should one have?
Are you interested in the consistency of fecés?
What are your first memories of feces and bowel movements?
Did you ever see animals, mother, father, etc., defecate?
Did you ever play with feces?
Did you ever play with your anus or the anus of another person?
Do you look at your feces after defecation?
Would it be nicer if human beings could live without defecating?
How often do you think of defecation of others?
Does sitting on the toilet diminish your interest in the esteem of others?
What happens if one cannot defecate?
Do you feel very bad when you are constipated?
Do you enjoy bowel movements?
Do you like to hold back bowel movements?

Psychoanalysis has often stressed the symbolic relation between money, possessive instincts, and feces. The relation is decidedly present, but this is only one side of the situation. The interest in money and possessions is closely associated with the wish for power. Furthermore, the interest in feces may very well be a symbol for possessive instincts. There is no reason why the intestines and the desires connected with them should be more important than human tendencies which express themselves in the muscular system.

e. Breasts. Nietzsche somewhere calls the woman's bosom useful and agreeable. Being a secondary sex characteristic, it is an important part of the body of a sex object. But furthermore, it is the organ by which the organism of the mother expresses its preparedness to care for the young. When the young is nursed it does not merely experience a gratification of hunger but it experiences protection and love also, expressed immediately in physical sensations. Since the mother also experiences corresponding impressions, the bosom becomes the expression of an important interhuman relation between mother and child, and it will also appear so in the sexual relation between man and woman. It is astonishing how little men know about the function of the breast. In a group of six men present in one session, no one had any clear conception about the connection between lactation and pregnancy and birth. The following questions may be formulated:

Have you been breast fed or bottle fed?
Can you remember being nursed?
Can you remember ever seeing anybody nursed? Siblings, or others?
What were your feelings about nursing? What are your feelings now?
What do you think of female breasts?
What do you think of nipples?
Do you want to handle breasts? Kiss them?
Do you ever want to hurt breasts?
Do you ever want to cut off breasts?
How do you react to horror stories of this kind?
Do you think breasts contribute to your beauty?
When did you first learn of the function of breasts?
What part do the breasts have in your sex play?
a. active; b. passive.
Do you get sexually excited when your breasts are touched by a man? woman? child?

f. Birth. We owe to analysis the insight that the thoughts of human beings are deeply concerned with the problem of birth. It is the beginning of life and miraculous in this respect. It is the most astonishing expression of the phenomenon of growth. It is a mysterious relation between one's self and another person, and thus it may become the symbol for the most important situations in life in general. No wonder that birth phantasies and their symbolizations play such an important part in every human being's life. Rank has formulated a theory that the trauma of birth is the deepest trauma in human life and that culture in individual life attempts to overcome this original trauma. Such statements are, of course, one-sided. I have often pointed to the fact that in psychic experience the one situation might be a sign or a symbol for another situation. An important event like birth might, of course, serve in similar capacity. There is no use denying the variety of life situations. In addition we have no immediate experiences of our own birth—at least they cannot be ascertained. We have experiences in relation to mother and father and their love. We have experiences about separation and about danger.

Every elaborate sign system or theory of symbolizations should take into consideration that it is very often difficult to find out what symbolizes what. There is no question that many patients symbolize their problems under the picture of birth. To start all over again, to regain one's independence from one's parents or from one's analyst, is very often seen under the symbol of birth. Tunnels, caves, houses, water from which one emerges may serve as picture material. The wish to go back to a position of security in the protection of the mother or of a former love object may appear as a wish to go back to the womb of the mother. Psychoanalysis has been one-sided in taking the body as the only constant of human life. The wish for security is as original as the wish to go back to the womb of one's mother. There are also practical problems connected with childbirth. Economic and social considerations originating in another sphere of psychological attitudes may influence one's wish of either having children or not having them. Since pregnancy and birth are connected with pain, discomfort, and danger, the woman's attitude toward these will be of importance. The following questions may arise:

Did you ever see the birth of a human being? an animal?
Did you ever hear someone tell of a birth?
What do you remember about the birth of your siblings?
Do you understand the mechanism of birth?
Where did you think children came from, when you were small? At the present time?
Did you ever think mating had something to do with it?
Did you ever think children came out by the mouth? anus? or a cut through the abdomen?
When did you first hear something about the uterus?
Do you think you are able to give birth to a child?
Were you ever afraid that you were not able to?
How many children do you want, and how many did you want?
Did you ever have phantasies about these topics?
What do you think of abortion? What are your experiences with it?
What do you think of birth control? Methods of birth prevention?
What do you think of operations which permanently prevent childbirth?
What is sperm?
Do you (men) think you are capable of having children?

Do you think birth is painful?
Are you afraid of giving birth to a child? by Caesarean section?
Are you afraid of dying in childbirth?
Do you or did you ever resent the fact that women have to bear children?
Should one use analgesia during birth?
Do you want to nurse your children? Have you done so? Did you enjoy doing so?
Do you fear that bearing children will spoil your beauty?
Do you fear that bearing children will make intercourse less enjoyable?
Do you believe that it would hinder any career that you planned?
Do you believe that children would hinder or aid your relationship to your husband (wife)?

g. Disease. L. H. Ziegler and J. Heyman have pointed to the incomplete information and wrong ideas human beings have concerning diseases. They have furthermore shown that such misconceptions might serve as the basis for symptom formation. A disease is not merely the experience of one person; it also implies a social situation of great importance. One cannnot go through the history of any human being without finding diseases as important turning points in their own attitudes or in the attitudes of others towards them. A case of anxiety neurosis who suffered from the lack of affection when he was healthy, but received a great amount of affection when he was sick, reacted with palpitations and even extrasystoles whenever he felt that his claims for consideration were too much neglected. I have found that operations have a very deep effect on children—tonsillectomy, for instance. It constitutes an enormous threat. The preceding chapters, especially Chapters 1 and 2, bring further material. The following questions point to the problems involved:

When did you first hear something about disease in your life?
Was anybody in your family ever sick when you were small? (Father, mother, siblings, others.)
Did you ever hear anybody in your family talk about disease?
Which disease was most talked about in your family?
What did your family think diseases came from? From masturbation? From too many sex relations? From overindulgence in eating? From constipation? From being dirty?

Which diseases were dangerous according to the opinion of your family?
What did your family do when somebody in your family got sick?
What were the measures taken?
In what way did the behavior of the parents change?
Which of your own diseases do you remember?
How did you like to be sick, as a child? At present?
How often did you play sick, to get something?
Did you suffer very much when you were sick?
How did you (and how do you) react to pain?
How often do you feel fatigued?
When do you stay in bed?
Do you like to stay in bed?

h. Food habits. There is a great tendency in human beings to punish themselves by dieting. In depressions, this is merely exaggerated. The depressive case punishes himself, for his aggression and oral greed, by not eating. I have seen at least one case which showed this connection from the other side. The patient developed, after dieting and in close relation to it, a depression. For the child, the food is the essence of life and is the inside of the body. Not eating is a destructive tendency directed against the body. Dieting may become the symbol and the expression of the denial of sex. Denying oneself the kind of food one likes is the most primitive type of asceticism. The appetite of children is almost insatiable. Left to themselves, they eat a great deal more than they can stand. The feeling of satiation is not a reliable guide. The child is prevented from his gluttony by the adult and by the pain and discomfort after culinary excesses. It is not apparent which kind of food is digestible and which is not. That must be found by experimentation. It is very often difficult to determine what kind of food is good for health. Human beings are, therefore, in a continuous quandary as to what they should eat and what they should not eat. They are mostly guided by contradictory ideologies, habits, personal complexes, and the symbolic value of the different foodstuffs in their final choice of food, although physiological needs and reactions constitute the basic layer.

Mrs. Sch., suffering from an anxiety neurosis, has in addition accepted a dietary system which restricts food to the utmost, the details of which are not of interest for us. She denies herself food in the same way as she denies herself the full gratification of a sex relation with her husband and the freedom of motility, but she tyrannizes her husband and son through her diet. Oral wishes and desires were obviously strong in her childhood. In primitive society, diet is very often regulated by the scarcity of food. In the progressing civilization, with plenty of foodstuffs at hand, the instinctual indicators of how much and how often we should eat and what we should eat are no longer reliable. The instinct has to be continually guided by scientific and intellectual reasoning, for which the data at hand are, in spite of the great progress made, still meager. The problem is well characterized in an article by R. E. Remington in the *Scientific Monthly,* 1936. Food habits are dependent to a great extent on our surroundings. Our adaptability to new food decreases rapidly with advancing age. The following questions may be asked:

What do you eat?
Which meal is the most important for you?
What food do you prefer?
Have your food habits changed?
How is your appetite?
How many hours can you go without eating?
Can you stand hunger?
How do you like milk?
How much do you eat?
Do you think you eat enough?
Do you think you eat too much?
In what way does food influence the organism?
What is the ideal diet, according to your opinion?
What do you think about a glutton?
Should one indulge in food or should one try to restrict the intake of food?
How do you feel after a good meal? After a bad meal?
How much water do you drink?
Do you drink with every meal?
How much should one drink?
Can you stand thirst?
Which is worse—to be thirsty or to be hungry?

4. *Attitude towards oneself as a psychic personality*

Thanks to psychoanalysis, we know a great deal about symbolizations of the body, and body functions. The implication in analysis is that one should merely consider the somatic functions as important, but the self and the body are not opposites. They are merely different sides of the same basic life function. It is, therefore, absolutely justifiable to consider all problems from the point of view of the self, its opinions, its goals and purposes. One can justly say that every somatic function of an organism points into the future and has a meaning in its being directed towards the outward world. Unfortunately, we know very little about the goals in human life and the systems of goals. The following questionnaires have, therefore, a still more preliminary character than the previous ones, but even in this incomplete form they have helped me and the patients to a rather considerable degree in coming to an orientation and to an increase of insight into the situation. I repeat a paragraph from a previous communication based upon the discussion in a group.

B., twenty-one years old, has a severe social neurosis which causes him to withdraw from contact with others, to have severe feelings of insufficiency, and his speech is actually hesitant. He occasionally stammers when he checks impulses of rage which are directed against those who, he believes, ridicule him. There were developed excessive ambitions to overcompensate for his feeling of being threatened. In school games he did not want to be on the losing team. His interest in auto races and all speed races involving motor-driven vehicles seems to make him feel that their force is added to his. He does not like sports in which he is dependent only upon his own ability.

E., twenty-one years old, with a basal metabolism of minus 23, has felt that he has no energy and no drive. Accordingly, he exerts himself too much, feels bewildered, and then gives up almost completely, until he becomes really inefficient. His sexual energy seems to have little vitality. There were no phantasies and sex impulses when he came for treatment. In spite of a rise in the basal metabolic rate to minus 8, under the influence of thyroid medication, he did not change until the psychotherapy had given him insight into his problem. Sexuality then awakened. The question is, where did he get energy with which to drive himself forward? One may draw the conclusion that human beings should gaily acknowledge their shortcomings. They should be taught neither to overcompensate nor to brush them out of their consciousness. Everyone should be aware of the necessity of having shortcomings. The ideals of general efficiency and striving to be blameless are wrong. One should accept it, if one is a minus variant as a personality. Minus qualities in ourselves and others make us human, and the attempt to be perfect only makes us into caricatures.

F., twenty-one years old, an anxiety neurotic with the fear of sudden death, has no problems of this kind. He lives in an emotional attachment to his mother and brother and expects protection from them against the dangers connected with his own lack of strength. It does not matter here whether this attachment to the mother is sexual or not, but it is important that he has no inferiority feelings in the ordinary sense. There is no reason to believe that there is only one fundamental problem which lies at the basis of neurosis. One should evaluate life situations as human problems in their varieties of expression.

C., twenty-four years old, suffers inferiority and guilt feelings because of obsessional sex drives against children and men, and obsessional aggressions, such as kicking and pushing. He had been forced into this situation by his mother, who overpowered him. If there are feelings of inferiority they are the result of a complicated sexual development. He is very much frightened by his impulses, the strength of which he overrates. Perhaps too much is expected of us in a moral way, and it should be acknowledged that there are impulses which go against the standards of society. One should be lenient with one's own immorality, especially if it harms no one. It is probable that tolerance of one's own impulses does not strengthen them, but reveals them as inefficient and weak; that is, if they do not fit into the structure of the personality and into society.

In W.'s case, nineteen years old, the fight against the father and the protection of the mother against the father (also sexually) are prominent. In his attempt to substitute for father he cultivates intellectuality. He denies himself sexuality because he condemns it in his father and mother. He wants to convince himself and others that he is superior to his father but he is only concerned in having others acknowledge his superiority. He is shy and self-conscious with people who, he believes, give him exaggerated attention.

Modern men suffer from the idea that they should be perfect. They expect health and are unduly perturbed and get excited by minor symptoms. (W. has palpitations when in bed.) There should be patience with one's body, and no fear of being weak and tired. People want to be highly efficient, show speed and energy, when they should have the courage to be slow and adynamic. It is easier to be tolerant towards oneself if no comparison is made with others. Humanity should be considered as consisting of varied types, and those types who are not so gifted are an important part of society as a whole. The imperfect human being is needed as well as the one approaching perfection, and there should be tolerance towards one's own stupidities. The stupid person is more than a mere background for the intelligent.

If humans ask of themselves speed of movement (C. and E.), of speech (B.), and strength (F.), why should one not ask to be beautiful in all the parts of one's body? The perfection sought for oneself is demanded of others, and intolerance ensues. Intolerance is greater towards the members of one's own family; they are expected to be ideal figures and without blemish. They cannot, of course, live up to these images. Parents have to pay dearly for every perfectionistic ideal they put into their children's minds. The child will soon measure his parents against the ideals implanted in him, and find them wanting. When the parents teach their children the suppression of sex, children retaliate by fighting against the sexuality of their parents. Asexuality belongs to the perfectionistic ideals. Sometimes it is expected that sexuality should be awakened only at the conventional signal. Perfectionistic ideals exist not only for physical functions but also for one's strivings, and can be positive as well as negative. One demands, for instance, from oneself and others: (1) absence of hate; (2) a continuous flow of love to one's love object; (3) continuous sexual impulses towards a socially acknowledged love object; (4) absence of promiscuous impulses or sensual impulses in general.

a. Opinions about ourselves

What do you wish that others should think about you?
What impression do you want to make?
Do you want to appear clever, handsome, strong, composed, blasé, experienced, naïve, unsexed, oversexed, or undersexed?
Do you want to be considered as religious?

Which impressions do you actually make in all these respects, according to your opinion?

In what way do others appreciate you?

What is the difference between the impression you make upon others and what you actually are?

How do you judge other people?

How often do you compare others with yourself?

To what type of persons are you particularly attracted?

Do you think you are capable of reading the character of other persons?

How often are you deceived by the mask of shyness of other persons?

How often do other persons want to appear different from what they actually are?

How often are other people unable to express themselves?

How often are other people self-conscious?

What do you think about people who are self-conscious?

Do you think that they are ridiculous?

Do you admire people who talk publicly?

Do you admire actors, salesmen, politicians?

Do you want to influence other people?

Do you want to influence a great crowd by personal contact, or do you desire to influence them in another way?

Do you want to be famous?

How important to you are the opinions of others about yourself?

b. Goals in life

What do you live for, socially, sexually, in the family?

What is the purpose of your life?

What is your destiny?

Why do you not commit suicide? (I have been told that a well-known psychologist submitted this question to the members of a psychological meeting. It is obvious that this question will mostly have to be asked in a modified way and very often will have to be omitted.)

Do you desire fame?

Do you desire success in love?

What does success in love consist of?

With how many women (men) do you want to have intercourse?

With how many women (men) should one have intercourse?

Which type of woman (man) is desirable to you?

What do you think of education?

What is your education?
Do you think your education is what it should be?
Are you well enough informed?
Which subjects did you prefer in grammar school, high school, etc.?
What are you interested in: your work and daily occupation, reading, writing, music, sports, active or passive, politics, science, psychology?
How did your interest develop?
What should you be interested in?
What should others be interested in?
What are your recreations: drinking, company, dancing, sex, art, games, sport, exercise?
Are you efficient?
Do you like to work or are you lazy?
Should one be lazy?
Are you satisfied with yourself?
Do you work on yourself?
Do you think you are what you should be?
Do you think you will ever be what you should be?
What are duties?
Which are your duties?
Who determines what is duty?
Where did you get the rules of your conduct?
Do you think you are responsible to God, to your family, to society?
Should one support oneself or should one take money: from the government? from one's parents? from one's brothers and sisters? from other children? from one's relatives? from one's husband? from one's lover? from one's mistress?
Should one give money to, or support, any one of these persons?
Should one obey laws?
How many laws have you broken so far?
What is the worst crime?
Should one be honest towards everybody?
Should one be kind?
Should one help others?
Have you been honest, kind, and helpful to others?
What is the worst deed you ever committed?
What is the best thing you ever did in your life?
What is sin?
Should one worry in difficult situations?

Should one tackle the problem?
Should one sacrifice one's self?
Did you ever sacrifice anything?
Should parents sacrifice themselves for their children?
Should children sacrifice themselves for their parents?
Should husband and wife sacrifice anything for each other?
Is one allowed to hate and punish others?
Do you believe in punishment?
Do you believe in revenge?
Should a man be masculine?
Should a woman be masculine?
Should a woman be feminine?
Should a man be feminine?
Do you want to have characteristics of the other sex?
What is feminine and masculine: in the body (face, hair, skin, eyes, chest, buttocks, legs)? In spirit and emotion (thinking, feeling, activity, reliability, friendship, love, postures)?
Do you want to be natural?
What does it mean to be natural?
Do you believe in authority, equality, subordination?
Do you want to be a leader, a follower, a comrade? Which are you?
In what form of government do you believe?
How much appreciation do you need?
Do you want to be admired?
Are you afraid of being an object of contempt or indifference?
Do you want to conform to others?
Do you want to stand out in good or in bad?
In what way are you different from others?
Describe a human being as he should be.

c. Work aspect of life. Human beings are always directed towards the world and are never merely passive. They are always constructing. We speak about work when the actions of an individual are of social consequence. We have to differentiate between the act of working and the product. When one goes through the biographies of human beings, one finds that at certain periods of their lives, the result of their activity is of greater consequence than at others. The work is an individual achievement, but it is also in very close relation to the social situation. It is the point where individual strivings, the social situation, and the other outward reality meet. The work history of an individual is, therefore, of particular importance. (Cf. the work of Charlotte Bühler.) One has said that every neurosis manifests itself in the erotic sphere. One might as well say that a neurosis manifests itself also in the sphere of work. The relation of the individual work to culture and surroundings is of fundamental importance. One should not see the work as merely a sublimation of otherwise dangerous instincts; one should see something fundamental in the human drive of re-creating the world. Every life consists of a series of achievements. It is difficult to formulate specific questions which one should ask.

What did you achieve in knowledge and education? What was your school record? What were your achievements in school?
What are the achievements of your life?
Are there periods in your life when you achieve more than at others?
Do you consider it as an achievement when you improve yourself?
Or does an achievement lie merely in action?
Do you want to achieve something in your narrow circle?
Do you want to organize?
Do you want to inspire?
Do you want to be a leader?
What would you like to achieve?

5. *One's social functions and relations*

It is obvious that the relation to oneself, the relation to one's own achievements, is a social function. Even our body is, as I have previously shown, a social function. To speak about social functions and relations, therefore, cannot mean that one speaks about a specific category of experiences, but merely that one approaches the experiences from a specific aspect. One's work, one's attitudes towards one's self, one's social aims, are not merely our own concern. They are everybody's concern. The previous questionnaires were concerned with sex from the point of view of the body, but even with the most worthless love object there is always something spiritual concerning sex. There are no sex problems which are not love problems, too. Impotency, for instance, is far from being a local embarrassment; it indicates a deep difficulty in the inner relation to other persons. The same is true concerning any other type of so-called sexual aberrations.

There is no question that the most complicated ideologies are built up around the problem of love. One may say that the erotic relation puts almost every individual before a test. Many try to escape through various avenues of flight from love and sex in a deeper sense. One may choose a style of life which does not give the opportunity of seeing a sufficiently great number of persons of the other sex. One might have the feeling that one has to take care of one's parents and siblings. One might demand too much from one's love object, and use the unavailability of such a precious object as the pretext for escaping love and sex altogether. The probability is that one can find in the majority of persons of the other sex human and sexual qualities which justify a deeper relation and which come out during the deeper relation. The general course is that when an individual falls in love, he starts to elevate the love object and avails himself in this way of possibilities of human and sexual discoveries about the other person otherwise not attainable. Women who get older without having made satisfactory sex contacts demand more and more from the man whom they might choose as sex partner. This is an escape. To demand wealth and beauty in the highest degree from one's sex partner is a method of escaping sex. It is a protective mechanism. Women who are ugly very often make much higher demands on their prospective mates.

One should generally have the attitude that every love relation is in itself extraordinary enough even when the participants are mediocre in every respect. One might avoid meeting persons who are eligible as mates. One might develop moral scruples of some kind. One might introduce social and financial considerations which are not valid. Finally, one might lose the desire. For instance, M., a patient with a severe hypochondriasis, occasionally has extramarital relations but very often he has no desires at all and is interested neither in the woman nor in sex. "At times, I have not the slightest desire for it." One might get overwhelmed by fear of venereal infection. One might have no erections. One might have a premature ejaculation. Women defend themselves by frigidity, sometimes coupled with dryness. One might develop an eczema or a lichen on the penis, as one of my patients did in connection with love problems. In women a psychogenic fluor might be protective. Finally, there might be sex relations which, although physically satisfying, remain unsatisfactory from a human point of view. Sometimes one wonders how the majority of human beings come, at least for a while, to full erotic satisfactions. In the relation between two persons outside and inside of marriage one very often sees that they are afraid to exhaust their sexual and human possibilities in the relation. Sexual inhibitions disturbing the sexual aspects are very common, even when both partners are fully potent. In addition, the difficulties of adapting oneself to another person in erotic relations are at first underrated, and then attempts at adaptation are often given up prematurely.

a. Love relations

What is love?
With which type of persons do you fall in love? (Size, complexion, body build, similarity to other persons, social standing, intelligence, moral qualities.)
Are you bound to such a type?
Can you choose outside of your preferred type?
Do you love at first sight?
How much time does it take until your feelings develop?
How long do your love relations last?
Do you think in the beginning of the end of the relation?
How often so far have you been in love?
How often should one fall in love?
Do you think it is right to have sex relations with somebody whom one loves?
Do you think it is right to have sex relations with somebody whom one likes?
With somebody for whom nobody cares?
With somebody whom one dislikes?
Can you be in love and continue to be in love without complete sex relations?
Do you think that casual relations are right?
How many casual relations have you had?
Are you afraid of losing independence in love relations?
Are you afraid that the love object may disappoint you?
Are you afraid that your desire may decrease?
Are you afraid of being deceived?
Are you afraid of being deserted?
How do you value unfaithfulness of your love object?
How do you value unfaithfulness to the love object?

What do you think about homosexuality, sado-masochism, and other perversions?
Do you want to be superior to your love object?
In what way do you want to express your superiority?
Do you want the love object to be superior to you?
Do you enjoy sex relations with a person whom you love?
How much emotional response do you expect from your love object?
How much verbal expression of the love of the other person do you expect?
Do you want to know every thought and experience of your love object?

b. Friendship. It is merely another aspect of the same problem of interhuman relations when we now discuss friendship. One should keep in mind that there are obvious relations between friendship and sexuality, mostly homosexuality. This was particularly true in the case of De B., who was dominated by his relations to his cousin, behind whom the figures of father and brothers loomed. His close dependence very soon changed into an immoderate hate. The struggle for superiority in friendships is very outspoken. Identification with the stronger friend may help in solving social tasks. Friendship may be one of the indirect ways of solving social problems. The following questions may be asked:

What is friendship?
What do you think of friendship?
Do you want to have friends? How many?
Can one have friends belonging to the other sex?
Can a friendship exist between two persons who have sex relations with each other?
How much sex can there be in the friendship of two persons of the same sex? Of opposite sexes?
How much should a friend know of one's own life?
How many good friends can one have?
How many close friends should one have?
How many acquaintances should one have?
Should one's friends be richer or poorer? Same or different social standing?
How much time do you want to spend with your friends? When married? When unmarried?

How much do you want to share your intimate friends with others?
In what way can one prove one's friendship?
What are your earliest memories of friends?
Did you have sex play with any of your friends?
Did you like to play with children who were poor?
Did you like to lead, or be led, in games?
Did your parents interfere with your playing with children?
Did you like to play with adults rather than with children?
Did you play with your brothers or sisters?
Did you want friends of your brother to be your friends, too?
Did you feel that your brother or sister had more friends than you had?
Did you like to put your arms around your friends and kiss them?
Did you ever hate your friends?
Did you ever wish the death of your friends?
Did you ever wish to kill one of your friends?
Did you ever hit one of your friends?
How often did you fight with your friends? Playfully?

c. Social situation. It is of course necessary to be oriented in regard to the patient's social situation and to appreciate the material and intellectual cultures which have surrounded him. The following questions may give a preliminary help:

What is the occupation of your father, mother, grandparents, sisters, and other relatives?
What is their present income? Capital?
What is their education?
To what race do they belong?
What is the history of your education and of your employment?
What is your opinion of the home in which you were brought up?
How many rooms did the family occupy?
With how many others did you share the room and the bed?
What are your remembrances of the furniture?
How many pieces were in one room?
What pictures were in the room?
Were there many vases in the room?
How often did the family change the apartment?
In what neighborhoods were the different apartments?

Did your family consider themselves as wealthy, middle-class, or poor?
Were you taken care of by mother, siblings, nurses?
How many servants were there in the house?
Were the servants treated as equals or inferiors?
Who were your playmates?
Were you allowed to play on the street?
Did the family interfere with your playing with other children?
What was the aim of the family as viewed by you before or after the fifth year?
Was the school to which you were sent considered as a high-class or a poor one?
How much money did the family spend on clothing?
Were you carefully dressed: at home; away from home?
How much money was spent on food?
Did the family claim to be educated and cultured?
What were the efforts made in this respect?
What were the books read by any member of the family?
What were the types?
What type of music did they like?
What was the attitude of the family towards sports, drinking?
In what way did the family regard manual labor?
In what way did they look at intellectual achievements?
What was the financial goal of the family?
What is the attitude of the family towards racial problems? (Jews, Italians, Negroes, Germans.)
What are the family religious problems?
Do the members of the family go to church?
Do they consider affiliation with a church a social necessity?
Is the family interested in politics? Actively?
Do they go to the polls?
Do they campaign?
Is the trend of the family conservative, liberal, radical? In politics? In art? In morals?
Who plays the most important role in the family?
Are father and mother autocratic, or do they listen to others?
Who are the people with whom you mix, and who are the people with whom you would like to mix?
Do you believe in separating the social layers and also the racial layers in social intercourse?

6. *Two special questionnaires on aggressiveness and death*

In previous studies I have made large use of a questionnaire on aggressiveness.[1] Criminals and children, neurotics and normals answered the questionnaire. It has proved to be valuable. It has, of course, to be modified when used with children. The work has been done in connection with Lauretta Bender and Sylvan Keiser. The questionnaire on death has been extensively used by Bromberg, Wechsler, and myself in normals, neurotics, psychotics, criminals, and children. It is obvious, from the previous remarks, that in order to come to an insight into an individual's problem we have to understand his aggression and his attitude towards death. In every psychoanalysis these problems come up again and again. As every one of these problems is fundamental, they overlap with almost any other problem. But such a questionnaire may keep the ramifications of the problem in the minds of the patient and the physician. The discussion of any one of these problems may become necessary at any time in handling the groups. We have generally found that in the attitudes towards death, two fundamental types should be distinguished. Hysterical patients fear death as removal from love objects; obsession neurotics and depressive cases, as interminable punishment. However, the idea of death may also serve all kinds of erotic gratifications. Thus, death may be, on the one hand, the representative of the most dreaded dangers; on the other hand, the representative of the escape from these very dangers, and of a gratification the withdrawal of which was threatened.

One should keep in mind that the questions offered cannot exhaust the manifold problems of human life. They merely serve, quite in the same way as the short remarks which introduce them, the general orientation of what may go on in a group; they hint what kind of material may turn up, and in what spirit the material should be handled. Only in exceptional cases will one be able to place one or another part of the questionnaire into the hands of the patient, or to use the one or the other section as a topic for discussion. The discussions are, after all, directed by the material a patient brings forward

[1] L. Bender, S. Keiser, and P. Schilder, "Studies in Aggressiveness," *Genetic Psychological Monographs*, Vol. 18, Nos. 5 and 6, pp. 357–564, 1936.

and by the associations which he himself and the others offer. However, very often the physician will be able to draw the conclusions from the manifold material, show the general principle and the way in which the general principle expresses itself in the individual patient. The activity of the physician in interpreting obviously cannot be small. In addition to his activity in interpreting, he will have to use the same methods of activity which are used in psychoanalysis if the situation demands it. Also, in group treatment the anxiety neurosis case, for instance, has to be led into a situation from which his anxiety drives him away. The principles of this activity are not different from the activity demanded by individual treatments. I have attempted to make the methods teachable. Other physicians can be present (generally not more than one), and the questionnaires have at least proved useful in conveying the general meaning of the treatment. As mentioned, it is too early to come to a definite conclusion about the technique and its results. It seems to me that properly applied it is in some cases even more efficient than individual psychoanalysis (the best method at hand). In many cases individual analysis remains necessary. I have the preliminary impression that cases with character difficulties and psychopathy are particularly fit for the method of group treatment.

SOME GENERAL REMARKS, ESPECIALLY ABOUT THE PSYCHOTHERAPIST

Psychoanalysis generally insists that the physician who does psychoanalysis should not make a physical examination of the patient. If he thinks that such is necessary, another physician should be consulted. This procedure has great disadvantages. The physical examination done by himself may give to the physician a much better view of the situation, and his knowledge of the patient may enable him to use better judgment concerning the case. I think, therefore, that the physician should examine his patient before he starts with psychotherapy. I do not think that gynecological or anal examinations are advisable. I further agree that in the course of an analysis it may not be advisable to repeat the physical examination. The man who conducts the psychotherapy is, however, in charge of the patient and should act accordingly. In many cases he will be of aid in physical treatment of a more or less complicated character. I have often been able to avoid mistakes by making a physical examination of patients who were sent to me for psychotherapy.

It is obvious that I am of the opinion that psychotherapy should be done by physicians. The problem of disease plays such an overwhelming part in psychotherapy that the psychotherapist should also have first-hand knowledge of organic disease. Even then he will not always be able to avoid mistakes, but on the whole such a preparation is necessary. I am, therefore, against lay analysis and lay psychotherapy. In many forms of treatment the physician of course has to rely upon a personnel that does not consist of physicians. The training of the personnel of a ward in which psychotherapeutic problems play a part is of paramount importance and should be done by a fully trained psychotherapist. I have a deep appreciation for the help offered by the nursing, occupational, and educational staff. However, I think that the final synthesis has to lie in the hands of the physician.

A particular problem is offered by the didactic analysis of normal persons and by the treatment of the behavior problems in children. I do not see any reason why a didactic analysis should not be performed by a lay person. A normal and healthy person, anyhow, has to decide for himself, and merely the suffering should be taken care of by the physician. In fact, didactic analysis has been done by lay analysts with considerable success. In children education and treatment are hard to separate. Behavior problems are decidedly problems of education. I cannot conceive of any education which does not have aims similar to those of psychotherapy in addition to the aim of acquiring knowledge. I do not, therefore, object to psychotherapeutic treatment being given to children by persons who are fully trained in education and also have had a sufficient psychotherapeutic training. It is very difficult to draw the border line between giving advice to and directing the adolescent, which is the task of the educator, and treating, which is the task of the physician. The criterion is the depth of suffering. The domain of the physician is human suffering and the methods of its relief, as far as the suffering is not unhappiness and unavoidable according to the situation.

Under the present circumstances, only the physician who deals with the physically ill and the psychotic as well as with the neurotic and psychopathic has a sufficiently close contact with these fundamental human experiences. The relation between body and soul is so close that one cannot know about the one without knowing about the other, too. The full knowledge of somatic function is a prerequisite for the psychotherapist. Statements of this type are, of course, largely dependent upon the social situation of the time. It is at least thinkable that a program could be outlined for the education of the future psychotherapist which is not identical with that for the physician, but this is not our concern here.

Official psychoanalysis demands didactic analysis from the candidate. It demands further control of the analyst in training through an older analyst when he sees his first few cases and, furthermore, neurological and psychiatrical experience. I have made my point of view clear concerning the training analysis. I would add that the more thorough the psychiatric training of the psychotherapist is, the better. The diagnostic difficulties in the field are great, and experience at least diminishes the chances of error. It is further necessary that the physician should have seen a great number of cases. He should know the possibilities of every method and should have experience in handling human beings. It is obvious that the hospital situation is the only one which offers such a possibility.

Obviously there are many things that are to be learned about psychotherapy. After all, this book is an attempt to show how much has to be learned about it. It is further advisable that the beginner should have the possibility of definite help.

If I did not think psychotherapy could be taught, I should not have attempted to write this book. One very often hears that one has to have a specific gift in order to be able to do psychotherapy. One also hears something about the personality of the psychotherapist. One thinks that the physician who has the right bedside manner will also be able to do good psychotherapy. Finally, one comes to the conclusion that psychotherapy is an art and not a science. One points to the so-called successful practitioner who plays the role of the good uncle and thus cures his patients. I think one should keep in mind that, as the preceding pages show, the psychotherapist will fail if his psychotherapy is based upon the display of what one calls personality. He has to try to help the patient to increase his insight, he has to know the technique, and he has to learn very much before he can do so. In spite of all the differences of opinion in the different schools of psychotherapy, we are in possession of a definite body of facts pertaining to psychotherapeutic technique. They can be learned, and they must be learned. It is obvious here, as in every other field of human endeavor, that differences in the specific endowment necessarily exist. This is, however, true also of the surgeon or the internist. It is obvious that the surgeon and the internist, even if they are "born" surgeons and internists, have to learn something before their capacities become useful. It is furthermore obvious that some measure of human reliability is necessary for every kind of responsible occupation. It is good to see these facts as soberly as possible.

One occasionally points to physicians who, although not considered very highly by the profession, or at least as one-sided, are very highly esteemed by their patients, who insist that they were benefited. It is rather obvious that these psychotherapists help to a better insight, at least to one part of the reality, and we should not consider their work as useless, although incomplete. With the improvements of psychological knowledge and psychotherapeutic technique and the possibility for teaching them, physicians as well as patients will demand methods of treatment which are better rounded.

Chapter 10

THE TREATMENT OF SPECIFIC TYPES OF NEUROSES AND PSYCHOPATHIES

• •
•

THE TECHNIQUE OF treatment of the various types of neuroses, psychopathies, and related conditions will be considered here. It is not intended to present a thorough discussion of psychological theories or complete clinical descriptions. Neither am I interested in the classification of the neuroses, but I shall arrange the material as it seems fit in order to discuss the problems of treatment.

NEUROSES IN WHICH A CONFLICT OVER AN IMMEDIATE SITUATION PREVAILS

ACTUAL NEUROSES

I have stated that I consider the Freudian theory of *actual neurosis* incorrect. However, there exists a group of neuroses in which infantile conflict is not of paramount importance and where the neurosis almost completely serves the present conflict. We may appropriately start with the so-called war neurosis.[1] The war neurosis

[1] This refers to the experiences of World War I. There is a great deal of literature on the dynamics of the war neuroses during World War II.

was a comparatively simple method of escaping the unbearable situation in the trenches. It served the tendency to self-preservation. It is obvious that there are varied reactions possible in such dangerous situations. The individual may react with his whole personality, especially when fright is involved, and more primitive mechanisms may mingle with the obvious attempt to escape the present danger situation. It is obvious that the technique in such cases cannot be an elucidation of earlier experiences in one's childhood, but that merely the present situation has to be considered. In military medical practice, the threat of the immediate pain of an electric current and the pain itself often were employed to force the patient to give up his symptoms. In some countries the promise was added that the soldier would not have to go back to the front. It cannot be denied that these methods, crude as they are, were effective. However, the so-called war neurosis and neurosis in general are very different from each other. The war neurosis originates from an attempt to escape a terrifying situation, the structure of which is simple. The method of escape is simple enough and the cure may equal the disease in primitiveness. Such a procedure is not applicable to the more subtle structure of neuroses which originate from less brutal and more complicated situations.

In some of the war neuroses and responses to catastrophes, like the earthquake in Messina, fright reaction develops. Fright and panic mean that one is overwhelmed by the situation and does not want to do anything any more. This may express itself merely in the psychic sphere, but phenomena in the vegetative sphere are not uncommon. If one compares neurotic reactions with sham death reflexes in animals, one might be justified in doing so in fright reactions. We deal, then, with the reactions to a clear-cut catastrophe in the outside world. It is obvious that therapy must give the individual the opportunity to recover from his fright reaction in a situation which is as simple as possible. The individual should not be forced into any activity.

See: Roy Grinker and John Spiegel, *Men Under Stress* (Blakiston, 1945); William C. Menninger, *Psychiatry in a Troubled World* (The Macmillan Co., 1948); A. Kardiner, *The Traumatic Neuroses of War* (Paul B. Hoeber, 1947); Thomas A. Rennie, *Mental Health in Modern Society* (New York, Commonwealth Fund, 1948); Emmanuel Miller, *The Neuroses of War* (New York, The Macmillan Co., 1940); and Therese Benedek, *Insight and Personality Adjustment, a Study of the Psychological Effects of War* (New York, Ronald Press Co., 1949). [L.B., Ed.]

Active psychotherapy will be indicated only if underlying conflicts interfere with the recovery and use the primary symptoms of fright as the basis for a neurotic elaboration. One may call fright reactions panic reactions. Adolf Meyer and Oskar Diethelm use the term *panic reaction* in all types of anxiety states which originate from deep-lying conflicts. The use of the term is not justified since it implies an oversimplification of the neurotic problem.

It is much more difficult to come to practical conclusions concerning compensation neuroses. Our psychological knowledge concerning these cases is very limited. In some cases, the wish for compensation is obvious. The symptoms serve the economic tendencies. However, I have seen hardly any cases in which this was the whole problem. The problem always remains, why do individuals choose this way in order to get an economic advantage? It is not easy, not socially acknowledged, and the bitterness with which the compensation fights are held very often points to a deep-lying problem of discord with society and the father image. Paranoid developments may follow; the life may center around the distorted social relation in which the childhood relation to the parent of the same sex is very often reflected. Sadger has pointed to the castration fears and the castration ideas in so-called traumatic neuroses. I should prefer to say that every severe trauma is experienced as a threat to the unity of the body, and some patients react to such a threat by almost completely disrupting the body image and developing severe hypochondriac symptoms. The sequence may be out of proportion to its trauma.

I have observed a man whose only claim to surpassing mediocrity was his ability as a baseball player. He admired his father merely because his father had told him that he was a good runner. After lifting a heavy weight, a hernia developed which made an operation necessary. The operation was not very successful. The patient had to wear a truss and could not play baseball any more. He developed an enormous fear that he might hurt himself again, was finally afraid of infection and germs, and developed a compulsory system of washing and avoidances in order to escape infection. He was convinced that his view was correct. The infantile material brought forward in a treatment which extended over months was scarce. The transference remained superficial and no cure was achieved. Such an instance merely shows the difficulties in treating cases in which a trauma has played an important part.

Some of the difficulties of the traumatic neurosis lie in the present situation. The trauma and its social consequences have to be carefully considered. It is generally acknowledged that it is helpful to the patient if the litigation is settled as quickly as possible. One will do well not to forget that patients suffer from a feeling of social injustice, and this may even be one of the conditions under which traumatic neuroses develop. A sincere attempt to understand the social situation is necessary. In many cases psychotherapy of a deeper type will be essential. It seems to me that group psychotherapy, not yet tried in this type of case, promises results. The severe paranoiac and hypochondriac pictures have the meaning of a psychosis. The difficulties of approaching the patient are great and the prognosis is not good. However, when treatment is requested, it should be tried and may meet with some success.

As mentioned, whenever repetition compulsion, in the sense of Freud, is present, it serves the present and the infantile needs of the patient, and one should try to understand the motives for the repetition. It is obvious that even in traumatic cases one is not always entitled to say that one deals only with a conflict in the present. Human beings, after all, always have a past. It has been found that there exists a tendency to have accidents, and many persons who are not handicapped physically in an obvious way suffer not one but a series of accidents. (Cf. Alexandra Adler.) The accident then serves basic masochistic tendencies of the individual as, by the way, many operations do. At any rate, one should not overrate the differences between neuroses with actual conflicts and those with infantile conflicts. The present situation has its full meaning only in the light of the past, and the past situation has its full meaning only in the light of the present.

The various psychogenic pictures one sees in prisoners accused of severe crimes have very often a simple structure, their nonsensical answers reflecting the popular idea of insanity (Ganser syndrome). Their stupors and depressions are, indeed, in very close relation to the wish of escaping the consequences of the crime. The symptoms disappear rather suddenly when the legal side of the case takes a turn for the better. There is a gradual transition from a psychogenic reaction, in which the patient is successful in hiding his problem from himself, to malingering. The problem remains as to what kind of person commits such a crime and chooses this type of escape. This is, of course, the problem of crime in general, with all the difficulties involved in the problem.

Among the actual neuroses Freud includes acute anxiety states, neurasthenia, and hypochondriasis. I am rather at a loss to accept these types of neuroses in this classification. Personality problems starting in early childhood are obvious in all the neuroses of this type. There may be the one or the other type of neurasthenia which occurs in connection with an acute difficulty in the outward situation, especially when financial difficulties arise; but the businessman who reacts to a business depression with headache, fatigue, constipation, diminished potency, sleeplessness, etc., had narrowed down his life, owing to unconscious motives, before the business failure occurred. His reaction reveals difficulties in adaptation which started much earlier. We shall, therefore, discuss the problem of neurasthenia later on. Hypochondriac pictures, based upon specific attitudes towards one's own body image, are rarely in connection with one's present situation. They reflect early attitudes, and as far as they do not remain in the background of the picture, are very often a serious sign indicating a deep-seated neurosis or a beginning psychosis. Hypochondriac neuroses and psychoses constitute, according to my opinion, a clinical entity. However, hypochondriasis may be a part of a manic-depressive or schizophrenic psychosis. I have seen anxiety states in which the present situation was of great importance, but I have never seen anxiety states in which the present conflict was not closely related to a conflict of the past.

This group of neuroses should draw our attention to the fact that the present situation should be carefully investigated and that the present conflict can be of great importance. The therapy will, therefore, have to give attention to the social situation. One should be aware of the situation of the past. It is, of course, necessary to take careful consideration in all these cases, but especially in the traumatic group, of the physical state of the patient. Physical residuals of head injuries, for instance, very often form the nucleus around which hysteriform pictures are built. The investigation of Otto Poetzl on war injuries in the first World War gives the deepest insight into this problem.

In the consideration of the psychological problems encountered in neurosis following head injuries, we have first to deal with the psychology of the trauma as such.[2] During the trauma the individual experiences a threat to the integrity of his body—a threat of death, disability, or deformity. At the same time he acknowledges the superior force of the traumatic agent which might become a symbol of the power of the parent. The individual may experience masochistic gratification in the trauma and might even have sought the trauma for a similar reason. When a head injury has occurred, unconsciousness may be followed by a period of organic disorientation with a severe disturbance in brain function.

We are interested in those cases in which the organic consequences are not prominent. There may be a more or less outspoken difficulty, on a psychogenic basis, in the reorientation of the body and the outside world (Kardiner, 1932). The terror of annihilation may be revived again; it may occur at the specific hour of the day of the accident or as a mere terror, or as a revival of the traumatic scene of the accident, in imagination, hallucination, or as a dream. Dreams may be an unchanged revival of the traumatic scene, or they may constitute a more or less symbolic interpretation of annihilation—e.g., drowning and catastrophes of other types—and finally there are often dreams of persecution. It seems as if the individual cannot get over the dangerous situation and again and again tries to become acquainted with it. This is the meaning of the so-called repetition compulsion which, according to Freud, is shown particularly by repetitive dreams in traumatic neurosis. He believes the repetition compulsion is connected chiefly with ego instincts and less with libidinous instincts.

There cannot be any doubt that the individual does not get over the entire situation which he has once experienced. Furthermore he may derive some masochistic gratification from his suffering. All his previous doubts and fears may express themselves as death fears. The terror may finally be replaced by the fear of lasting defect in the intellectual, and in some cases even the sexual, sphere. One may speak of this as fear of impairment of the body image.

When the organic signs of headache, vomiting, dizziness, and vasomotor phenomena are present they add to the insecurity and terror. Hypochondriacal and neurasthenic signs will be more out-

---

[2] The rest of this section was reprinted from Paul Schilder, "Neurosis Following Head and Brain Injuries," Chapter 12, in *Injuries of Skull, Brain and Spinal Cord,* ed. by Samuel Brock, 2nd ed., 1943. [L.B., Ed.]

spoken when the body image is changed—e.g., after a craniotomy.

It depends upon the previous structure of the personality whether the individual will overcome the continuous threat of annihilation or whether a more chronic neurotic picture will occur. Difficulties in memory may lead to a deep fear of loss of integrity of one's mind or personality. Hysterical pictures may express the wish that the suffering should be compensated for by the love and appreciation of others around one. The hysterical symptom emphasizes the suffering in its social aspects, and its demands arise frequently in connection with previous deprivations of love; these symptoms are often related to the need for emotional and financial compensation. Hysterical syndromes are frequently built upon somatic compliance, i.e., a somatically impaired function. All these reactions are based not only upon the present situation, but also on the past of the individual. However, in the case of traumatic neurosis following head injuries, the head injury with its psychological consequences is an indispensable factor in the total development. In cases in which compensation comes to the foreground, the feeling of social injustice is of paramount importance.

It should be kept in mind that many individuals with traumatic neuroses in general, and especially those following head injury, suffer not only from their neurosis but also from typical organic consequences of the trauma. Many persons can and often do force themselves to work even though they suffer and work under great difficulties (Riese, 1929). There is no reason why one should expect anyone to put forth a great amount of self-sacrifice and effort under conditions of distress which surpass the average difficulties encountered in working. It may be necessary to remark that organic symptoms often can be overcompensated for by an effort, but the necessary effort may be very great. The diagnosis of neurosis is unjustified merely because the individual gives in to symptoms instead of making extraordinary efforts. One should also be reminded that ability to work as such is not a sign that the individual has no symptoms. Furthermore the organic consequences of head injuries are increased almost always by work; this may have a bad influence on a concomitant neurosis. If one deals with neurotic manifestations, one has to keep in mind the symbolic significance of work. It frequently symbolizes sadistic aggression which the individual does not want to exercise in order not to be exposed to counterattacks. Tools and machinery may produce additional fears. Phobic reactions may be connected with scenes reminding him of the accident. Work means also that the individual is independent and strong and has no further claim for consideration of others. Finally it may mean that the individual is no longer entitled to compensation. Under such conditions it can readily be seen that the advice to go back to work is of very great psychological significance and should not be lightly given. In the great majority of cases there will be no special reason to push the patient back to work as long as he has complaints, irrespective of whether or not there are organic residuals. When there are no organic residuals and the patient continues to complain, the advice to go to work has to be considered as only part of the total psychotherapeutic program.

It is preposterous to believe that neurosis of any severe degree can be cured by changing the external situation alone. It is true that among the traumatic neuroses the compensation factor may play a more or less important part. This will partly depend on the type of the neurosis. In general we may expect that the compensation question will be less outspoken in the acute terror reactions, will gain a greater importance in the neurasthenic hypochondriac reactions, and will find its greatest role in hysterical reactions which demand attention and love. It is generally conceded that the medical-legal complications connected with compensation might increase the neurotic symptoms. However, in most cases the root of the neurosis lies deeper, and a neurosis which consists merely in the claim for compensation is obviously malingering, or at least very near it. It is usually acknowledged that a speedy settlement of the compensation question is preferable. Riese (1929) and Schnyder (1936) emphasize that even after lump-sum settlement, difficulties of neurotic character often remain. On the whole it is advisable that the physician who treats a patient with traumatic neurosis should be aware of the compensation element, but he should not approach the patient with the idea that the main question is whether the patient is entitled to compensation or not. Even the individual with traumatic neurosis who demands compensation suffers and has the right to be treated as a patient. It is therefore advisable to approach the patient as one would any other neurotic patient. Psychotherapeutic procedures should consist of the procedures usually followed in such cases, i.e.: winning the transference, working through the transference, breaking the transference. The physician should listen to the complaints of the patient and let him express himself as freely as possible.

Psychoanalysis has taught us that we are more certain of building up the transference of the patient correctly if we are not too active. According to the character of the case it may be advisable to use forms of short psychotherapy or the classic techniques of psychoanalysis. It is more important that the patient understands than it is for him to get advice. I think it is essential that the patient should also have a clear understanding of the physical findings in his case. There is no reason why the whole problem should not be discussed with the patient freely and in intelligible terms as soon as he shows any interest in it. In many cases it may even be advisable to see that the relatives and individuals close to him should have a similar understanding. It will depend upon the skill of the psychotherapist to decide at which part of the treatment the situation should be discussed with the patient. According to the general rules of psychotherapy, active therapy can only be started when a positive transference has been gained.

As mentioned above, the advice to go to work is very active therapy. Moralizing, scolding and threatening have no place in the therapist's scheme. In some cases it might become advisable for the physician to take active part in shaping the total reaction of the patient. In the majority of cases it will not be necessary to help the patient gain an insight into his own psychosexual development and go systematically into childhood experiences. In many cases this will be unavoidable, as in other forms of neurosis. Group discussion and group psychotherapy have never been tried systematically in cases of this type. This seems to be a method for the future. At the present time there should be a planned psychological approach to the patient. At any rate the physician should know his own attitude towards the social problems involved and should especially guard himself against the negative countertransference, which is often shown by those who have written on compensation neurosis. It might be well for the physician to be aware that he is not a referee to decide on compensation questions and that his chief task is to help the patient to understand himself so that he can find a way out of the neurosis.

ANXIETY NEUROSIS

I have previously discussed the fundamental problem of anxiety. In anxiety neuroses, difficulties in sex adaptation are obvious. However, in the last group of seven cases I have treated, there were two in which there were no obvious disturbances on the physical side of sex relations. The successful sex act, on the other hand, had no manifest influence on the symptomatology. The situation is clearly indicated by an observation made several years ago, in which the anxiety neurosis was the reaction to marriage with an unloved and unlovable husband. Because of the husband, sex relations took place more rarely than the patient wished. After a successful intercourse the patient always felt better. She was finally free from symptoms when she met a young man with whom she fell in love without knowing it. When she realized the depth and the danger of her affection, she broke off the platonic relation and the symptoms returned.

It is the psychosexual situation which is of importance. There are no simple relations between anxiety and physical satisfaction. The infantile problems of anxiety neurosis cases center around the Oedipus complex. The early attachment to the parent of the other sex is frequently obvious. Many variations are possible. The Oedipus attachment may, for instance, persist in too strong a way. In other cases an attachment to the parent of the same sex, or a sibling of the same sex, might introduce early homosexual attitudes and a distorted superior and inferior relationship. In other cases, the dominance of the parent and the sibling of the other sex might push the boy into a dependent situation; the mother and the mother image would be experienced as men; and the fight against this relation might lay the foundation for anxiety states. Fear of the love object plays an important part. It may even arrest the sexual development before any sexual adaptation in the sense of the Oedipus complex is reached. In one of my cases which is particularly difficult to treat, aggressive attitudes of the parents were experienced as a threat of dismembering and were answered by violent counteraggression.

Anxiety is a phenomenon which may originate from experiences of very different types.[3] In the earliest stages of its development the

[3] The rest of this section on anxiety was reprinted from Paul Schilder, "Types of Anxiety Neuroses," *International Journal of Psychoanalysis* 22:193–208, 1941. [L.B., Ed.]

child is threatened particularly by the loss of equilibrium and by the physical forces of gravitation. Only gradually does it learn to orientate itself in space and to appreciate the definite importance of the vertical and horizontal directions. It is very probable that at this stage of development the love object represents among other things an insurance against the danger of falling. The love object in this respect is a supporting figure. However, the child also reacts with anxiety when its supply of food is not assured. For the child, moreover, food means the inside of its body, since according to the notions of young children the inside of the body consists of the food which has been ingested. Direct threats against the integrity of the body are probably experienced only at a later stage. They are closely related to the child's aggressive impulses directed against the bodies of other people. At this level, fear of dismemberment in general will become important, and later on, with the awakening of genitality, this will culminate in the theme of castration. During this whole course of development the love object will offer protection against deprivations and will on the other hand be feared as a possible aggressor. The fear of losing the love object will come into the foreground when sexual development has reached a higher level. When there are hostile impulses towards the love object they will be reacted to with feelings of guilt. At the earlier levels there will be fears of counteraggression on the part of the love object, which is also hated; and the insecurity connected with the dread of its loss will be increased by the guilty feeling which forces the subject to identify himself with the person whom he has killed in phantasy.

If we consider the variety of the situations which, in the course of development, provoke anxieties, we shall not be astonished at finding a great variety in the types of anxiety neurosis which revive the various types of developmental anxieties. We must further take into consideration the fact that any anxiety will contain all the possible anxieties, though in various degrees and proportions. It must also be remembered that, in spite of the deep regressions which we have described, the typical case of anxiety neurosis has reached a level of heterosexual adjustment, in the sense of the Oedipus complex, and that it has one point of fixation in the genital relation to the parents. From the clinical standpoint, this distinguishes a case of anxiety neurosis with regressions going to fairly primitive levels from cases of obsessional neurosis, although cases with space distortions very often show obsessional trends. It is characteristic of neurotic anxiety in contrast to psychotic anxiety that the former is always accompanied by some appreciation of the love object.

The various types of anxiety are connected with different attitudes towards death. In a case of anxiety neurosis with only a moderate degree of aggressiveness, a type of death will be pictured which means merely separation from the love object. When the regression goes deeper, a fear of death may be replaced by a fear of dismemberment and annihilation, and the idea of death will be colored by these ideas. Walter Bromberg and I have shown that various types of concepts of death exist and that the idea of death changes with the type of neurosis and with the type and degree of regression.

I think that an insight into the problems which have been discussed here is of fundamental importance to a deep analysis of cases of anxiety neurosis, and it will be understood that the fundamental trends discussed in the various types of cases must find a reflection in the type of transference and in the analysis of the transference.

It is obvious that at least short psychotherapy, in the sense discussed above, is necessary. Short psychotherapy, in which hypnosis is used, often is successful. A great number of cases need an extended treatment either in group psychotherapy or in analysis. Even in severe cases, my results with group psychotherapy are satisfactory. Activity, not only in interpretation but also in pushing the patient into situations connected with anxiety, is essential.

HYSTERIA

Anxiety neuroses in which infantile problems are of importance have often been classified as anxiety hysteria. However, the psychological structure of anxiety neurosis is rather characteristic. The hostility against the love object is of importance. The danger of being separated from the love object, or of being attacked by the love object, plays the leading part. It is true that the Oedipus complex in most of the anxiety neurosis cases is as well developed as in hysterias, and the transference is, accordingly, strong with the positive transference prevailing. It seems to me that the heterosexual transference of obviously genital character is still more outspoken in hysteria cases. One should speak about anxiety hysterias only when anxiety is combined with typical conversion symptoms and is based upon the typical hysterical attitudes which are described in this paragraph. It is not necessary to discuss here in detail how close the hysterical symptomatology is in relation to infantile sex problems in connection with the Oedipus complex. That does not mean, of course, that pre-Oedipus fixations and conflict situations do not play any part in the hysterical symptomatology. However, they are of less importance and subordinated to the genital situation. The actual conflict very often originates in an erotic conflict. The attitude of the hysteria case stresses suffering and physical disease. Organic weaknesses and minor ailments are very often used for the demonstration to others of suffering. This often resembles the attitude of the sick child who received attention and love from the parents when it was suffering. The importance of early organic diseases for the genesis of the conversion symptom should be stressed. The hysterical person is one who needs love. In the anxiety neurosis, the wish for protection plays a much greater part. The anxiety neurosis case stresses the aspect of danger; the hysteria case, the aspect of suffering from lack of love. The relation of the hysteria case to its surroundings is, therefore, very close. He or she is seductive in the sense of wanting love from everybody. The ability to revive the infantile love object of father and mother in almost everybody around is appalling. The hysteria case is, accordingly, turned towards the world in general, and has lively interests. The difficulty lies in the fact that neither the animate nor inanimate objects give a lasting satisfaction. It is in relation to the great interest in the world that imitation of persons or of symptoms in the hysterical symptomatology plays such a great part.

Furthermore, the symptomatology of hysteria depends, to a great extent, on the surroundings and on the present social trends. As far as I can see, the symptomatology of anxiety neurosis has changed very little in the last forty or fifty years. The symptomatology of hysteria has undergone deep changes. Spectacular pictures and spectacular attacks have become rare and are at the present time to be found mostly among uneducated people and Negroes. The hysterical patient today may develop headaches, may complain about weakness and sickness and organic symptoms. He may complain, furthermore, about pain. The great hysterical attacks, the long-lasting dreamy states, the contractures, etc., have become rare. Since the hysterical patient has, in connection with his lively interest in human beings, such a lively interest in the world, he may deny himself this interest in his symptoms and develop amnesias, which merely testify to his great interest in the situation which he forgets.

The hysterical hallucination and the hysterical dreamy state so closely related to daydreams, the sexual contents of which are hardly veiled, do not constitute a deep negation of the everyday reality. It is difficult to appreciate the sexual disturbances in the narrower sense. Hysterical impotency in men shows, in severe cases, a complete absence of sexual urges. But these cases are rare; I have no complete understanding of them, and the reports in the literature are meager. Much more common are cases of impotency in which intercourse is not possible with a valued love object and is possible with a degraded love object. Frigidity or lack of interest in intercourse in hysterical women is common and comparatively easy to influence. Even in their affliction and sufferings, hysterical patients mostly retain their close relation to the world.

Psychogenic depressions of hysteriform type are very common at the present time. In the severer cases of these types one will very often find a more marked hostility towards the love object and also especially against the persons who substitute for the parent of the other sex. Some of the mechanisms may remind us of the mechanisms of true depressions.

During the treatment of hysteria, positive transference finds a more or less strong expression. The patient has to understand it in relation to the present situation and to the past. The patient also has to become aware of the degree to which he is dependent on his former love objects. Symptomatological results are comparatively easy to reach with almost any method. They are rather useless if insight is not reached. Short psychotherapy, with or without hypnosis, may be applied if the case is not too severe. It is of special importance that the physician have insight into the nature of the positive transference and the necessity of analyzing this transference.

It is interesting that hysteria has been the starting point in the modern approach to psychotherapy. The number of communications concerning hysteria in modern psychotherapeutic literature is small. My own material concerning deeply understood cases is insufficient. The ease with which a preliminary therapeutic result can be reached very often constitutes a difficulty for a deeper understanding. Cases in which the hysterical symptomatology persists, on deeper analysis, very often show mechanisms which we would hesitate to call hysterical. One of my patients, for instance, complained of the weakness of the left side of her body connected with paresthesias and pain in the abdomen. This had developed while she was repulsing the approach of a lover who was sitting at her left and seemingly tried to put her hand on his sex parts. The patient, thirty-three years old, was a typist and very efficient in her occupation. The weakness in the left arm appeared during her typing and made it impossible for her to go on with her occupation. In her family were eight other girls. She was the fifth. In spite of this, she remained ignorant of sex and pregnancy for a very long time. Once she heard her father say that a girl had been stepped on, on her toes. When her employer stepped by chance on her toes when she was seventeen, she was afraid that she might be pregnant. Once, during her menstruation, her father scolded her. The menstruation stopped and she had a pain in her abdomen similar to the pain she now had. She always wanted to have as many children as her mother had. Her mother has, at the present time, shaking and weakness on the left side.

She always felt that she had to work for the family. When she made good money her family took it away from her, especially her brother-in-law, whom she even wanted to kill. The patient loved her father dearly. There was no material concerning obvious hostility towards her mother. She was very jealous of her younger sister, whom her father preferred and when she was small he had taken into his bed. The patient had always had sex desires but she felt she should not give in to them. The man who made advances to her proved to be married. She was always particularly proud of her ability to make money and was proud of her typewriting. She thinks that typewriting is a very graceful occupation.

The patient has been treated for a very long time with great difficulties. It was very difficult to get any free association and the material was scarce, although she dreamed profusely. The result of the treatment was unsatisfactory and the improvement, especially concerning typewriting, was insufficient. There are doubtless hysterical mechanisms in the case. The left side has served for sex gratification as well as a defense against sex, but owing to her typewriting her arm was also her weapon of aggressiveness and superiority in the family. The case has, therefore, at least strong relation to occupational neuroses in which the organ which serves the social purpose of activity and aggression becomes the center of attention and pride (loaded with narcissistic libido). The disturbance concerning the body image therefore goes deeper than one sees in hysteria. Although the structure of her personality and her attitude towards sex are hysteriform, the symptoms seemingly have deeper roots. The patient has said, "My disease is this man's fault. I have sacrificed myself."

Early disappointment in the relation to the parents plays a leading part in the structure of hysteria.[4] Later traumas bring this early disappointment into the foreground again. In the early relations to parents, organic disease plays a very important part. It makes the individual still more dependent upon the parent. It also concentrates the love of the parent on the child. Organic ailment is, therefore, of fundamental importance for the whole psychology of hysteria. It reinforces the masochistic attitude in the person afflicted. The affinity of the hysterical patient to organic disease and trauma has to be considered from this angle. Hysteria thus becomes the expression of suffering from disease in its human and social aspects. It stresses helplessness of the child and dependence on the love of the parents. From this angle it becomes understandable that the actual cause of the hysterical difficulties in women is often to be found in erotic disappointments, whereas in men the social conflict and an accident play the most important part. At any rate, the person afflicted with hysteria addresses himself to a highly organized social structure. The hysterical patient acknowledges reality, but he cannot get a definite hold on it. Therefore, he is curious, eager, and full of interest in human beings.

The passing hysterical symptom is thus based upon the same mechanism as the lasting hysterical symptom and the hysterical personality. However, even the passing hysterical symptom is only possible when the individual has reached the level of the Oedipus complex and also the level of a lively interest in the outward world. The individual takes refuge in the symptom when the erotic or social situation becomes too prohibitive.

On the basis of this discussion it becomes obvious that attitudes which lead to hysterical symptoms are facilitated by organic disease. However, it is of fundamental importance to note that such atti-

---

[4] The remainder of the discussion on hysteria is from Paul Schilder, "The Concept of Hysteria," *American Journal of Psychiatry* 95:1389–1409, 1939. [L.B., Ed.]

tudes asking for erotic and social help are present only in those organic diseases which are not too severe. In general, they will be found in chronic diseases or in the beginning or at the decline of an acute disease. If the organic disease is at its height or completely incapacitating, the individual will get the full social recognition for it without hysterical symptoms.

However, one should not speak of hysteria when the patient merely has an attitude of neglect towards organic symptoms, as is true in very many organic cases, or when the individual does not put up a particular fight in the face of organic disease. One should stick to the definition that hysterical symptoms are the expression of the attitude of love towards the parents in a symbolic form. As in all products of unconscious thinking, many tendencies are condensed in the hysterical symptoms. However, whatever the share of pregenital and destructive tendencies in the hysterical symptom may be, it is less than the share of tendencies in immediate connection with the Oepidus complex. This is, after all, the definition of hysteria. We speak of the hysterical character in individuals who easily develop hysterical attitudes or who retain such symptoms through a longer span of their lives. I have also observed hysterical symptoms in schizophrenias; however, they were merely in connection with those parts of the personality which had obtained a fuller adaptation to reality. One finds, accordingly, hysterical phenomena in almost every type of neurosis and psychosis.

It is difficult to decide when the Oedipus complex makes its appearance. Many analysts believe that genitality and the Oedipus complex make their appearance before the third year, and my own observations point in the same direction. Hysteriform phenomena have been observed in children at the age of one year and a half. However, it seems to me that the structure of these cases is not identical with the structure of cases of hysteria. They probably represent comparatively simple emotional outbursts in which aggressive and destructive impulses prevail. The conversion connected with these outbursts is different in its mechanism from one of strictly hysterical type.[5]

I want to emphasize again that the hysterical conversion is not the only expression of psychological problems in the body. There exists a neurasthenic obsessive, depressive, and schizophrenic conversion.

[5] Cf. Patrick Mullahy, *Oedipus—Myth and Complex* (New York, Hermitage Press, 1948). [L.B., Ed.]

Every level of psychological adaptation has its own way of expressing itself in the body. One should not only stress that the conversion symptom is an expression of psychological tendencies but one should also stress that the conversion symptom very often uses, as a pattern, physiological and anatomical sequelae of organic diseases. The organism has not only a life dependent on the psyche, but also one of its own, and every organic disease has an influence on, and brings into the foreground, specific behavior patterns and tendencies. The unity of the psychophysiological organism is dependent upon the soma as well as upon the psyche. The structure of the conversion symptoms finally cannot be understood unless we get a clear insight that individuals know about their bodies, that they have their price in specific parts of their bodies, and that the image of the body they carry within themselves is to a great extent dependent upon how much attention a specific part of their bodies, and their bodies as a whole, receive from other persons. In hysteria, in which the social and human relations to other human beings are so outspoken, this becomes especially evident. The body image of the hysterical case has been built upon its love relation to the parents. Organic disease again modifies it in connection with the attitude of the parents to the organic disease, in addition to the immediate changes which are provoked by the organic disease.

It is necessary, in order to treat any case of hysteria and for that matter any case of organic disease, to have an insight into the fundamental problems of hysteria. If one understands them, it is not difficult in many cases to show the patient his problems, and to help him to a better adaptation in his situation. The problem of hysteria is fundamentally one of social contact with other human beings under the aspect of suffering. It is not sufficient to study the psychosexual development of the hysteria case, but one has to widen the problem into that of interhuman relations. If there has been a basic difficulty in the family relations of the child, long-continued psychoanalysis or group psychotherapy is necessary. In other cases the correct attitude of the physician will help the patient to regain his full adaptation to his love objects and to society, which he has abandoned under the stress of a situation in the present which revived difficulties encountered in childhood.

Physicians often have misjudged the depth of suffering of the patient afflicted with hysteria. They have seen in such a patient the helpless individual who, like a child, leans upon the stronger person. They have blamed the patient for his struggle for love and his tendencies to imitation. This mistake has found a classical expression in the theories of Babinski, who had to make an artificial separation between the hysteria which is purely of the pithiatic type and so-called physiogenic disturbances of so-called reflex type. Hysteria is a form of human suffering which affects the psychophysiological person. It is only when we understand the seriousness of the problem that we can help the hysterical patient to a fuller social adaptation for which he struggles. Hysterical symptoms, organ neuroses, and organic diseases are forms of human suffering closely related to each other.

ORGAN NEUROSIS AND ORGANIC DISEASE

One should not talk about organ neurosis unless there are changes in the function or in the physiology and anatomy of the organ which can be objectively demonstrated. As Chapters 1, 2, and 4 have demonstrated, psychological problems may lead to changes in the organism which might be facilitated by the state of the organ (somatic compliance). This term was at first used by Freud for hysterical symptoms which are based upon an organic disease of minor degree. The term *somatic compliance* comprises, thus, two different aspects. (1) The psychological experience of the abnormal functioning of the organ attracts the conversion into this direction. (2) Such an organ may also be more available concerning the tendencies of conversion. In exophthalmic goiter, asthma, eczema, gastrointestinal disturbances, and many other diseases, psychological problems can be of paramount importance. (Cf., again, Dunbar's books.) Besides the hysteriform mechanisms, all kinds of deeper motives can be found. In all these cases the relation to one's body should be particularly studied. One should give special attention in all these cases to the attitude of the family towards disease in general and towards the particular organ. Mechanisms of identification may play a very important part.

One should neither overrate the chances of psychotherapy nor underrate its difficulties. Somatic treatment will often be necessary, irrespective of whether the symptom has a psychogenesis, when further physiological and anatomical changes have taken place. Outward circumstances very often will necessitate the choice of a shortened form of psychotherapy. Even then, it will be necessary to give attention to the infantile material. Success will often depend on the ability of the physician to bring forward infantile material, even when only a short time is available. Agnes Conrad has reached satisfactory results with such a method in exophthalmic goiter cases. The therapeutic results of psychotherapy in asthma are far from being satisfactory, although a few cases analyzed with good results are reported. Cases unsuccessfully treated are very often not reported. Similar considerations are valid for organic cases in the narrower sense. The optimism of G. Groddeck is not justified. At the present time we have to be modest and conscious of the limitations of the psychotherapeutic approach, although psychotherapeutic efforts should always be made.

The psychotherapeutic spirit is particularly necessary in the treatment of chronic organic diseases, as, for instance, tuberculosis, in which the attitude of the physician will very often be a deciding factor in the success.

We also have not much reliable data about psychological problems in connection with surgery. The importance of the psychological preparation for an operation is so far not sufficiently appreciated. If one considers that it is possible by hypnonarcosis, or anesthesia preceded by hypnosis, to reach a deep anesthesia with a smaller amount of gas, one may think of the possibilities of using psychological preparation in surgical cases, to an extent which has so far not been appreciated.

Hypnosis has been successfully used to induce sleep during childbirth in order to make the birth painless. It is necessary to prepare for this treatment during pregnancy. In the hyperemesis of pregnancy, therapeutic results have been reported. My own efforts in this respect, not very numerous, have not been successful.

Our knowledge about the psychological factors involved in the genesis of organic diseases is limited. The studies of Agnes Conrad, G. Draper, and Franz Alexander and his co-workers give some preliminary hints. Otto Fenichel stresses too much the narcissistic attitude of the sick person towards his illness. Psychoanalysts too often neglect the inner laws of the organism and disease. Freud himself has been much more cautious in this respect.

It cannot be emphasized enough that the psychotherapeutic approach to the organic case has to take careful cognizance of the organic problems. Physical and psychological findings have to be checked again and again in relation to each other. The field is at the present time still in the experimental stage.

NEURASTHENIA

The term *neurasthenia* is not very popular in American literature. This may be in connection with the fact that after the communication of G. Beerd (1880), the connotation has been used rather uncritically. It is, however, a rather well-defined complex of symptoms with a rather definite meaning. The obvious symptoms are fatigue, inability to work, headaches, constipation, spermatorrhea, prostatorrhea, difficulties in potency (especially ejaculatio precox), and sleep disturbances. The symptom complex may appear more or less suddenly or may develop in a chronic way. The neurasthenic conversion is a counterpart of the hysterical conversion. Whereas in the attitude of the hysterical case the organ is always in close relation to the outward world, the interest of the neurasthenic case is directed more towards the body as such. Although the neurasthenic very often has reached a superficial sex adaptation, his sexual organization is labile and difficulties in potency arise easily; they are very closely related to deep-lying anal and oral complexes and to aggressive instincts which are inhibited by fatigue. Neurasthenia inhibits work and whatever may be expressed by work and working. It is a restriction of social functioning. Homosexual components are very often outspoken in neurasthenic pictures.

It is obvious that the treatment of neurasthenic cases is difficult. Although it is usually simple to get a superficial view of the present situation, insight into the infantile situation is in no way easy to reach and very often a protracted treatment is necessary. The relation of the pictures to masturbation is in no way simple, although some younger patients relate their neurasthenic symptoms to masturbation. In some of these cases it is obvious that the masturbation has served rather primitive attitudes, of the type characterized above. Impotency in relation to neurasthenia is a symptom not easy to treat. Impotency of the neurasthenic type may at first appear as the only symptom. At closer inspection it becomes obvious that the impotency is far from being the only symptom and that it is in connection with deep-lying adaptation difficulties. The work of Wilhelm Reich affords further details. I have pointed especially to the close relation of neurasthenic symptoms to the processes of the construction of the body image, particularly in early childhood.

Physiotherapy is very often used in cases of this type. Sanitariums frequently specialize in this. Such an approach may be successful because of the symbolic value inherent in massage, exercise, and hydrotherapy of any kind. The problem of the neurasthenic still remains in the psychological sphere, and the physician should have an insight into this. The physician treating neurasthenics should be fully aware of the physiology of fatigue and sleep. Patients very often have taken fantastic connotations from popular books. The physician should also have knowledge of food habits and diets and should be aware that his accurate understanding of the physiological side of the problem is indispensable for the discussion of the patient's ideologies concerning his body. No type of psychotherapy can evade that. It is a fact that even heavy mental or physical overwork does not produce neurasthenic symptoms. Fatigue provoked in this way disappears very quickly. In the psychological sphere fatigue is, according to the appropriate term of Kurt Lewin, *psychic saturation,* and revolt against a too simple and monotonous reality. In many cases the patient has to be led to a deeper understanding of the situation, either by short psychotherapy or by psychoanalysis. Group psychotherapy can be used. Hypnosis is mostly useless.

HYPOCHONDRIASIS

It is often a matter of taste whether one wants to call a symptom neurasthenic or hypochondriac. In comparison with the neurasthenic, the interest of the hypochondriac in his body and his physical symptoms is still greater. The relation of the hypochondriac's symptoms to the world is still less outspoken than the neurasthenic's symptom. Psychoanalysis speaks merely about the overloading of the body with narcissistic libido and does not give much help in the understanding of the genesis of this overloading. It further justly stresses that the hypochondriac organ is treated like a sex organ. I may add that the hypochondriac organ has no relation to the sex parts of another person. The hysterical globus or clavus very often points to the sex parts of a specific lover. The various sensations in the body of the hypochondriac have merely a relation to himself and to his own sex organs. The leading symptom in hypochondriasis is the hypochondriac sensation. The hypochondriac fears concerning a particular organ or disease are less characteristic. It is almost impossible in cases of real hypochondriasis to get any considerable amount of transference. Also, the material proffered is so meager that a psychological construction is very often not possible. It was not possible in my cases. Accordingly, the results are poor in severe chronic cases, of which I have treated a comparatively large number for a long duration. I consider these cases as specific types of neurosis.

It is interesting that the patients often appear as well adapted as persons suffering from a chronic organic disease. They may even retain some sex activity and some amount of work may be performed. I have observed such a case for several years. There is only one important fact in the early history, namely, that he had heard that his mother, who died when he was only several months old, suffered horribly with terrible fits. One of his sisters died a very painful death when he was seventeen or eighteen. He saw her several times in a hospital. He married early, but his marriage was annulled. Subsequently he got his satisfaction by rubbing his legs against women in the subway till he ejaculated. He gave up this practice after several years and had sex relations only occasionally. He had an inexhaustible wealth of physical complaints. His heart palpitated, he fainted, his legs became so cold that he could not walk, his body felt heavy, when he ate he had terrible sensations in his stomach. He had had an abdominal operation which, so far as I could ascertain, was based on a wrong diagnosis of organic disease. He had been checked up physically with all the modern methods medicine has at its disposal again and again; with the exception of extremely bad teeth, nothing had been found. Psychotherapy brought only slight and temporary relief.

DEPERSONALIZATION

Depersonalization is a state of the personality in which the individual feels changed in comparison with his former state.[6] This change

[6] This section on depersonalization is reprinted from Paul Schilder, "The Treatment of Depersonalization," *Bulletin of the New York Academy of*

extends to the awareness both of the self and of the outer world, and the individual does not acknowledge himself as a personality. His actions seem automatic to him; he observes his own actions like a spectator. The outer world seems strange to him and has lost its character of reality. We find, therefore, in this picture changes of the self, or depersonalization in the narrower sense, and changes in the environment, or feelings of unreality, alienation of the outward world, or "derealization." Pictures of this type occur in a great variety of clinical conditions. The picture has been observed as a passing phenomenon combined with *déjà vu* in the normal. It may appear in connection with organic diseases of the brain, especially before and after epileptic attacks. It has been observed in depressive psychoses and schizophrenia. In the beginning and in the phase of disappearance of severe neuroses it is not uncommon.

However, this picture occurs also as the dominant symptomatology of a very severe and chronic type of specific neurosis. Patients of this type complain year after year about their changed experience concerning the self and the world. Cases are on record with a duration of twenty or thirty years.

The philosophical and psychological interest which these cases offer is considerable. H. Taine was the first to use the picture as proof for his philosophical theories of perception. Besides the complaints of changes in perception and emotions there are complaints concerning the experience of one's own body and about changes in the perception of time and space. Accordingly, the philosophers have used every one of these complaints as proof that this particular function is the most important one in our relation to self, body, and world.

The various authors have stressed different sides of the psychological problems. Reik stresses the constant self-observation which, according to his opinion, is based on sadomasochistic attitudes. Oberndorf puts the main emphasis on the erotization of thought and especially upon the wish to adopt the way of thinking of the opposite sex. Other authors stress the exhibitionistic and voyeuristic components in the picture. Bergler and Eidelberg are of the opinion that there is a strong tendency to anal exhibition, and this exhibition is transformed into an increased tendency to self-observation. I am inclined to stress the fact that the patient with depersonalization has

---

Medicine 15:258–66, 1939. See also articles on depersonalization by Iago Galdston and K. Haug. [L.B., Ed.]

been admired very much by the parents for his intellectual and physical gifts. A great amount of admiration and erotic interest has been spent upon the child. He expects that this erotic inflow should be continuous. The final outcome of such an attitude by the parents will not be different from the outcome of an attitude of neglect. Dissatisfaction has to ensue even if the parents live in a state of continual admiration of the child since every such relation does not consider the child as a total human being but merely as a show piece. The dissatisfaction and deprivation of the child has to express itself in an increase of aggressive and submissive tendencies. These combine with sexual tendencies to sadomasochism. Finally, by identification with the parents, self-observation will take the place of the observation by others. The self-observation will be blended with sadomasochistic tendencies. The individual will at first be able to admire his body as well as his thinking. Since such a detachment from the love object cannot remain satisfactory, the self-adulation will be followed by hypochondriac signs. To the denial of vision in the sphere of perception is now added the loss of admiration of oneself. The individual, however, does not completely give up and will at least enjoy the self-observation which represents the sadistic components as well as the voyeuristic and narcissistic (self-admiring) ones. The patients, furthermore, preserve their intellectuality in this way and are able to continue their activities in the social and physical world, which may appear outwardly successful although empty of emotional satisfaction for the individual. Depersonalization is the neurosis of the good-looking and intelligent who want too much admiration.

It is understandable that a neurosis of such depth will need a psychotherapy of long duration. The best observers in this field agree on this point. Oberndorf, for instance, has treated his cases for a long time; and Bergler and Eidelberg write as follows: "We think that this absolute pessimism concerning the treatment is not justified; however, it is a prerequisite for the therapy that one knows the mechanisms and starts on the right point. Moreover, a very long time is necessary. While the analysis of a more severe case of obsession neurosis takes at least two to two and one-half years, at least double the time is the requirement for the treatment of depersonalization. It does not seem to be very hopeful if one demands half a decennium for a treatment. However, '*amicus Plato, magica amica veritas.*'" The experiences of C. P. Oberndorf and myself are, however, better.

Some of my cases were treated with individual psychoanalysis; some of them were treated in group psychotherapy.

Psychotherapy in depersonalization cases takes a great amount of time, is technically difficult, does not always remove all problems, and does not protect the patient from relapses. However, there is no question that every case of depersonalization needs a great amount of psychological help, and there is no reason to be pessimistic concerning psychotherapy in these cases. The treatment has to be psychoanalytic or has to utilize psychoanalytic insight.

Considering the difficulties of the psychotherapeutic approach, one might ask what could be done for these patients by medication. I have occasionally tried benzedrine in depersonalization cases; however, the results were temporary, and the psychotherapeutic approach was in no way helped by the medication. Guttmann and Maclay have studied the influence of mescaline on depersonalization symptoms in so far as they consist of changes of the surroundings (derealization) but not of the self. However, this improvement was of short duration, not lasting longer than one day. The authors come to the conclusion that it may be used as an adjuvant for psychotherapeutic activity. A drug which brings a relief of short duration is obviously not of great therapeutic value with such chronic problems. It is usually not very helpful in psychotherapy when one proves to the patient, by the temporary relief with drugs, that he can feel better. Drugs which allow the patient to come to a deeper insight by increasing the transference situation and changing the state of consciousness help the psychotherapeutic approach much more than drugs which merely relieve symptoms. Sodium amytal may act in such a way. It has not been tried in depersonalization cases. I have, myself, tried to use benzedrine as a help in the psychotherapy of the neuroses. However, as mentioned above, such results were not achieved in depersonalization cases.

The modern methods of treatment for schizophrenia have only been tried occasionally in severe neuroses. B. Glueck mentions in one of his publications a case of severe obsession neurosis which was improved by insulin treatment. In the series of cases treated in Bellevue, one case of severe obsession neurosis reacted only temporarily to the treatment. At Bellevue we generally found the application of metrazol therapy simpler from a technical point of view and decided, therefore, to make an attempt to treat this particular type of neurosis with metrazol. The depersonalization cases constitute a comparatively well defined group of neuroses. The psychotherapeutic approach to these cases is difficult. Results obtained in such a group with metrazol might be of use in evaluating the treatment for neurosis in general. We have followed the technique of L. von Meduna.

In most of our cases the first signs of improvement appeared after the first three or four injections, and in the majority of cases the symptoms disappeared after about six to ten injections. We find it advisable, however, to give two or three more injections after the symptoms have cleared up. The symptoms may disappear without further psychotherapy; even then, the individuals always have unsolved problems. I am, therefore, of the opinion that every depersonalization case which is treated with metrazol needs extensive psychotherapy even after he is free from manifest symptoms. We have acted accordingly in all cases in which the outward circumstances made the application of psychotherapy possible. This is the same point of view which Orenstein and myself have taken in respect to insulin and metrazol treatment of schizophrenia.

One may, of course, raise the question whether the results of this treatment of depersonalization are merely due to psychological factors connected with the treatment. The patient experiences indeed terror and fright and even a threat of death. The transference is increased when he regains consciousness. However, it seems to me that such psychological phenomena are obviously the reflection of deep-lying changes in the organic functions. Furthermore, experience shows that deep-lying neurotic pictures cannot be influenced by mere fright. I am, therefore, of the opinion that organic changes in the brain function connected with metrazol treatment have a therapeutic effect on the depersonalization neurosis.

SOCIAL NEUROSIS

We have seen that in depersonalization the amount of interest an individual receives in his early childhood is of great importance for his later relation, not only to himself, but also to others. The patients with a social neurosis, although they seem to seclude themselves from their surroundings, have a very close relation to other human beings. The patient who fears to blush, blushes in the presence of everybody. The patient who gets shy is shy irrespective of whether he cares for the person or whether he does not. In one case, analyzed rather deeply in individual analysis, the patient had been inordinately spoiled by his mother and kept dependent and passive. He developed sadomasochistic attitudes which he later transferred to his social relations. In his relations to others, he wants their love and their admiration. At the same time he protests against his being dependent upon them. His shyness and his fatigue protect him against failure and make him independent again. At the same time, however, they increase and intensify his relations to other human beings. His difficulty with an acne at the time of puberty, which might have been partially determined by psychogenic factors, and his fatigue make action, aggression, and sadism impossible. When he is shy he starts to sweat and to shake. The mother, who had given him so much love and admiration in his childhood, is herself shy. Since his father was aggressive and active and not liked by the mother, fatigue and inactivity allow him to evade the dangers of not being liked by the mother. Before puberty he had been rather active and energetic. Sadomasochistic trends could be followed in detail before his third year. He very easily gets dependent in an abject way on his chosen love objects, who are small and obviously helpless.

The basic difficulty in the social neurosis lies, therefore, in an early social relation with too much admiration by father and mother, with a subsequent attempt to re-establish similar relations to other persons and symbolizations of these fundamental sadomasochistic relations in contacts with other persons. A deep dependence on the parent of the same sex, with subsequent revolt, may have a similar result. One often has called persons of this type schizoid or introverted, but I have pointed out before that these terms do not mean very much. Persons of this type have an extreme interest in the social reality and other human beings, but this interest remains undifferentiated. Neurasthenic symptoms are common. The social difficulties may be accompanied by somatic symptoms like blushing, sweating, tremor, but the somatic symptoms are not always obvious. Fatigue is a very common symptom, and the inner relation of this syndrome to neurasthenia is very outspoken. We may generally say that in the cases of neurasthenia, hypochondriasis, depersonalization, and social neurosis, we deal with a group in which the relation to one's body or one's psychic personality is disturbed. They all observe either their body or their mind. They very often repeat an attitude love objects have displayed towards them. Primitive interest in the body, in the oral and anal functions, is characteristic. Sadomasochistic trends are added. Homosexual revolt is not uncommon. The genital Oedipus relation, although present in the majority of these cases, is very often rather severely disturbed by the primitive drives. Even though cases of social neurosis are not uncommon in women, it seems to me that they are much more frequent among men, from whom a greater amount of social activity is demanded. The two cases of social neurosis I have lately observed among women were both intellectually outstanding and professionally active. It is perhaps not uninteresting to note that Charlotte Brontë, to whose aggressiveness her letters and *Jane Eyre* sufficiently testify, was extremely shy. We have to consider that it is also obvious that neurasthenia is more common among men. Depersonalization seems to be equally divided between the sexes. Neurotic hypochondriasis prefers men, according to my material.

Although the treatment of social neurosis is in no way a simple task, my results have been very satisfactory in psychoanalysis and especially in group treatment. In some less severe cases in which I could utilize the knowledge gained by cases observed for a long time, short psychotherapy has been successful. It is essential that the patient should not withdraw from the socially difficult situation. In some cases he has to be brought back to it by definite orders. In particularly trying social situations benzedrine, which intensifies interhuman relations and gives the feeling of being appreciated and loved, is useful. The use of alcohol, which has a similar effect in minor degree, is dangerous. The transference situations in neurasthenia, depersonalization, and social neurosis are rather similar. Owing to the impairment of the Oedipus situation, the positive transference is not so dramatic as in cases of hysteria. The resistances are generally strong; the negative transference, the distrust, rather outspoken. Oral and anal elements color the transference. This group, including stammering, can be contrasted to the hysteria anxiety neurosis and organ neurosis group in which the genital elements and the positive transference prevail.

STAMMERING [7]

It is obvious that according to the characteristics given above, stammering is merely a type of social neurosis expressing itself in speech. It is not necessary to repeat here how much stammering depends on the social situation and what painful feelings of shyness may be connected with stammering. It is obvious that stammering hits an organ which is particularly important for social contact and communication. The aggressiveness of the stammerer is obvious. It is not even necessary to go back into the early history. Very often the beginning of stammering is in connection with an aggressive act committed by another person who was stronger, which made the retaliation of the aggressiveness impossible. The act of stammering, consisting of "tonic occlusion" and clonic repetition, reflects the interplay between aggressive impulses and their inhibition. Freud has pointed to the similarity of the noises made by the stammerer to the noises during defecation. While anal components may be present, they are certainly not the only etiologic factor.

The general attitude of the individual towards those around him is of very great importance. The tempo of speech is increased, another sign of the aggressive tendencies. The stammerer also wants to answer immediately. Furthermore, he wants to give great attention to the formulation of his speech. Organic factors, as seen in stammering in encephalitic cases, may play an important part in the increase of impulses. Anal impulses may also be present in these cases. They are obviously secondary to the impulse disturbance in connection with speech. Brought into a short formula, we find in stammering a disproportion between the verbal formulation at hand and the impulse. This disproportion may be due to an increase and speeding up of the impulses either on an organic basis or from psychological motives, or it may be due to slowness of the formulation, or to a too great emphasis on the formulation. The knowledge of this basic problem is necessary in order to understand the various methods of treatment of stammering which have been devised. The order to slow down the speech and not to hurry with the answer is indeed of great importance. Every stammerer is a potential orator who

[7] See J. L. Despert *et al.*, "Psychosomatic Studies of Fifty Stuttering Children," *American Journal of Orthopsychiatry* 16:100–33, 1946. [L.B., Ed.]

wants to attack with his speech. Demosthenes developed from a stammerer into a violent political agitator. One should keep in mind that his stammering already indicated his violence.

It is wrong, therefore, to put the emphasis in such cases on an organ inferiority which has been overcome. I do not see any reason why speech training based on the understanding of the basic psychological situation should not be done. Smiley Blanton advises against giving any attention to the speech as such, and relies on the psychological understanding, preferably by analytical methods. (Cf. also the book of I. H. Coriat.) The psychoanalytic understanding, stressing the oral and anal components (sometimes the urethral components are present) and the aggressiveness in relation to early family situations, has finally to come to the understanding of the symptom as impulse disturbance and has to take into consideration the mechanics of the symptom. Stammering is much more common in men than in women, which is probably in connection with the fact that the social demands on boys and the aggressiveness asked from them are so much greater. It has been stated above that neurasthenia and social neurosis are also much more common in men than in women.

Short psychotherapy may be sufficient in simple cases. Hypnosis has been useless in my hands in cases of this type. I have no psychoanalytic experience of my own sufficiently extensive to judge the therapeutic results of psychoanalysis. Favorable results have been reported. Negative components probably play a very great part in the transference. Activity is, according to my opinion, unavoidable in the treatment of stammering also if psychoanalysis is used. It is obvious that group psychotherapy properly conducted will have a very beneficial influence, even if, as in the procedure of Greene, the point of view of education, exercise, and regulation is emphasized more than the insight in the total situation. I consider group psychotherapy, in cases of stammering, as the method of choice, and prefer group psychotherapy which tries to progress to the deeper human aspect of stammering.

TIC

Stammering is very often connected with movements of all types outside of the oral sphere. The movements serve a specific purpose. Very often they signify an additional effort when the expression by the mouth is blocked. They may facilitate the breaking through of the speech impulse through the tonic occlusion of the mouth. They constitute a symbolic expression of aggressiveness. Although these movements are ticlike, they differ in one important point from the tic. The stammerer seeks in his speech and in his movements a close relation to the world. Stammerers generally do not stammer when they are alone. The tic patient also suffers when he is alone, although the tic frequently increases when the patient is under social stress. Basically, the tic does not express any relation to the persons around. The tic very often expresses the fact that the individual has given up his interest in the world and has concentrated as much as possible on his own body, thus cutting off his relations to the world. In other words, tics are very often the motor counterpart of hypochondriasis. The tic patient very often is infantile, vain concerning his body and his intellect. His sexual development frequently has remained severely hampered by his enormous want of admiration and by his great interest in his own body. One speaks at the present time, therefore, about narcissistic components in tics.

In a very persistent tic concerning the gait, in which the patient interrupted the gait movements by torsion and flexion in the hip, the symptom had a very complicated genesis. The patient in his early childhood had the opportunity of watching intercourse between his parents, "boiling with rage." The mother once complained that the father hurt her leg. Sleeping in the same bed with his father, he once touched his father's penis with his leg. His first queer movements occurred when he approached a woman cousin in whom he was interested. He swung his legs in a wide circle in order to impress her, but the tic developed into its full strength only in connection with the obsession that there might be either dirt or something valuable on the street, and he had to turn around in order to look for it. The patient has an inordinate vanity concerning his appearance. He spent, especially in puberty, a considerable amount of time before the mirror. He is also very anxious that his bowels should be clean. He complains bitterly that, owing to poverty, he can eat only trashy food. He is also greatly convinced of his intellectual capacity. He does not like to do clerical work, but he says he was successful in interviewing persons as to their capacity for jobs. His success consisted merely in the fact that he liked this type of occupation.

It is obvious that the tic shows a power and strength in his leg comparable to the strength of the father's penis. Furthermore, the tic also serves his vanity. He wants to turn around to see the valuable objects coming from his bowels. In a secondary elaboration, the tic allows him to be the center of attention on the street and he achieves a prominence in this way quite different from the humble position he holds in life. In spite of the obvious relation of the tic to the Oedipus situation, the interest of the patient in himself is overwhelming. He wants to be able to admire himself, also his bowels. This overshadows even his wish for social recognition. The wish for social recognition, expressed in the primitive motor way, brings cases of this type in close relation to the social neurosis, although their object relations are more superficial than the object relation of the social neurosis case. The patient was in some degree benefited by group psychotherapy, in which he still participates.

Exercises before the mirror, which have been recommended by H. Meige and E. Fendel, not only proved useless in this case, but even increased his symptoms. I have seen good results by such exercises in other cases. The patient has to stand before the mirror, put his finger to the muscle which tics, and refrain from ticking—at first for a short time, from two to five minutes, according to the severity of the tic. Such sessions have to take place about twice a day. It is advisable that the physician be occasionally present at one or the other of these sessions. After the patient is reasonably sure that he is able to suppress the tic for a given length of time, he is asked to suppress it for a longer period. A scheme has to be devised in which the tasks are increased according to the specific symptomatology of the patient. This method seemingly is based upon the utilization of the narcissistic relation one has to one's mirror image, and to the increase of libidinous tension in an organ which is touched by one's hands. It is obvious that such activity can be combined with methods which are of a more searching character. The mirror method, combined with local touch, also has a decidedly physiologic aspect, since it is also efficient in cases of tic in which the organic origin cannot be doubted. Even in such cases, something can be reached in the psychotherapeutic way, the influence of psychological factors on so-called extrapyramidal motility disturbances being particularly strong. One should keep in mind, however, that there are tics, especially torticollis cases, which need organic treatment, and operation may be the only real help. (Cf. Hassin.)

Deep hypnosis, with complete relaxation, has given Otto Kauders and myself good results occasionally. If the hypnosis is not deep, one should try to reinforce it by drugs. It is advisable to let the patient sleep a sufficiently long time till the effect of the drug has worn off. Stammering and tic are difficult psychotherapeutic problems. The hysterical counterparts of stammering and ticlike movements on the basis of hysterical psychology share the greater accessibility of hysterical symptoms.

OBSESSION AND COMPULSION

It is obvious that a complete discussion of the different types of neuroses cannot be given here. It is merely intended to give preliminary help in facilitating the practical approach. We owe to Freud the insight that the fundamental characteristics of obsessions and compulsions are based on anal-erotic, urethral, homosexual, and sadistic trends. He has further described the character of the obsession neurotic case. It is identical with the so-called anal-erotic character. We find that patients of this type are parsimonious and insist upon orderliness and cleanliness. Superstition and a tendency to believe in the magic power of thinking very often are present. The patients show, furthermore, a very outspoken hate against their love objects or ambivalence. In different types of obsession neurosis, the proportion of homosexual, anal, aggressive, and magic patterns may vary. In some cases the relations to phobias are rather outspoken. One of my cases has suffered from a particular fear of being touched or bitten by dogs and cats, but he also had to watch continually and could not eat food when his mother had tasted it. The anal and aggressive patterns in this case were particularly outspoken. Magic thinking entered the picture only so far as he overrated the dangers of dirt and infection. In a hypochondriac case after a hernia operation, the general belief in the dangers of dirt, infection, and bacteria was also present and connected with compulsive washing.

In hysteria, the disturbance in the sex function is very often obvious. Obsession neurotic cases frequently show no obvious disturbance in their form of intercourse. They may even have full orgasm. They do not repress in the same way as the hysterical patient does, and their remembrances concerning the first few years of their life are often astonishingly complete. In hysteria, repression prevails; in obsession and compulsion we deal with a defense mechanism which tries to displace the accent from the original desires which come out in the obsession and compulsion. The infantile impulses may come out in the obsession and compulsion almost unchanged. However, symbolizations are not uncommon. One may say, at any rate in a schematic way, that whereas in hysteria, repression (forgetting) is paramount, in obsession neurosis, displacement plays a more important part, and hand in hand with it goes the tendency to consider one's thoughts and actions as not belonging to one's personality. Also, the structure of the superego is different in obsession neurosis and in hysteria. In hysteria, the superego is strong enough to keep experiences out of the consciousness, to a great extent. The superego has, therefore, no particular reason to use other devices to make the material innocuous. In the obsession, the forbidden material of the aggressive and anal type comes continually into the foreground. The individual has, therefore, to devise methods in order to make this material less dangerous. Freud in his later writings has drawn attention to psychic acts which try to isolate the dangerous material. One patient, for instance, forces objects back which remind her of sexual experiences, either by saying a formula or by making movements of pushing with her hands, or by looking, or with all three methods combined. Another method is the undoing, to make an action or a thought invalid by doing or thinking the opposite. One might say that in hysteria the enemy is kept out of the fortress (the "consciousness"). In obsession and compulsion neurosis, the enemy is in the fortress. One has either to push him out or to isolate him, or one must counteract every one of his actions.

In the last few years I have become more and more interested in obsession and compulsion neurotic cases in which organic signs point to an organic background for the increase of aggressiveness.[8] The particular activity of such patients, originating at a very early age, has led to an emphasis on the act of exploring holes and pushing something into something else. Some features of the so-called anal erotism could be thus explained from the motor side. Since individ-

[8] In "The Organic Background of the Obsessions and Compulsions," *American Journal of Orthopsychiatry* 94:1397–1413 (1938), Paul Schilder has discussed this problem in more detail with reports of case histories. [L.B., Ed.]

uals of this type are active in a way which disturbs the adult, the adult retaliates and the child comes into danger situations. To such situations the child may answer with an increase in reactive aggressiveness.

These patients often displayed a particular concern with problems of space, geometry, arithmetic, impact, and motion. Configurations in the outward world which are not closed provoked fears of an obsessional character, or they provoked reactions which restituted, directly or in a symbolic way, the inner equilibrium of the outside world. In the aggressive actions the distance in space did not count any more. One of my patients, for instance, felt that she had kicked objects and persons far away and might have provoked accidents and deaths of thousands in this way. It is technically of great importance to know the symbolic meaning of space and to interpret it to the patient. It is also obvious that these patients who check their motor impulses continually, finally no longer know which impulses they have followed and which impulses have remained without action. Accordingly, possibility and reality are no longer clearly separated. The patient disapproves of his violence and blames himself. There is an obvious feeling of guilt, very often in connection with the fear of direct retaliation by a father figure. The problems of right and wrong become paramount. There is, in addition, the continuous doubt.

In such cases, the insight into the structure of aggressiveness will be of paramount importance. It is obvious that aggression gets its shape by experiences in connection with early childhood situations in which the reaction of the parents to the aggressiveness plays a very important part. The reactions of the parents may not express themselves in actions concerning body openings of the child. But the aggressiveness of the child must, nevertheless, have an influence on its attitude to body openings.

One would expect that cases with a partially organic origin of the increase in aggressive impulses might be particularly difficult to treat. My experience shows the opposite. Properly handled, these cases react very well to psychoanalysis as well as to group psychotherapy. The primary aggressiveness and the reaction concerning one's own aggressiveness and defense against the primary symptoms are very often closely interwoven with each other. The compulsion to move one's toes and to kick and the tendency to curse God were such primary expressions in one of my cases. He felt compelled to throw away shoes and objects which he wore during outbursts against God. This is seemingly a reaction against the primary impulse, but it has taken over the energies involved in the first act. The structure of these cases may become very complicated.

In these cases there is direct evidence of a change in motor drives.[9] My own studies have shown me that about one-third of the obsessive and the compulsive cases show organic signs pointing to pathology with the same localization as that found in encephalitis. These changes may be constitutional, or they may be due to lesions in fetal life, to birth traumas or to toxic and infectious processes of unknown origin. F. Kehrer has recently pointed to the coincidence of true obsessions and compulsions with chorea and ticlike hyperkinesis. It is of great psychological interest that the motor factors in obsession neurosis show the relation of drives to perceptions and also prove an excellent approach to the fundamental therapeutic problem in obsessions and compulsions.

Freud has stated that the system of conscious experience has perception and motility as its basis. According to him, access to motility is through consciousness. Consciousness and motility are the nucleus of the ego in the psychoanalytic sense. Psychoanalysis has given attention to the more complicated functions of the ego and has neglected the study of the primitive motor functions in connection with problems of the ego. The work of Smith Ely Jelliffe and E. Stengel is an exception to this general neglect of organic motor functions. The general psychoanalytic literature does not sufficiently emphasize motor problems in relation to obsessions and compulsions. (Cf. the work of P. Federn, E. Bergler and G. S. Goldman.) The more general discussions of Nunberg and Fenichel mention Freud's fundamental discussion of the defense reactions in obsession neurosis, i.e., isolation and undoing, but do not stress the motor elements in the psychology of obsession neurotics.

I have shown previously that in many obsession neurotic cases there are neurological signs which point to parts of the brain which have to do with the distribution of impulses. These include tremor of the eyelids and arms, propulsive speech, rigidity of the face, lack of convergence of the eyes, convergence of the arms and elbows,

[9] Reprinted from Paul Schilder, "The Structure of Obsession and Compulsion," *Psychiatry* 3:549–60, 1940. [L.B., Ed.]

minor changes in the postural reflexes. In some cases the symptomatology points to an increase in the motor impulses.

Furthermore, there are a great number of cases of encephalitis which show obsessional phenomena, partially in connection with palilalia and palinphrasia. Coprolalia has been observed in tic cases. My own material contains a case in which a tic was converted into a compulsion to curse and use obscene words.

Most of the theories of instincts do not take into consideration that motility is an outlet for the needs of the total personality. Every instinct therefore has access to motility. Sexuality in the narrower sense carries with it its own activity just as well as the ego instincts. Also the conscious organization of the ego in the analytic sense is, of course, an organization with motor implications. Besides these more organized forms of activity and motility we often have to deal with changes in functions which are partially related to motility, as for instance in the changed drives of postencephalitics. Activity and motility are directed towards other persons. Sooner or later they lead to problems of superiority, inferiority, and to problems of aggression and submission. Sexuality has motor outlets as well as the ego instincts and the ego, and aggression may be connected with either of them. It has been shown that an increase in motor drives leads to aggression when considerable enough. Aggression may come from sexual, genital, and pregenital drives, internal drives or motor drives proper, or external drives. The drives in connection with the organization of the total personality, or the ego, stand in between. Aggression is a quantitative increase in activity beyond the usual which leads to a fight for superiority as well as to a destructive attitude towards persons and objects. If one uses this formulation one would say that normal sex activity does not include aggression. Aggressiveness in connection with internal drives is called sadistic. One may have the opinion that in sadism an admixture of external aggression and internal aggression can always be found. One may have the opinion that internal aggression is sufficient. One may say furthermore that the phenomenon of sadism occurs when sexuality is added to external drives. I am indeed of the opinion that sadism may start either in the internal or the external sphere. At the height of the aggression coming from either sphere, an admixture of the other sphere probably does occur. Furthermore, it has been stated above that strong external drives blend with internal drives partially by way of symbolism.

Although in the majority of cases the anal drive is dominant, I do not doubt that there are cases in which the neurosis is chiefly based upon oral and genital drives and their transformations. My own material does not contain instances of this type, but Hitschmann has stressed the importance of urethral tendencies. The question remains why these drives become the basis for an obsession. We have comparatively little indication of a particular constitutional strength of these internal drives. It seems that these internal drives are closely connected with aggression.

The internal drives are never isolated. They are in close relation to factors of interhuman relation and defense or the ego in the psychoanalytic sense. The ego, as well as the internal drives, has its own motility. Out of the interaction of the interhuman relation and the internal drives, problems of superiority and inferiority, activity and passivity, aggression and submission, arise. Conflicts between the ego and internal drives will finally lead to an expression in the motor sphere. There, expressions in the motor sphere are more the result of general human problems than of the increase in motor drives described above.

The obsession-compulsion neurosis in which motor phenomena are of proven importance and the obsession-compulsion neurosis in which the internal drives are paramount lead to very similar pictures. One cannot even say that compulsions have a closer relation to external drives. In the long run, motility belongs to every part of the personality structure.

Some patients derive a part of their aggression from preceding attacks of others. Aggressiveness is therefore experienced by the patients as reactive aggressiveness. The patients even experience an aggressiveness based upon increased external drive as counteraggression. Obsessions and compulsions come from a double source: from the fear of the patient of being attacked and from the continued preoccupation with such fear; and from the defensive measures against dismembering, castration, poisoning, and contaminations. Attack and counterattack are not tolerated by the total organization of the personality of the patient.

Aggression and submission are closely related to each other. By projection and identification either one may play both parts at once. It seems more than plausible that aggressiveness and increased destructive tendencies are an answer of the child to the fear of destruction and to the fear of being pushed into the inferior role. Since the threatening forces which demand submission are still present and are incorporated into the personality by the projection, a strong but dissociated superego will force the individual to develop strong feelings of guilt in connection with aggression. The feelings of guilt will be increased when the individual becomes aware of his normal or reactively increased internal drive. Alexander and Bergler have particularly pointed to the fact that a very severe superego puts unjust demands upon the individual. Finally, the individual succeeds in evading exaggerated demands. These authors, as well as Federn, have described in detail the complicated reactions and counterreactions between internal drives, interpersonal drives, and the superego. It seems that the individual demands from himself absolute exactness, isolation of the obsessions from other parts of the psychic life, and absence of doubt. I have shown above, in discussing the motility of obsession neurotics, how the increase in motor drives makes it impossible to act as a unified individual. Drives fight continually against the forces which counteract the drives. The drives, both internal and external, are also a part of the personality and try to devaluate the severity of the demands of the superego.

There is a decided difference between cases of this group and the group of cases in which one gets the impression that attitudes of the parents and the formation of the Oedipus complex are the main factors in the genesis of the compulsion and obsession neurosis. Actions and attitudes towards the child's body openings and its body in general, the varied interests of the parents in the sex parts and in the anal region, and, furthermore, the aggressiveness and the severity and the moral standards of the parents have to be chiefly considered. It is difficult in these cases to decide how strong the constitutional factors are which accentuate, for instance, anality. In the majority of obsession neurotic cases, the patient, although deeply involved in the primitive phases of object relations, has developed to the stage of the Oedipus complex. It seems to me that the present tendency in psychoanalysis to emphasize that so many persons do not even reach the Oedipus stage is not justified in the majority of cases. As I see development, in the majority of cases the individual develops in his relation to the outward world, especially to the love objects. However, this development loses its influence and power when too many primitive attitudes interfere. These are primitive attitudes not only concerning sex, but also concerning social relations. Freud himself finally stressed the diffusion between death instincts and sex instincts in the obsession neurosis. I think that the description I have given above is more appropriate.

I have stressed the importance of an insight into the spatial problems and of physics for the deeper understanding and for the practical handling of such cases. I may add, from a general point of view, that spatial problems play an important part in every type of neurosis. Since I have discussed this problem in detail on another occasion, I refer here merely to the technical aspects.

In some comparatively rare cases the fear of continued torture and an endless continuation of it in time may form a part content of the obsession. Otherwise obsession neurotics treat time like a valuable object, like money, feces, from which they do not want to part. The possessive tendencies of the obsession neurotic cases have been brought in connection with their anal erotism, but they must also have close relation to the aggressive impulses. One not only wants to take away from others but one also wants to keep objects of all types for oneself.

Since the world of the obsession neurotic patient is dangerous, he needs a special security. He may ask questions continually. He may, on the other hand, repeat again and again what he has said in order not to be misunderstood. He must, furthermore, have definite standards concerning right and wrong. He will always be insecure concerning the exactness of his connotations. In the psychoanalytic treatment we have to reckon with these factors. We very often shall have to demonstrate to the patient that his logic and punctiliousness are an escape from reality and that he uses them as a resistance in analysis to escape from free association. It is also obvious that we cannot give in to the patient when he demands sterile logical discussion, further explanations, and repetitions. It is perhaps the most important instance for the technical necessity that questions and demands of the patient in every psychological treatment should be considered as the expression of his psychological situation and especially of the state of resistance and transference. I see no reason why the patient should not be told when he makes errors of fact and of reasoning. This is particularly important, since important psychological problems are connected with these errors.

The analyst and the psychotherapist not only are allowed to but must reason logically. A sharp differentiation should be made between a formalistic logic and the logic which means adaptation to the reality. The distinction may be difficult. This consideration is also valid for any other type of neurosis. It has special importance in the treatment of the obsession and compulsion neurotic cases. It is also obligatory that the patient be made aware of the processes of defense going on in him. He should also learn what the consequences of such a defense are. Such an interpretation includes not merely the contents but also the formal characteristics of the patient's thinking. It must mean something definite when a patient considers a thought occurring against his wish and not belonging to him. We must interpret neurotic symptoms quite in the same way as we do dreams, interpreting not only the contents of the dream but also the formal characteristics of the dream. There is no question that experienced analysts act in this manner, but the necessity of continuous activity in analytic treatment is not formulated in the analytic literature. One may also discuss these problems under the heading of resistance and negative transference. This indicates that resistance and contents are merely two sides of the same psychic process. The resistance in obsession neurotic cases often appears in the intellectual sphere. The negative transference often uses the same procedure. If one analyzes obsession neurotic cases, or uses an analytic approach in group psychotherapy, one is immediately struck by the fact that there are two phases of the resistance. The one is more in connection with specific situations and symptoms; the other pertains to almost any approach to reality. One also receives the impression that these are two types of resistance not so different from each other.

One may call the widely spread type of resistance character resistance. One arrives, therefore, at the preliminary formulation that the individual may be satisfied with one or the other attitude in relation to his drives. They seem socially acceptable. There is no suffering connected with them, either socially or individually, and we may call such formations character. However, if such a character formation hinders the patient's insight and approach to reality, he should be made aware of the processes of defense going on in him. He should learn what the consequences of such a defense are. We find resistances in connection with character in every neurosis. If one merely removes the symptom and leaves the structure of character intact, the danger of recurrence of symptoms is greater. In many cases the patient not only has to give up his symptoms but will have to change his whole system of adaptations or, in other words, will have to change his character. There is a certain definite character type in connection with every type of neurosis. However, the similarities between a symptom and the character do not prove that they are identical. It is characteristic of an approved part of one's character that it has a social value and contains insight into important structures of reality. The greater difficulty concerning character resistances is in connection with their partial usefulness. From a more general point of view I think that even a neurotic symptom very often shows a part of the reality otherwise hidden. Freud has acknowledged this point of view concerning paranoiac cases only. The analysis of the symptom alone is therefore not sufficient. The character has to be analyzed, too. Whenever analysis takes place, resistances are present. Otherwise, analysis would not be necessary. The negative transference in obsession and compulsion neurotic cases is mostly very stormy. It may sometimes be difficult to handle.

The obsessive and compulsive character is based upon the same interplay between external, internal, and interpersonal drives as neurotic symptoms. However, in the neurotic symptom, the internal or external drive breaks through more or less transformed, according to the mechanisms described above, and the ego of the patient continues to defend itself against the drive. When the individual makes peace between the ego and the drives, character trends appear. The obsessive character is the sum total of compromises between the ego, superego, and the id. In some of these patients very far-reaching character disturbances may appear. The individuals may be misers, hoarders, cruel moralists, collectors, and so forth. The individual may even be of the opinion that his impulses are all right, and he may follow them more or less openly. L. Bender and I have shown that in children, drives of which the child approves are in the foreground. We have called this particular type of infantile urge an *impulsion* and have stated that this form is in close relation to the obsession and compulsion neurosis of adolescents. The interpersonal relations and the superego in children have not led to an organized defense. Of course therapy is concerned not only with symptoms but also with character. The relation between the two is continually changing. The fundamental problem is the change in the internal and the external drives and the organization of a defensive reaction. If this defensive reaction is weak then the picture is that of an impulsion. Then the impulsion may be a symbolic expression of a deeper wish. If the counterorganization is strong enough it leads to the formation of a symptom and varying conflicts between the symptom and total personality. The individual may himself allow impulsions. However, these impulsions may be more symbolic than the impulsions of childhood. If the impulsions can be brought into harmony with the interpersonal relations, we speak about obsessive character. The obsessive character may be more or less approved by society. This will reflect indirectly on the attitude of the individual towards his personality and character. There is a complicated play between what the individual allows himself of forbidden drives in symptoms, impulsions, and character trends and what the ego and superego of the patient demand and forbid. The parts of the personality may vie for domination in the total personality and may try to cheat each other.

In some of the cases it is probable that the difficulty starts with a disorganization of the external drives. In another group of cases the family situation provokes a change in the internal drives. This change may be facilitated by constitutional elements although we do not have definite proof of this. The change in the internal drives will change the external drives, and any change in the external drives will have repercussions in the internal drives. All drives finally end in motility.

We have reason to believe that the neurotic individual with obsessions and compulsions feels attacked by motor forces in the outer world and by aggressive attacks from other individuals. This attack from other individuals can originate in their motility or in their poisonous excreta like sputum, feces, and urine. If the individual is in danger of being pushed into an inferior, dependent position and if his integrity is threatened, he will answer with aggression of external and internal kind. Both may be reinforced by constitutional and organic factors.

The treatment has to be based upon the insight of the patient into the way in which his internal and external drives have made their appearance in all important life situations and human relations. In order to gain this insight, the full armamentarium of psychoanalytic technique has to be used, and the patient must be shown in every instance in which way the content of his experiences is the expression of the mechanisms described above. He will be helped if his experiences are revealed in group therapy. Individual interviews however will be necessary at given phases in the treatment. I have found it advantageous to have the patient draw whatever comes into his mind or to draw his dreams. The analysis of the contents of the drawings must go hand in hand with the analysis of the form. It is of particular importance that the patient understand the relation of his symptoms to his motility and aggression. It is furthermore necessary that the patient should conceive of his motor drives not as isolated phenomena but as part of a total situation between him, his love objects of the present and past, and society.

FRIGIDITY AND IMPOTENCY

I discuss these topics under a separate heading, merely because of their practical importance. They are not entities, even in the loose sense with which we speak about different types of neuroses. They are only symptoms which occur in connection with different types of maladaptation. It is justifiable to consider also, with Wilhelm Reich, the type of orgasm, the depths of satisfaction, and the release of tension after the intercourse, and to speak about an orgastic impotency when this release of tension, often experienced as sleepiness, is not sufficient. The patient with impotency or frigidity very often assures us, as many other neurotics do who complain about one specific symptom, that they are all right otherwise. Even when no other symptoms are present, one very soon finds that one deals with more or less severe deviations corresponding to one or the other type of neurosis and character deviation described above. The prognosis and the treatment will then be adapted to the underlying neurosis or character deviation.

In impotency we find one type, which is hysteriform, centering around the infantile relation to the mother and to the woman who demands deeper appreciation. Another type centers around preoccupations connected with the pregenital problems. This is the type which has clinical relations to neurasthenia, social neurosis, and hypochondriasis. The therapeutic problem is usually much more difficult. One may find among such cases persons who have repressed their genitality so early that its development has already been seriously crippled in childhood. I have had the impression that in some of these cases organic factors of unknown type play a part. Even then, they may be amenable to psychotherapy. Combinations of psychotherapeutic procedures with hormonal treatment have often been tried. I do not see any fundamental objection to such an attempt. I have done it myself and sometimes have had the impression that the hormonal treatment helped in the success. The difficulty lies in the fact that the hormones which have been available up to a very short time ago were far from being reliable. If they are, we should be aware that the problem of impotency is basically a problem of sexual adaptation in the psychic sphere and that the interrelation of these psychological factors to the hormonal situation is certainly not simple, if it exists at all. The field needs much more investigation before any reliable procedure can be found. In cases in which there are obvious changes in the gonadal function, an organic therapy of course is indicated. I consider local treatments in the form of massage of the prostate and passing a sound as senseless, unless one deals with obvious infections as, for instance, after gonorrhea. The so-called prostatic enlargement is merely the consequence of the deviation in the sex function of psychic origin. The effect of local urological treatments is often harmful from a psychological point of view. Its suggestive influence is counterbalanced by the psychological dangers incurred. It is important to keep in mind that most of the disturbances in potency are of psychogenic nature. The impotency of the presenile person very often is not the expression of organic involution but the expression of the specific psychological problems which are merely expressing themselves in an organ system, the vitality of which may be diminished. Even the organic impotencies in diabetes, tabes, etc., are often in their final expression dependent on psychological factors. It is obvious that deeper forms of psychotherapy should not be used in cases with organic components, and one will generally refrain from endocrine treatments if one conducts a deeper form of psychotherapy. In some cases it may be necessary to refer the endocrine treatment to another specialist.

The problems of frigidity are still more complicated, owing to the fact that the function of the clitoris in the normal sex relation is not very well known. We expect that the female orgasm should occur without particular mechanical irritation during or before intercourse. It is possible that the stimulation of the clitoris during intercourse plays an important part in the final satisfaction. It is a special problem in female frigidity that seemingly early clitoris masturbation plays an important part in its genesis. According to our general principles we would ask, of course, what this clitoris masturbation means psychologically, and would not merely consider clitoris masturbation as habit formation. The great prevalence of frigidity in women is probably due less to the fact that the female sex organ is more complicated and more exposed to psychological misinterpretation in early childhood than to the fact that women are under a continuous social pressure to repress their sexuality, a factor which starts to be effective long before puberty. Otherwise, the same considerations are valid for frigidity as for impotency. Pain phenomena in the sex organs which disturb cohabitation, as far as they are not strictly organic, have a meaning very similar to that of frigidity in general.

The treatment for impotency, and frigidity as well, needs the activity of the physician in so far as he has to insist on intercourse when the treatment has been far enough progressed. The difficulties in giving such advice have been previously discussed. The patient has to know what he or she wants and has to act accordingly. If the person has merely one love object, one of course has to raise the question whether the impotency and frigidity are not due to shortcomings of this object in a sexual respect. Such an investigation is only possible in extended psychotherapy. The advice to change love objects should not be lightly given. Very often the love object, who seemingly is the potent partner, has to be treated, too. One often will find at the basis of sex difficulties of a couple, ignorance of one of the partners, or neurotic attitudes which isolate the individual from the partner, finally leading to an insufficient consideration of the other partner's needs.

Urologists often recommend rest in cases of impotency, and especially in cases of ejaculatio precox, on the theory that an irritation exists in the genital tract. Theory and practice are equally wrong. Only in the beginning of psychotherapy do we have to advise the patient not to have intercourse, when we do not want the patient's attempts at intercourse to impair the development of the transference situation. When a transference is sufficiently established and when some preliminary insight is gained, there is no reason why we should advise the patient to refrain from sex activities. There are some cases in which one may forbid intercourse for a longer time if one is reasonably sure that the patient will not obey the order. Such a procedure has this advantage: the patient does not feel that he is under an obligation, and an eventual failure may be less depressing. The patient may also profit by his feeling that he is acting against an order. However, if the advice to continence is too faithfully followed, the patient has to be told that the time of waiting is over and that he is now allowed to make attempts. If the permission is not sufficient, the patient has to be urged to have intercourse. One may object to this procedure on the ground that it is insincere and tricky. It often is an efficient procedure, although I prefer not to use it, and to adhere to the basic rule of modern psychotherapy of not saying anything to the patient which one does not believe oneself.

It is very simple to explain to the patient, after a sufficient transference is established, that he may now attempt intercourse, that there is so far no necessity to do so, that he may fail, and that such a failure should not be discouraging. Later on, one may tell him that it is necessary for him to have intercourse and to face the possibility of a failure. In many patients, the resistance against attempts is great, and they insist that they want at first to be sure of their potency. Obviously, they never can be. All kinds of evasions are used. The patient may confess to having aversions and fears concerning prostitutes. He may pretend not to have an opportunity of finding any other love objects. He may also protest against another person being merely a technical tool. Any one of these objections may have a deep justification. Psychotherapy has to find out where these doubts originate. Very often they are simply pretexts invented in order to escape any sex activities.

In the course of a psychotherapy the patient has to know what he wants. If he wants to be a saint and he can stand it, it is not the task of the physician to discourage him. However, saints usually do not come for treatment of impotency. The task of the physician cannot be to impose morals on the patient, but he has to help the patient find the morals fitting to him. The patient has to know for what he needs his potency. It is obvious that the technical knowledge of sex problems is necessary in order to give help and advice to the impotent patient. It is, for instance, obvious that many patients are not sufficiently oriented about the female sex parts and the technique of intercourse. Patients with premature ejaculations should know that shortening of the interval between two sex acts may improve the situation considerably. However, no discussion about the technique of intercourse will do the patient any good unless the psychotherapy reveals to the patient his deeper attitude towards sex.

It has been justly pointed out that the basis for an exaggerated need for sex activity is not very different from the basic problems of impotency. In cases of so-called nymphomania (exaggerated sex demands of women) and satyriasis (exaggerated need for sex activity in men) the psychological situation has to be investigated. The local genital situation hardly ever plays any part.[10]

NEUROSES AND BEHAVIOR PROBLEMS IN CHILDHOOD

These remarks have obviously a preliminary character. A full discussion will be given by L. Bender later on, on whose work the following remarks are oriented.[11]

In order to treat children one has to understand them. One must regard children as personalities and not infringe on their right to express their personality. Children with behavior difficulties and neuroses have been faced with problems too difficult for them. One of the greatest difficulties a child can be confronted with is lack of love. Children need, helpless as they are, a great amount of love which considers their needs and not the needs of the adult. So-called spoiling means merely that the adult satisfies his erotic and aggressive needs on the child. Love means caresses, stroking, and, by derivation, clothes. The child also needs food, and assurance that he will get it. It needs help in securing motor equilibrium. It needs, further, an opportunity of displaying its activities as far as they go. Children react to deprivation and insecurity with aggressiveness, since they experience them as aggression against themselves. The aim of psychotherapy of the child is, therefore, to find the sources of deprivation and insecurity, to remove them when they are in the outside world, and to help the child in the understanding of its position when the insecurity is merely due to unsolved conflicts.

[10] Many new insights into the problems of sex behavior have resulted from the Kinsey reports, even though the research method of Kinsey did not include psychological evaluations. [L.B., Ed.]

[11] In *Child Psychiatric Techniques* (Springfield, Illinois, Charles C. Thomas, 1950), Lauretta Bender has included the writings of Paul Schilder and other associates on the therapeutic, as well as diagnostic, approach to children. [L.B., Ed.]

Even the most casual psychotherapy will have to study the relation to father, mother, and their substitutes, and to siblings. The child is in danger situations and reaches, therefore, for love objects which guarantee not only instinctive satisfaction, but also other securities. Everything which endangers the relations to the love objects endangers the total existence of the child. It sees, naturally, the problems not only in relation to these love objects, but also in relation to their bodies and to its body. One has, therefore, to give full attention to the sexual problems of the child and its relation to its body. Ward routine, in the sense characterized above, discussion, and adaptation will be useful in a great number of cases. Play technique is extremely helpful. It is obvious that education is an important part of the total situation of the child. I consider, as previously mentioned, Melanie Klein's technique in child analysis as violent and arbitrary. It is a one-sided projection of the problems of the child into one system. I do not deny that it may be helpful in a more or less symbolic way, the child using its one-sided approach more as a model and a symbol that difficulties can be solved and that dangers can be eliminated.

In difficult cases, I favor much more the cautious approach of Anna Freud, who takes the total situation much more into consideration. In the majority of cases, especially when a ward is sufficiently organized, complete analysis in younger children will not be necessary. Without having sufficient experience, I am convinced that treatment in groups and in surroundings in which other children participate is the method of choice, even if a deep analysis should be necessary. But group treatment, in any event, has to be supplemented by individual discussions. The educational and social situation should be carefully considered. When the child is older, the play technique has to be more and more replaced by an association technique or its modifications. When the children are around eight, nine, or ten it will very often be advantageous to have the child invent stories or continue stories, or to express itself in relation to pictures and art productions. The older the child gets, the closer will the technique resemble that used in the adult.

The younger child reacts to difficulties in the situation by a change in behavior. It becomes a "bad" child. Aggression, shouting, hitting, restlessness, violent acts against other children, especially siblings, become its most important weapons in the fight. It may use urination and defecation as weapons against the adult, and the child already clean may wet and soil the bed again. Obviously, urination and defecation not only serve its aggression but also the erotic needs of the child. It may also cling to erotic gratifications of another type, especially in masturbating but also by displaying a great interest in the sex parts and the erogenic zones of other children. It is obvious that the masturbation, sometimes starting in the first few months of life, serves an immediate somatic urge as well as being the expression of erotic problems in connection with the relation to the parents. It does not interest us specifically whether the Oedipus complex is already developed at a very early age, as Melanie Klein states, or merely later on, as the classical analysis holds. I am more in favor of Klein's opinion. The strong urge of even small children to give and receive love is striking in direct observation, and in long-protracted analyses of adults I have often found evidence of very early tender relations in the sense of the Oedipus complex.

When the child becomes older, after five or six, its behavior difficulties take a different aspect. Precocious sex behavior, urination and defecation at improper occasions may still be present. Its defiance is better verbalized now; outbursts of rage, crying, not eating, lack of attention in school, become more and more outspoken. Its aggressive behavior may concentrate on specific persons and situations. The underlying problems are basically identical with the problems of the younger child. The Oedipus complex finds a more or less familiar expression. Lying and stealing may become the leading symptoms. They may, of course, have a very different meaning. The child by lying may express its superiority. It may want to appear more important, to get more love; it may hide behind the lying a more or less terrifying problem of another kind and finally may find symbolic gratifications according to the contents of the lie. Stealing has to be considered from a similar point of view. It may be the expression of the wish for compensation for impairment of any kind. I may remind you that according to the psychoanalytic interpretation in the so-called kleptomania, the individual regards the object as a symbolization of a penis. The individual may want to hurt the person from whom the object is taken, or may wish to impress others. Very often the forbidden act forces the parents to give more attention to the child. The punishment may be desired in this respect and may at the same time relieve the feeling of guilt which may have originated with deeper-lying sexual conflicts. This is, according to Freud, a rather common occurrence. Juvenile criminals may commit crimes in connection with unconscious feelings of guilt.

The child may also, if the home situation becomes unbearable or does not promise any deeper satisfaction, run away from home, or, under similar circumstances, not go to school. If the motives for running away or for truancy are obvious, we may speak about a behavior problem, even if the deeper motivation is hidden. If the child runs away from home without conscious motivations, we talk about fugue and speak about a neurotic symptom. The border line is often not very sharp. One may also call enuresis, soiling, and difficulties in eating, neurotic symptoms as well as behavior problems.

Among the neurotic manifestations in the narrower sense, anxiety plays the leading part. The child accustomed to overprotection and erotic gratification does not want to be left alone and reacts with anxiety. If by too intimate relations to the parents or by visual participation in parental sex relations the erotic demands are increased, anxiety is liable to appear. It is generally a danger situation for the child when his sex demands—either by inappropriate behavior of the parents or by a seduction of adults or other children—are inappropriately increased, since sooner or later the point is reached where such gratifications are no longer sufficient. The erotic situation has to be carefully investigated in every case in childhood in which anxiety becomes obvious. The most common types of specific infantile neurosis are the phobias in which a specific fear, especially concerning animals, is observed. Since Freud's analysis of little Hans, we know that the animal which provokes fear is a substitute for the father in relation to the Oedipus complex. Anxiety dreams of a similar content may have the same meaning and may be the first signal of the approaching infantile neurosis.

Conversion symptoms can occur at a very early age. Continuous crying, not eating, and vomiting belong in this category. Children are particularly prone to develop habits in motility like tics and shaking under an emotional stress. This has partially to do with the fact that the motility in the child is as yet not well organized and many difficulties may arise in the process of organization. Symptoms of this kind may be used later as the basis for the formation of tics and, therefore, should not be treated lightly. Restlessness and inability to sit still have to be considered from a similar point of view. Obsession neurotic difficulties are comparatively rare but may appear in the rather early ages of five or six. In the majority of cases, obsessions at this age manifest themselves in compulsive behavior, in particular fastidiousness and neatness, and in an urge to count. Fears that something might happen to the love objects are very often early signs of an obsession neurosis. Signs of this kind indicate that a thorough psychic treatment is necessary.

It is necessary to give particular attention to the physical state of the child. An increase of aggressiveness and of problems connected with it may be associated with an encephalitis. Difficulties in the nutrition of the child on an organic basis may have the same effect as deprivation due to the family situation. Diseases and deformations, difficulties in walking and learning to talk are the basis of symptom formations in the motor field and in the field of speech. Children who do not talk or who develop stammering often have an organic lesion or inferiority which, in connection with the situation, leads to the difficulty. Itching diseases may lead to an overvaluation of skin sensations, aggression, excessive masturbation; all these factors will be effective only in connection with the total life situation. Every organic disease of the child—and there are so many—is not only a physical problem but also a severe psychological problem which has to be dealt with. It is probable that the majority of conversion symptoms take their origin from actual diseases experienced in childhood. Somatic treatment may add further difficulties. An enema is not only a physical treatment but an important psychological event in a child's life. The proper evaluation of physical illness is important not only for the handling of the child during the illness but also for the understanding of subsequent neurotic symptoms. One should ask which gratifications originated from the organic disease, which were the deprivations in connection with the disease, and which are the reactions to deprivation and gratification.

The child, like everybody, wants to do justice to the situation. It compares itself with other children, and if it does not do so itself, the parents do. If there is any disability in the child we therefore deal not only with the problem of this defect, but also with the problem of adaptation to the disability. Very valuable remarks about this point are to be found in the writings of Alfred Adler and his pupils. There are disabilities concerning motility and especially concerning speech. They have to be studied and treated carefully, and one has to avoid pushing the child into situations for which its equipment is not sufficient. Very great difficulties may arise from congenital reading disability, which has been carefully studied by S. T. Orton. I agree with him that one deals with an organic difficulty due to an underdevelopment of specific parts of the brain. If the condition is not recognized in time, the child is put before a task which it cannot solve, feels unjustly attacked, and reacts with more or less far-reaching behavior difficulties. It may compensate for the reading disability by an increased interest in the optic and mechanical world. Such a compensation is, of course, desirable if the child and its surroundings appreciate the defect in the correct way. The compensations should not remain in the realm of an escape.

The correct appreciation of specific learning difficulties is of importance. It is possible that such learning difficulties may be exaggerated by situational difficulties. Very often an organic delay or impairment is the nucleus around which the difficulties of the situation crystallize. Insight into the nature and structure of reading difficulties may thus give valuable hints of how to approach the problem of specific shortcomings and their opposite specific abilities in the child and, of course, in the adult also. Everybody should know his intellectual and other capacities, which are, after all, an important part of the reality of an individual. If there are more or less severe shortcomings, the individual has to face them, whatever they may be. There is in every human being much intrinsic value for which he can be appreciated by the community and can appreciate himself.

PSYCHOPATHY

Psychopathic individuals are those who are halfway contented with themselves but suffer from their relation to society. They harm others and suffer from the reactions of others. E. Kahn's book enumerates and describes the various types of psychopathic personalities. L. Bender stresses emotional deprivations in infancy in psychopathic children and compares them with similar personality deviations associated with an organic background. We may also say that psychopathy is the problem of a character formation which is not sufficient for the social tasks of the individual.[12] It has been mentioned that

[12] See the work of William Goldfarb, H. Cleckley, and Ben Karpman on the dynamics of the psychopathic personality. See also the symposium

neurotic symptomatology cannot be separated from character formation, and we find, therefore, character formations which are in close relation to hysteria, compulsion neurosis, or stammering, but without any definite symptoms from which the patient suffers. Other character formations might lie in the direction of manic-depressive psychosis or schizophrenia but without psychotic symptoms. However, the variety of attempts to find an adaptation to the demands of oneself and of society is almost inexhaustible. Characters are the crystallizations of such attempts, and we can speak about psychopathy when this attempt has not been very successful from the point of view of society. It is obvious that this pattern formation takes place at an early age, that constitutional characters and organic changes are of importance, and that the relation to father and mother is of decisive influence.

We are here merely interested in the technical problem. The character is a system of defense and adaptation which has been codified and incorporated into the personality to such a degree that it can be maintained without very much renewal of the cathexis, since psychic energy has become bound to the character structure as potential energy. It offers, of course, great resistance to analysis. The individual knows that in giving up his character he will come into a state of chaos and suffering and does not want to take this risk. We also expect the same resistance, although in a lesser degree than in the normal, in a psychopathic case. Since the neurotic suffers, he will be more amenable to the analysis of his character. These differences are diminished by the fact that almost every so-called normal has one or another neurotic symptom, and psychopathic personalities almost always show neurotic symptoms of more or less severe degree, by which they suffer. With the exception of cases with compulsions and obsessions, neurotic symptoms may be treated in psychopathies with short psychotherapy. If one wants to change the character deviation as such, a deeper form of treatment will be necessary in the majority of cases. Hypnosis is then useless. The general principles of treatment are the same as in treatment of neurosis except that special attention has to be given to the resistance coming from the character.

Wilhelm Reich has pointed to this particularly, and he has drawn the conclusion that one should start every psychoanalysis with the

---

(Ben Karpman, Chairman) on "The Psychopathic Delinquent Child," *American Journal of Orthopsychiatry* 20:223–65, 1950. [L.B., Ed.]

analysis of the resistance and the negative transference. In neurosis, as well as in character deviations, it will depend entirely upon the patient which problem of analysis is taken up first. An analysis of the resistance as such is impossible according to the discussion given above. Reich has justly pointed to the importance of the so-called impulsive character. These are persons inclined to sudden change in their behavior. They give in to their asocial impulses without hesitation. He is of the opinion that in such cases the father and mother had fundamentally different attitudes and goals. The individual is thus prevented from getting a unified attitude towards the social reality. This factor indeed plays an important part in the genesis of psychopathy.

It seems that psychopathic reactions also are more common in children of parents who show sudden outbursts of temper. Quarrels between father and mother may have a similar influence in impairing the possibility of adaptation to the family, and to society later on. In one of my cases the patient was afraid of the father, who, although generally kind, went into violent rages from which the patient escaped by locking himself in the toilet. The mother displayed an aggressive tenderness towards him as the oldest son. His attachment to the mother was very great. His attitude towards the father was that of antagonism. In the earlier and in the later experiences there was a mixture and succession of sadistic and masochistic tendencies, masochistic attitudes prevailing. He also expected a complete gratification irrespective of what he might do or might not do. This latter attitude is seemingly in connection with the fact that at any rate his mother loved him and wanted to give him whatever he needed. His phantasies and dreams otherwise centered around situations like being castrated by the Ogpu. He was amiable and humoristically inclined, which probably had very much to do with the discrepancy in the attitude of the parents since even if he was threatened by the father his mother loved him and nothing could happen to him. He was not able to work steadily and he lost one position after another. In his sexual life he remained bound to his dead mother and had never had any deeper interest in any person of the other sex. He was impotent before he came for treatment. He had premature ejaculations. Even when he had full erections he failed in finding the female sex opening. He was not very much concerned with this difficulty, taking it smilingly. He took it as a matter of course that without any particular effort on his part everything would come in order. During the treatment he succeeded in a reasonably good sex adaptation. He had the same attitude about his lack of earning capacity, until his poverty became too oppressive. It is obvious that in such a case the patient will lose his feeling of well-being during the treatment before he can adapt fully. I have found that patients of this type profit particularly from being in groups. Incidental symptoms of psychopathic individuals react rather quickly to any type of psychotherapy which is halfway rational. If one wants to influence the character or the psychopathy as such, one has to dig deeper.

I may merely make a short remark here about so-called schizoid personalities and schizoid psychopaths. These terms are used today so widely that they obliterate the insight into the various character types. One is entitled to use these terms only concerning persons who, in their whole attitude of shyness and withdrawing, show a deep lack of interest in other persons; in their tendencies to delusions and hallucinations and in their inclination to paranoiac reactions, they show a decided similarity to schizophrenic pictures. The difference lies merely in the fact that the schizoid psychopath still retains a closer relationship to the world, and even if he gives this up under the stress of circumstances, and goes into psychotic pictures, he returns to the reality again. Some of these cases are based upon constitutional factors; in others early experiences are paramount, and there is no reason why group psychotherapy or psychoanalysis should not be tried.

Janet has used the term "psychasthenia" for a group of varied cases, and this term has found its way into the literature without becoming more definite. As it is generally used, it excludes hysteria and includes almost everything else, but means especially cases of social neurosis, depersonalization, obsession neurosis and compulsions, and those types of psychopathies which are not of particularly aggressive character. I cannot see any particular reason to adhere to this term; but I do think that in the field of neurosis, discussions about classification and terminology are rather useless. One should try to describe the types faithfully, but should be aware of the great difficulties in making sharp distinctions. In the choice of the therapeutic methods the classification of neuroses does not help. We have at any rate to ask for the depth of a neurosis. We may also raise the question of how far the character is involved. When a short psychotherapy is tried or a preliminary analytic investigation is undertaken, one very soon sees which type of transference and resistance is prevailing.

Janet's term "psychasthenia" is in close relation to his theory that many cases of neurosis are due to lack of psychic tension or a lack of psychic energy. Janet treats these cases accordingly by bringing them into situations where not much energy is spent. Such a theory neglects too much the actual life problems of the patient, does not give him sufficient insight, and leads to a therapeutic attitude which restricts the life of the patient and hinders his final adaptation. It is only justified in cases in which the psychotherapist feels that he is helpless. This is fortunately only a very small percentage of cases. It has been justly pointed out that there are many schizophrenics among Janet's psychasthenics. In some of the schizophrenic cases it is justifiable to simplify the life situation of the patient to the utmost. Such a procedure, however, is not justified in the great majority of neuroses. There are cases which have progressed so far in their neurosis that they cannot stand any attempt to give them a deeper insight. The physician's task is difficult. He no longer has any possibility of leading the patient out of his neurosis and must restrict himself to consolation, guidance, and advice. He may then try to make the life situation of the patient as agreeable as possible without too much impairing the life of the more active members of the family. A neurosis of almost any type may in this way become inaccessible to a deeper curative approach. The physician then functions like the narcotic which alleviates the pain and discomfort of the otherwise incurable sufferer.

PERVERSIONS

All perversions have a complicated psychogenic structure. They are the outcome of infantile conflict situations which led to difficulties in adaptation and a rather rigid pattern formation. Since the perverted person does not object to his perversion, unless it leads him into serious social difficulties, which may also appear as a moral conflict, perversion and psychopathy belong very close together. The importance of constitutional factors is difficult to appreciate. It does not seem that the constitution prescribes the subsequent form of perversion; it offers merely the possibility of reacting to specific traumatic situations in a more specific way. One has again and again tried to bring homosexuality in connection with the biologic facts concerning hermaphroditism and intersexes. As far as I can see there is no justification for such an assumption. Furthermore, we have no definite proof of a hormonal genesis of homosexuality. I agree with O. Schwarz in this respect. As long as our biological knowledge is incomplete, we should keep in mind the psychological side of the problem; and, as I can say from my own observations, some cases of homosexuality can return to heterosexuality under psychological treatment. I have the impression that the proper handling of puberty situations can achieve very much, even in short psychotherapy. Any approach which does not frighten the adolescent can be useful. In all perversion cases of long standing or those in which the problem was overwhelming in earlier childhood, more elaborate methods of treatment will be necessary. For the basic understanding of the problem of perversion, one should keep in mind that the full development of love relations to the other sex is always disturbed when, in the early relations to the parents, a part function of the body has been stressed too much or when aggression and submission interfere with the natural situations of dependence and mutual help. In the treatment of the adult the sexual ideology should be fully discussed; but this is, after all, necessary in every treatment.

CRIMINALS

The psychoanalytic approach to the problems of criminals and of crime has been discussed lately by Alexander and Healy. The psychoanalytic approach has to remain incomplete, since the social structure is of paramount importance in the genesis of the criminal and of the crime. Therapeutic results so far reached are less encouraging than one would wish. I think that an approach by groups stressing the ideologies and possibilities for adaptation comparable to those of the modern psychiatric hospital should offer possibilities. If our general therapeutic approach is helpful, it should be of use in the approach to the cure of the criminal. However, crime is so closely bound to the structure of society that we do not have the right to look at the criminal apart from society; and the question has at least to be raised not only of how one should cure the criminal, but also how one should cure society.

The classification of criminals into psychotic, neurotic, psychopathic, and normal criminals is, of course, the basis on which treatment has to proceed.[18] The criminal who has a psychosis obviously does not need treatment different from other psychotic patients. Two subdivisions of these should be recognized: those who become psychotic and who in their psychosis continue previous criminal attitudes, and those whose criminal acts are committed merely because of the psychosis. I saw, for instance, a schizophrenic case who killed his wife and his three children with a hammer in order to give them eternal life. Whatever the deeper motivation of such a crime may be, it is a crime of a psychotic individual and of a completely different meaning from the crime of the so-called criminal in the narrower sense. It would be easy to multiply instances of this type. A case of such structure has, of course, to be committed to an institution and treated like any other case of schizophrenia.

A neurosis as such will rarely be the direct cause of a crime. There are, however, cases in which the neurosis as such is the crime-producing factor—for instance, in kleptomania and especially in shoplifting. It may sometimes be difficult to draw the border line between neurotic shoplifting, and the shoplifting which is done purely on a criminal basis. Such cases naturally need the same treatment as any other neurosis. Sometimes it may be sufficient to discuss the more obvious mechanisms; sometimes deep psychotherapy will be necessary.

The psychopathic group, that is, individuals who, besides the fact that they commit crimes, show a more or less deviant character formation, will need the same treatment as other psychopaths. It is known that the treatment of psychopathic personalities is among the most difficult tasks in psychotherapy. The psychopath has no manifest conflict between his superego and his ego. He has reached some sort of equilibrium which is acceptable to him from the point of view of his personality. The problem of psychotherapy will therefore first be to make the individual feel sick and then to cure this illness. However, individual psychotherapy in these cases may often be in vain, and one will have to change the environment so that it fits the situation. The noncriminal psychopath can often exist only in an

---

[18] The rest of the discussion on the treatment of the criminal is taken from Paul Schilder's, "The Cure of the Criminal and the Prevention of Crime," *Journal of Clinical Psychopathology* 2:146, 1940. [L.B., Ed.]

environment which is made easy or strictly regulated. He may need a helping hand throughout his lifetime whether he is analyzed or not analyzed. Criminal psychopaths have to deal not only with their psychopathy but also with their crime, and the penal institution will be very often an environment which drives the psychopath deeper into his conflicts.

Now we come to consider sex criminals. They have generally the same basic psychology as the perverts. There is no question that the most difficult problems of psychotherapy are involved, for instance, in the treatment of any perversion. However, many analysts and I myself have occasionally had good results in the treatment of homosexuality and other perversions. Although homosexuality is technically a crime, it is one of the crimes which are only persecuted under specific circumstances. Voyeurism, exhibitionism, are obviously sex crimes of minor importance. Sex offenses against minors are of a greater social importance although the minors play a more active sexual part than is generally supposed. (Cf. L. Bender and A. Blau.) The newer psychoanalytic attitude towards perversion insists that the perversion not merely is the persistence of an infantile sexuality but is the result of an infantile neurosis. The treatment of perversions and the treatment of neurosis are therefore very similar; however, it is again necessary to make the patient suffer directly under his perversion if success is to be reached.

We are of course fundamentally interested in those criminals who are neither neurotic, psychotic, psychopathic, nor defective. About 80 per cent of all criminals belong to this group. There are, for example, shoplifters who make a business out of shoplifting. The Gluecks reported that some of the girls began to lie and steal almost from babyhood. Reformatories often show women who merely could not get along with harsh parents. Most of the women show illicit sex influence as the chief form of their adolescent and early misbehavior. In the vast majority of cases, sentence to the reformatory was not the first experience these women had with legal authorities and institutions.[14]

Superficially it would appear that criminal action gives pleasure

[14] There is a great deal of newer work on the psychological and psychoanalytical analysis of crime and the criminal and their treatment. See Ben Karpman (1939), John Bowlby (1946), the book edited by K. R. Eissler (1948), Melitta Schmideberg (1949), Arthur N. Foxe (1950), and Paul Reiwald (1950). [L.B., Ed.]

and satisfaction to the criminal individual. He may steal, may be truant, may get illicit sex pleasure, and may show his strength and power. This is particularly true about the aggressive criminal, especially the holdup man and the murderer. Alexander and Healy stress particularly the oral passivity and dependence.[15] However, Karpman has justly protested against the overemphasis on oral tendencies. In the material of Sylvan Keiser and myself which deals with holdup men and in which aggressive action was in the foreground, the passivity expressed itself in anal trends. D.M., for instance, feared throughout his life sexual attack in the anus by boys. He traced this fear back to repulsion to enemas at five years of age. However, he is also interested in women's breasts. He always felt weak because of a heart ailment which incapacitated him and made him physically inferior to other boys. With a pistol he feels courageous, strong, and virile. Accompanied by another boy he held up and shot a female subway agent. At five years of age his mother burned to death in his presence when she tried to take him away from a fire.

In the foreground is a fear of passivity, which means to be hit, to be beaten up, or to be attacked. Analytically one may talk about castration fear. It is partially a fear and partially a wish to be in a female masochistic position. It is possible that his wish to suck the breast and his fear of the insertion of the penis have a similar basis. The gun is again an embodiment of masculine force and aggressiveness. The question again arises, why did his problems result in action? We are inclined to believe that there are two outstanding psychological traumata in early childhood. First was the death of his mother, which must have severely impaired the personality structure; and secondly, the long-lasting debilitating disease during childhood. There may still be other factors which cannot be defined psychologically that prevented a structuralization of the ego in an analytic sense and in addition permitted him to go through with a criminal act.

It would be easy to increase the number of instances. Physical weakness, early illness, and generally debilitating disturbances in childhood are important factors in the picture. The aggressive individual, pushed out from the company of other boys by his weakness and by his fear, has to build up his own group; and by his violence he substitutes for his weaknesses. The psychological mechanisms which

[15] See Edmund Bergler's discussion of this subject (1949). [L.B., Ed.]

have to do with passivity, anality, possible orality, and the overcompensation are not the only ones which are of importance. Sickness has a terrifying influence. There may be other early threats which hinder the organization of the personality and thus make it possible for the overcompensatory actions of aggressiveness to break through in violent criminal action. The criminal is isolated and tries to create his own society which admires him for his criminal action. It seems to me that aggressive criminals have generally a lower I.Q. than other groups of criminals.

Feelings of guilt are, of course, common in criminals. However, they are mixed with the fear of punishment. Freud has postulated the idea that the infantile feeling of guilt precedes the criminal action and is, in this respect, its cause. This cannot be substantiated. It is important to keep in mind that the criminal feels that he does not get from society what is his due, and indeed the majority of criminals come from the lower economic strata. Furthermore, their family background shows frequently fights between the parents, broken homes, and social desolation of every kind. This is particularly true about the "normal" criminal, in whom we are particularly interested.

To be sure, individual therapy will very often have some effect. However, the criminal's conflict is not only with the family but with society as a whole. Furthermore, family and society have also not succeeded in building up a reliable ego and superego structure partially in connection with the biological handicaps. Individual therapy, although helpful even when driven very deep as in psychoanalysis and allied methods, will be very often insufficient. It will be necessary to give to the boy not merely individual attention but one must build for him his society and his group. Only then may we expect that the individual will have a chance of not relapsing and not becoming a chronic offender. Enlightened prison administration has always aimed towards this goal by arranging for group activities of all kinds. However, group recreation, group work, and even football and baseball are only a small part of what can be done in groups. Our staff at Bellevue put the emphasis on group psychotherapy, which helps the patient increase his insight. One has to discuss with the individual his problems in an analytic sense in the presence of others. The problems of any one individual will objectify the problems of another individual present in the group. The group discussion on the fundamentals of human life will give the prisoner a clearer insight into his ideologies.

ADDICTION

Addiction is among the most difficult problems of psychotherapy. We are, of course, primarily interested in the character of the addict. It is astonishing how little is known about the basic difficulty in the alcoholic. My own and Frank J. Curran's studies have led me to the conclusion that the alcoholic has a psychological structure very similar to the structure of the cases with social neurosis. The alcoholic suffers deeply from a social insufficiency. He is not capable of coming close to other human beings and is conscious of it. He has high claims and expects special favors and appreciation and love. He wishes his body and his intellect to be loved by himself as well as others. Appreciation by his own sex is particularly demanded. In his earlier stages he wanted to have this appreciation, especially from the parent of the same sex. This constant social tension is relieved through alcohol, which gives the individual the feeling of being loved and being lovable. Only then is he also able to give love to others.

In the alcoholic hallucinosis the patient feels continually criticized by others and fears to be castrated and cut to pieces. This is an exaggeration of the same fear which plays a part in the alcoholic outside of his psychosis. S. Rado stresses, therefore, correctly, that the relation between ego and superego is disturbed in the drug addict. Oral components of sexuality may be of importance. However, the underlying feelings of guilt, insufficiency, and dissatisfaction with oneself are overwhelming. It is rather interesting that thus we come to an insight into the psychological relations between depression and addiction. The passing relief by alcohol is accompanied by the release of homosexual, oral, and sadistic tendencies and has naturally to be followed by an increased feeling of guilt and an increased dependence on alcohol. We may in general say that drugs, of which alcohol is merely one instance, reinforce the tendencies which have led to the need for intoxication, and make them more obvious. The homosexuality and vanity of the alcoholic become the more obvious, the more he is addicted.[16]

[16] See studies on alcoholism by E. M. Jellink. [L.B., Ed.]

An acute alcoholic intoxication gives the individual the desire to be loved and appreciated.[17] He feels as an individual accepted by others because of his capacities, appearance, and sexual qualities. At the same time he feels ready and willing to give the same appreciation to others. The perceptive and intellectual spheres are impaired. Hand in hand with this impairment and increased self-confidence goes a lack of inhibition which leads to a breaking through of sexual striving otherwise repressed.

This basic pattern varies with the total situation. There may be a lability of the perceptive and intellectual inhibitory (cortical) mechanism. This may lead to more or less dissociated breaking through of sexual and aggressive impulses. The social situation may demand particular drinking habits. Early experiences in childhood may have enforced one or the other variation in sexuality, which then appears during the intoxication. For similar reasons violence may break through. The total situation will determine the psychological picture of the acute alcoholic intoxication, the basic pattern of which, however, is a heightened feeling of one's being connected in love and admiration with other human beings so that one can even allow oneself the breaking through of one's sexual impulses. An underlying anxiety that one's social perfection may merely be assumed unjustly is never completely absent and may lead to self-assertion, irritability, aggressiveness, and the attempt to bully others. The psychological gain by intoxication points to the personality structure of those who need this psychological gain badly. These are human beings with feelings of great social insecurity and social tension.

The acute alcoholic intoxication is different in persons who are chronic alcoholics than in those who are intoxicated for the first time. It seems that in the chronic alcoholic the acute intoxication brings forward more primitive material with a corresponding increase in anxiety. Such an acute intoxication in the chronic alcoholic leads him imperceptibly to delirious and hallucinatory episodes in which he experiences primitive sexuality in a distorted form and feels particularly threatened in his social function. The threat does not remain in the sphere of social insecurity but extends from there to sexual threats and even to the threat of dismemberment and castration. Society has

[17] The rest of the discussion on alcoholism was reprinted from Paul Schilder, "The Psychogenesis of Alcoholism," *Quarterly Journal of Studies on Alcohol* 2:277–93, 1941. [L.B., Ed.]

become completely hostile and destructive, and the patient may not even blame his community for the attempt at destroying him.

The chronic alcoholic person is one who, from his earliest childhood on, has lived in a state of insecurity. This insecurity in childhood was necessarily in relation to the family, parents and siblings. The child has felt ridiculed and pushed into a passive position, sometimes by threat, sometimes by corporal punishment, and sometimes by deprivation. This threat may come from both parents or from one parent only. In men the threat by the father seems to be more effective. It seems that help and consideration from the other parent cannot counteract the tendency to submission and the direction of a severe superego which takes over the part of the punishing and repressing parent. The punishing parent is particularly intolerant toward sex in any form. The community is experienced as an agent similar to the restrictive parents. Individuals are generally ready to submit to these influences in a passive and masochistic way. Men generally blame themselves for their femininity and have to seek redress in ideals of heightened masculinity and strength. In women, paradoxically, this process may be similar, or the women feel that they are not capable of fulfilling their feminine functions. The characteristic of the alcoholic is social tension, with the tendency to give in passively to the assumed pressure or to react by overcompensation.

Alcoholism reverses this process. It gives social security and acceptance as long as the intoxication lasts. With the wearing off of the intoxication the underlying tensions and terrors reappear in increased form and demand renewed drinking.

The alcoholic is dependent upon his society, since he has a striving for social acceptance beyond the norm. The sociological and economic factors in alcoholism should therefore not be underrated. To be sure, no problem is merely an individual problem. Human beings live in communities. However, alcoholism is, even beyond this, a problem of society. Not only is there the problem of social competition, in which the alcoholic does badly, but society continually exposes the socially insecure individual to the temptation of a seemingly easy escape by encouraging drunkenness. Alcoholism is not only a problem of individual treatment but of social attitudes, and it seems, therefore, that individual treatment has to be complemented by offering to the alcoholic a social group in which competition is diminished and in which the use of alcoholic beverages is not foisted upon the patient. It seems, indeed, that all modern treatments of alcoholism stress the community factor.[18] However, beyond that, the alcoholic needs a deeper understanding of his problem, which very often is only possible by continued and intensive psychoanalytic work. The basic psychology of the alcoholic is preordained by the psychological effect of the acute intoxication, and all forms of alcoholic intoxication and patterns of chronic alcoholism center around the psychological effect of the drug. In some types of chronic alcoholism the personality difficulty is chiefly in the sphere of sexual adaptation. In others, the family situation or community situation seems to offer the chief difficulty. However, these variations are merely facets of the same basic problem. The best prevention of alcoholism will lie in an attitude of the parents which does not increase the insecurity and passivity of the child and guarantees a reasonably free development of sexual adaptation. If the family, and later on the community, do not stress superiority, perfection, and blamelessness and offer beyond that friendly help and understanding, individuals will not need alcohol as an escape from insecurities, but may be able to enjoy it as a method of heightening one's appreciation of oneself and of others on rare occasions of festivity.

The difficulties in the treatment of cases of this sort are enormous. It is necessary, in most cases, that the patient should not have the possibility of getting the drug, which throws him back more and more on his psychological problem. The foregoing remarks may show the direction in which increased insight in the alcoholic has to go. Hospital routine and temporary relief from difficult situations may be of help. Short psychotherapy, eventually with hypnosis, may be helpful. In the long run, deep psychotherapy will be necessary. I have evidence that the final cure of the alcoholic lies in his contact with a group. Alcoholism is, after all, a disease in social relations. The final technique has to be worked out. It is obvious that there must exist some hope that the patient may gain the esteem of a group, if it is worth his while to make the effort necessary for recovery. We are as far from the solution of this important problem from a psychological point of view as from a social point of view.

We know still less about the other types of drug addiction. As far

[18] See *Alcoholics Anonymous, The Story of How One Hundred Men Have Recovered from Alcoholism* (Works Publishing Co., 1939). [L.B., Ed.]

as I can see, the basic deviations of the personality are identical in any kind of drug addiction. If the tension between ideals and fulfillment becomes too great, the individual tries to escape by taking the drug which relieves the specific tension. It seems that the inability of the person who becomes a morphine addict, in adapting to the world, is still greater than in the alcoholic. But we do not know the specific difficulty in the adaptation. At any rate, we have to investigate the libidinal situation. E. Glover particularly stresses the difficulties in the ego formation, without saying clearly what he means by it. Every difficulty in adaptation based upon libidinous regression has, anyhow, to change the fundamental mechanisms of adaptation. In the few cases of morphinism and cocaine addiction into which I have had the possibility of a deeper insight, the desire for praise and admiration was still greater, and still less satisfied, than in alcoholism. The inability to adapt in this respect leads the morphinist still farther away from the social world, and he does not even keep up a semblance of the social relation which one finds in the sociability of the alcoholic when he is intoxicated. The person who takes morphine and opiates lives, indeed, in a private world of painlessness and happiness as long as the action of the opiate lasts. The activity of the alcoholic is absent. Psychologically we find, therefore, sufficient hints as to the particular danger of the alkaloid intoxications in the psychological structure of the picture provoked by intoxications. According to my opinion, the structure of the intoxication in the addict reflects the structure of the personality which has led to addiction.

The withdrawal of alcohol does not generally lead to severe difficulties, although I am convinced that its withdrawal in severe cases of alcoholism may be one of the factors which determine the outbreak of a delirium. In morphinism, the patient needs psychic help during the period of withdrawal. I believe that unless the patient suffers from a severe disease of the heart, the drug should be withdrawn in a few days. Hypnosis, in connection with barbitals or without them, is very often an effective help against the withdrawal symptoms, especially sleeplessness and restlessness. The help afforded during the abstinence period is not yet the personality treatment which the morphinist needs. This treatment is difficult and does not provide sufficient results in the majority of cases. It is advisable to keep the addict under control and every six months to put him in a quarantine in order to determine whether he takes the drug or not. Even then, one should not be too optimistic. I have no experience about the efficiency of psychoanalysis or group treatment in these cases. The various methods of somatic treatment invented to facilitate the withdrawing of the drug from the patient are not our concern here. It is easy to withdraw the drug; it is difficult to cure the addict.

Cocainism by sniffing is seemingly a less severe disease. Its relation to homosexuality is very outspoken and on the surface, and its effect on latent homosexuality is striking in so far as it very soon makes the perversion manifest. It seems that even when homosexuality and homosexual fixations were not manifest in childhood, homosexuality might be produced by cocainism. (Cf. H. Hartmann.) This fact is of importance for the understanding of drug addiction as well as of the effect of drugs. The two problems have a very close relation to each other.

Chapter 11

PSYCHOANALYSIS AND PSYCHOTHERAPY OF THE PSYCHOSES AND THE PSYCHOLOGY OF SHOCK TREATMENT

1. THE INFLUENCE OF PSYCHOANALYSIS ON THE UNDERSTANDING OF THE PSYCHOSES [1]

FREUD'S FIRST contribution to psychoanalytic psychiatry was contained in an article written in 1896. The case was one of paranoid schizophrenia with mechanisms similar to the mechanisms of hysteria. The therapeutic result was incomplete. Subsequently Freud's interest was for a long time directed towards other problems. In the meantime after 1902 the attention of Bleuler and Jung was more and more drawn to psychoanalysis, and they found "Freud's Mechanisms" not only in neurotic conditions but also in psychoses, especially in dementia praecox. Jung's *Diagnostische Associationsstudien* began to appear in 1904. The studies contain many references to the psychoses. In 1907 there appeared Jung's *Psychologie die Dementia Praecox,*

[1] Reprinted from Paul Schilder, "The Influence of Psychoanalysis on Psychiatry," *Psychoanalytic Quarterly* 9:216–28, 1940. [L.B., Ed.]

the first systematic attempt to interpret psychoanalytically the psychology of dementia praecox. In 1911 several papers of Ferenczi applied psychoanalytic thinking to paranoia and the psychoses, and Freud himself published his psychoanalytic remarks on the autobiography of Schreber. Bleuler's work on schizophrenia appeared in 1911, and Jung's *Wandlungen und Symbole der Libido* was published in 1911 and 1912. From that time the psychoanalytic literature has shown a deep and continued interest in the problem of schizophrenia.

Freud's first paper on manic-depressive psychosis, *Trauer und Melancholie,* appeared in 1917. A study by Abraham (1911) had preceded Freud's articles. Abraham's investigations of the earliest pregenital level of libido and of the developmental history of libido (1924) contained his further contributions to the subject. Freud returned to this topic in *Group Psychology and the Analysis of the Ego* (1921). There are numerous contributions to the psychoanalytic psychology of manic-depressive psychoses from this time on. Freud made only casual remarks about other types of psychosis in his papers on the general connotation of neurosis and psychosis. In one he wrote that the state of mental confusion is a conflict between the ego and reality.

The psychoanalytic literature on psychoses, with the exception of manic-depressive states and schizophrenia, has been rather scanty. Ferenczi and Hollos, and I have written on general paresis. Epilepsy has been studied by Maeder (1909) and Clark (1917). In 1925 I tried to give a general outline of the relation between psychoanalysis and psychiatry. Rickman published *A Survey: The Development of the Psychoanalytic Theory of the Psychoses 1894–1926* (1926, 1927).

The preceding notes are intended merely as bibliographic help in approaching the problem of the changes that Freud's contributions have wrought in psychiatry. At the time that Freud started his studies of psychoses, psychosis was considered only from an organic standpoint. The personality of the mentally sick person was not considered as a subject of any particular interest; furthermore it was not believed that the psychotic manifestations could be expressions of the personality.[2]

---

[2] See also the articles by the Association for Research in Nervous and Mental Disorders, 1928, and Leopold Bellak, *Dementia Praecox, the Past Ten Years' Work* (New York, Grune & Stratton, 1948).

The psychiatric world was fascinated by the problem of clinical classification. Kraepelin had shuffled and reshuffled clinical entities and was strongly opposed by the school of Westphal-Ziehen and Auguste E. Hoche. Finally, with the second edition of Kraepelin's book, there emerged the psychiatric opinion that there are only two essential types of psychoses: those which end in deterioration, later called dementia praecox; and those which do not end in deterioration, later called manic-depressive psychosis. Kraepelin adhered to the psychology of Wundt. Accordingly, he assumed that the supposed organic processes in dementia praecox and manic-depressive psychosis influence either the apperceptive and will functions or the emotions. The problem of personality did not exist for him. Under the influence of Stransky he believed that in dementia praecox not only apperception, will, and emotions deteriorated but that there was also a dissociation of emotion from thought content present, the so-called intrapsychic ataxia. Manic-depressive psychoses were considered to be based on quantitative exaggerations of moods and affects. These concepts culminated in the clinical entity called "mixed states," in which part functions of elation and part functions of depression were supposed to be present at the same time. This is real mosaic psychology. Personality problems of psychotics who suffered from better-known organic afflictions were likewise neglected. The symptomatology of psychoses was considered the result of the disturbance of the mosaic of brain functions and brain cells, comparable to the effect of sitting down by chance on the keyboard of a piano and thereby provoking a senseless noise.

It is the merit of Freud and psychoanalysis to have introduced a psychological point of view which is fundamentally different. Human beings were observed no longer as a more or less artificial hodgepodge of sensations, feelings, representation, with perhaps some sprinkling of apperception and will, but as personalities in life situations. Thinking had no specific place in Wundt's scheme. Freud had the temerity to assert that even a human being afflicted with a psychosis is still a personality with life problems. Although Freud did not write about the organic psychoses, his casual remarks show that he was of the opinion that it was possible to apply the libido theory and psychoanalytic interpretation even in organic brain disease. Consider, for instance, his remarks in his "History of the Psychoanalytic Movement" (in *Basic Writings of Sigmund Freud,* p. 949):

So far as I know, Bleuler, even today, adheres to an organic causation for the forms of dementia praecox, and Jung, whose book on this malady appeared in 1907, upheld the toxic theory of the same at the Congress at Salzburg in 1908, which though not excluding it, goes far beyond the libido theory.

While this statement is somewhat ambiguous since it seems to make a differentiation between psychoanalytic and psychological understandability of symptoms and the question of organic versus nonorganic, it closely approaches a principle which I would formulate as follows: Regardless of what may happen to an organism and its brain, it remains an organism in a life situation with a continuity of life problems.

I believe this also to be the deeper meaning of Freud's basic idea of the interpretation of dreams. Dreams have a meaning because they are experiences in the continuity of the life history of a person. One cannot deny that there are organic factors in sleep and dreams. It is rather amusing that one has in these days to defend the attitude that there is anything organic in organisms.

Bleuler thought there were two series of phenomena in schizophrenia: organic processes which have nothing to do with psychology, and other processes that are the reactions of the personality changed by the organic process. Ferenczi and Hollos made the same mistake when they considered an organic nucleus in general paresis to be unapproachable by their theories. A second principle of psychoanalytic psychiatry and of psychopathology in general may be formulated by stating that the possibility of understanding a symptom as the expression of psychological tendencies does not prove that this symptom is psychogenic in character.

In so-called psychosomatics, similar mistakes are common. By this I do not mean to say that organic symptoms cannot be the consequences of psychological conflicts; however, it is not always easy to prove such connections or to understand their true meaning. Especially in schizophrenia and manic-depressive psychosis does the evidence speak against psychogenesis as the decisive causative factor. Freud never made any optimistic statements concerning the curability of dementia praecox and said nothing definite against the possibility that organic factors might be operative. "In the spontaneous kind it may be supposed that the ego ideal is inclined to display a peculiar strictness, which then results automatically in its temporary suspension." (*Group Psychology and the Analysis of the Ego,* p. 109.)

The first principle, the continuity of the life problem, has had a deep and lasting influence upon psychiatry. No one, even the most reactionary, ventures today to consider psychoses merely as senseless conglomerations of symptoms unrelated to personality. Among German psychiatrists, Kretschmer was a leader in this trend. He contributed to overcoming the mechanical Kraepelinian and even more rigid Hocheian psychiatry. In France, despite the efforts of Claude, a psychology of the total personality is only beginning to be accepted.

From these general remarks we may turn to the more specific problems of psychoanalytic psychiatry. We have agreed that psychotic patients should be considered from the point of view that they are human beings with conflicts. However, we all have conflicts. What is the specificity of the conflicts of the psychotic?

Freud justly always tried to find specific mechanisms in different types of neuroses and psychoses. The different types were correlated with definite stages of psychosexual development or, in broader formulation, with specific phases in the development of the child. In a given neurosis or psychosis the individual regresses, under the stress of a current conflict, to an earlier stage in his development. This regression is prepared for by a definite weakness due either to constitution or to early experiences or to a combination of both, and constitutes a so-called point of fixation. The development of the child is envisaged by Freud to progress through well-defined stages. It is sufficient to mention the narcissistic, the oral, the anal phases and the phallic phase centering around the Oedipus complex and the genitals. These, in Freud's opinion, were psychobiological stages of development. The arrest of energies, the flowing back of energies to points of fixation, the breaking through of energies at the point of fixation, were seen by Freud as biological and physiological processes. This is essentially what is called the libido theory.

There are two propositions of Freud that are of fundamental importance: first, that there are psychological stages of development in childhood, characterized by specific sexual attitudes; second, that in neuroses and especially in psychoses the individual regresses, at least partially, to these various earlier stages of development. It is the great merit of Freud to have discerned these developments not only in their psychological aspects but in their biological and physiological aspects as well.

Although there are historical forerunners of Freud's concept of regression (especially Meynert), it is, in its entirety, an original conception of great importance. One might justly say that no modern psychiatrist should dare to approach this subject without accepting these fundamental concepts.

It is generally accepted that the regression in psychoses is particularly deep and that in schizophrenia a regression takes place to the narcissistic stage. Unfortunately the term *narcissism* is loaded with ambiguities. The narcissistic stage of development is considered a stage in which libido is directed exclusively towards one's own body. However, this concept of a phase in which there is only body and no world is self-contradictory. Freud was never clear about the use of the term *narcissistic phase*. Narcissism is, according to him, the final synthesis of isolated autoeroticisms. Psychoanalytic literature generally considers primary narcissism the most primitive stage of libidinal development, consisting of the concentration of libido on one's own body.

It would be preferable to describe a stage of incomplete differentiation of body and world in which the connotation of the body is in no way more distinct than the connotation of the world. There cannot be much doubt that we deal in schizophrenia really with a return to such a lack of differentiation between body and world. This regression does not take place in all spheres of experience. There are forces counteracting the regression and trying to maintain or regain a better appreciation of the world. It is, furthermore, of importance to note that regression and symptom formation are determined not merely by the point of fixation deepest in individual development but also by accessory points of fixation corresponding to experiences in somewhat later stages of development. Oral, anal, and homosexual trends then come to expression. Ego and superego mechanisms, partially preserved, interfere continually with the free expression of primitive sexual tendencies. I do not doubt that the superego in the course of regression also undergoes severe changes, returning to a primitive, less unified organization.

It is very difficult to argue about terms that are as badly defined as the psychoanalytic term *ego,* even if one leaves Rado's latest formulation out of the discussion. According to Freud, the ego is an organization which has to make peace between the different strivings. It is also the organ which, through sensual impression and by consciousness, has access to motor action. Sensual perception and motility are, in schizophrenics, certainly not disturbed in the same way as in general paresis, which should be considered as a disturbance of ego functioning. Sometimes *ego,* in the psychoanalytic sense, means almost the same as total personality; sometimes it means the organ of conscious action and the sensory motor system; and sometimes it refers to the part of the personality which, under the influence of the superego, conforms with society and directs one's behavior in a given situation. If Alexander, therefore, asserts that the ego function in schizophrenia is impaired he does not say very much. It seems much more likely that the ego in schizophrenia is either overpowered by id conflicts or it tries assiduously to dam back the stream of libido about to break through at lower levels of development. Nunberg has described in this connection a hyperfunction of the ego in certain paranoiac conditions.

At any rate we owe it basically to the work of Freud, Bleuler, Jung, and Meyer that the schizophrenic is seen as a human being with conflicts. In comparison with Meyer's formulation, psychoanalysis is at an advantage in that it is not satisfied, as Meyer, Campbell, and their followers are, to assign banal current and past conflicts as sufficient causes for schizophrenic psychoses. Psychoanalysis places the emphasis on elucidating the developmental history of the individual afflicted with schizophrenia.

Being interested merely in fundamental principles, it will be easier to formulate the basic problems of manic-depressive psychosis. There is the general opinion that the point of fixation lies in the oral sphere. It cannot be denied that in manics as well as depressives, oral tendencies are very strong, so far as we can judge, from earliest childhood. But quite in the same way as in schizophrenia, it is hardly possible to find precise early experiences, or from a sufficiently early time, to be made specifically responsible as points of fixation. Abraham correctly emphasized early relations to love objects, not exclusively in the oral sphere. If one studies a sufficiently large amount of material one becomes somewhat skeptical about the exclusive importance of oral aggression in manic-depressive psychoses. One finds an aggressiveness of enormous strength related to all parts of the body, and the cannibalistic phantasy is of perhaps no greater importance than other destructive impulses. The researches of Melanie Klein into destructive impulses of early infancy, experienced actively and passively in relation to every body aperture and every part of the musculature, seem to offer an appropriate basis for the understanding of manic-depressives as well as of certain schizophrenics. It is only possible in exceptional cases to point to the actual instance responsible for the increase in motives of destruction and dismembering. Freud combined the theory of pregenital sexuality in depressions with the assumption of a particular severity of the superego: a strong Oedipus complex. The regression in pathological depressions must, therefore, be of a very specific and partial character. The severity of the superego reflects the general tendency to destructiveness which finally is directed against the ego. According to Freud the self-reproaches against one's own person are due to the fact that the love object has been taken into the ego by identification. However, the love object is not only in the ego but also in the superego and probably also in the id. Identifications are always reflected in all three psychic systems. I doubt, furthermore, that the self-reproaches of depressives are often primarily directed against the love objects. The contention of Freud that those predisposed to depression choose their love objects narcissistically has never been substantiated. It is true that they have been attacked before, and their aggression is counteraggression. They have good reasons to blame themselves for their terrible hostilities.

Freud has conclusively demonstrated the severe changes of the superego in the manic-depressive psychosis. It is a cruel superego, and finally the individual gets tired of blaming himself and starts to love himself. All problems seem to disappear at this moment; nevertheless, he has not forgotten that he has been hurt and that he has suffered. Much of the content of the manic phase consists of complaints, of part misery and persecution. The individual emerges victoriously.

In every phase of the elation the manic patient is aware of the human value of those around him.[3] When the depressive patient attacks he is aware that he deals with a person. The manic-depressive patient is capable of loving and of being loved.

The basic points in the psychology of manic-depressive psychosis are rather well established. The value of psychoanalytic therapy has been emphatically stated by Freud and Abraham. Patients who are

[3] See Bertram D. Lewin, *Psychoanalysis of Elation* (New York, W. W. Norton & Co., 1950). [L.B., Ed.]

not cured by psychoanalysis derive at least considerable benefit. A considerable number of cases remain refractory to psychoanalytic treatment.

Freud considers mental confusion as a conflict between ego and reality. It is more correct to formulate that in states of confusion the individual has lost an ego apparatus and is therefore not able to maintain full contact with reality although he strives to do so with all his inner force. Helplessness and perplexity result. When the ego apparatus for the finer elaborations of perceptions is deficient, forms appear in perception and in representation which correspond to the condensation and symbolization of the dream. This is not the sphere of every personal problem which is affected in dreams and in schizophrenia.

One suspects that some confusional states might be understood in relation to earlier childhood experiences. However, it is difficult to elucidate this problem without introducing a new fundamental conception. In schizophrenia the individual is concerned with his innermost problems; the disease attacks the center of the personality (the id). In the manic-depressive psychoses the problems dealt with are somewhat less personal; they lie closer to the superego, are further away from the nucleus of the personality. In mental confusion, structures are affected which are still less personal and belong to the perceptive part of the ego in its final elaboration. I may add that in agnosia, aphasia, and apraxia we find the problem in layers still further in the periphery of the personality.

In agnosia and aphasia we see the perceptive function of the ego apparatus disturbed. Poetzl and I have repeatedly demonstrated how remarkably similar are the products which appear instead of the proper functions of language and gnosis to products that emerge from the system of the unconscious. These phenomena take place in a sphere which belongs to the periphery of the ego circle. What we usually call system of the unconscious or mechanism of the unconscious does not involve functions distant from the nucleus of personality, but this nucleus itself. In these nuclear phenomena we are usually able to point to the repressive forces responsible for the incompleteness of psychological development, which thus remain in the unconscious and infantile sphere. In other words, we know the motives of repression. We do not know the motives which hinder the completion of language development in aphasias. We do not know the difficulties which lead to the same arrests of development in the peripheral ego sphere of thinking (amentia). I do not believe the developmental arrest or regression in the periphery of the ego to be due to a psychological function which we can understand with our present methods of approach.

Therefore we classify amentias and dementias, including mental deficiency, agnosias, aphasias, and mental confusion, and organic toxic phenomena in general, as a disturbance of ego perception. Schizophrenia is classified as libidinal regression, while manic-depressive psychosis is classified as partial regression and particularly as reaction formation in the superego due to the well-developed Oedipus complex.

One sees that one comes in this way to a psychoanalytic classification of psychosis which is also acceptable from the point of view of clinical psychiatry. It is my opinion that misunderstandings might be avoided if one kept in mind that what is true in the one branch of science has to be true in another branch of science. Freud himself unfortunately was always against the infusion of psychoanalytic knowledge into psychiatry and psychology. His attitude was understandable when there was general hostility to psychoanalysis in psychiatric circles.

It is not difficult from a similar point of view to understand the epileptic psychoses, with their particular type of confusion and signs akin to aphasia; alcoholism, with its particular libidinal regression, superego formation, and organic confusion. It will not help in either of these groups to speak merely about "psychosis." In each, one has to find the specific mechanism in the field of the perceptive ego and in the field of libido.

If one follows such a classification, one will probably be averse to the classification of mental disorder which E. Glover has developed. He defines as an ego system or ego nucleus any psychic system that represents a positive libidinal relation to objects or part objects, that can discharge reactive tension, and in one or the other of these ways reduce anxieties. He places strong emphasis on projection and introjection. He is however not far from a fundamental error often to be found in psychoanalytic theory: that the world appears to an individual only as the result of systems of projections and introjections. Such a theory is always based upon a neglect of the function of the perceptive ego systems as characterized above. One is reminded of the error of Schopenhauer, who considered the world not as perception but as representation or image.

Closely related to this error is the overrating of anxiety and guilt: "Anxiety is the alpha and guilt the omega of human development." In *Civilization and Its Discontents,* Freud tried to prove that guilt is fundamentally anxiety. Anxiety is only one of the important emotional reactions of human beings to current and past difficulties. There are insecurities which can hardly be classified as anxiety. There is incompleteness of experience, which urges to completion; there is dizziness, and there are tensions; furthermore, there are strivings which are positive, based upon interest in the world and its variety. It is at best one-sided to stress that human activities are merely due to the wish to escape from terror and destruction. If one does not appreciate that human beings live in a world which they perceive and in relation to which they act, one will always be inclined to underrate genuine interest in the world, and will underrate the positive side of emotions. Our perception of the world is not merely due to projection and identification. Anxiety is only one of our manifold reactions.

The neglect of the external world (perception) and the overrating of the body as if it were independent of the outward world is deeply imbedded in psychoanalytic thinking. Systems which deny the importance of the world will always emphasize displeasure, fear, and anxiety. The recent emphasis on ego problems corresponds to an intent to overcome this deep-seated difficulty in the structure of psychoanalysis. The attempts at reconstruction have not been radical enough in my opinion.

In the organic psychoses we find changes which remain in the periphery of the ego. We have some understanding of these changes from the point of view of the psychology of the total personality. The indestructible center of the personality is aware of the change. A case of general paresis, for instance, is aware of the impairment of his thinking and judgment and reacts to this incompleteness with grief and despair. Patients who suffer from organic impairments in thinking and perception experience helplessness, perplexity, fear, grief, and also anxiety. Pierce Clark has shown the considerable libidinal problems to be found in amentia (mental deficiency). The change in the motor impulses occurring in encephalitis is only fully understandable if we use the psychoanalytic approach (cf. Jelliffe).

One might say that it is of no great importance whether one understands the psychology of organic processes or not in order to be ready to fulfill our tasks as psychologists and analysts. However, they reveal important aspects of human experience. It seems to me that the psychoanalytic approach to organic problems in the field of brain disease is of fundamental importance for organic neurology and neurophysiology. The influence of this work is even at the present time considerable. The approach to organic cortical syndromes, as well as to subcortical syndromes, has profited by psychoanalytic understanding. Our approach to the neurologically sick and crippled has become psychologically more efficient.

One should not generalize about the psychology of psychosis. The psychology of different types of psychosis shows fundamental differences. However, there is no question that psychoanalysis has changed fundamentally the attitude of the psychiatrist in his approach to patients and the problem of psychosis. Only on the basis of this approach will organic therapy reap its full benefits. This is probably even true in cases with severe organic changes.

Only through psychoanalysis has the mentally sick person emerged as a revealing source of deep human problems. Freud and psychoanalysis have not only given to the psychotic his place in the system of humanity but have also elevated humanity by increasing its insight into one of its most fundamental manifestations.

2. PSYCHOTHERAPY OF THE PSYCHOSES

Epilepsy [4]

Although epilepsy is fundamentally an organic disease, psychological factors have an influence on the genesis and the manifestations of this disease. There is no question that anger and fright have an influence on the attacks. If we can diminish the epileptic patient's difficulties in adaptation we shall help him. When the process of epilepsy merely provokes general feelings of discomfort, these feelings may be converted into conversion symptoms and can then be subjected to psychotherapeutic procedures. According to my opinion,

[4] See also W. G. Lennox: "Psychiatry, Psychology and Seizures," *American Journal of Orthopsychiatry* 19: 432–46, 1949. [L.B., Ed.]

in most cases of fugue, so far as they are not frankly psychogenic, psychogenic factors of the type described play an important part. The epileptic dreamy states and the violent emotional outbursts are very often also dependent on the situation. In cases in which the organic process is mild, psychotherapy may create conditions under which the organic process does not become manifest. Organic treatment of epilepsy should never be neglected. The psychotherapy can be merely considered as an aid for the organic treatment. It may be of preliminary help in understanding the epileptic if one stresses his enormous and deep-seated aggression, which is probably in connection with his readiness for motor discharge. During the epileptic attack and its equivalent, the patient gives the world up completely and builds it up all over again. This is experienced, as Pierce Clark has pointed out, as a return to the womb of the mother and rebirth. The loss of consciousness and life is symbolically expressed by the dismembering motive, which is also in connection with the muscle activities and the aggressiveness. One may expect to find the same motives in the adaptation difficulties of the epileptic, which are considerable. One should make the diagnosis of epilepsy only when there are definite manifestations in the form of attacks. Psychopathic individuals with a psychology reminiscent of the character changes observed in the epileptic should not be called epileptic, and they offer a much better opportunity for psychotherapy.

Toxic States and Organic Brain Diseases

I want to stress the fact that toxic and infectious delirious states are very much dependent upon the situation. By medical and nursing care which keeps the patient in contact with reality and its problems, and gives him an insight into his physical disease, delirious reactions can be prevented. This is, of course, not always true and depends on the strength of the organic factors. I have mentioned that every operation needs a psychological preparation. How far this preparation should go depends on the psychology of the patient. I believe that many postoperative psychoses can in this way be prevented.

Cases of brain tumor and general paresis have to be considered merely from the point of view of organic treatment. In the more chronic cases of organic damage of the brain in which the organic damage is at first mild, as in senility and arteriosclerosis, the organic deficiency may provoke the release of tendencies based upon the life history of the individual, and psychotherapy may become imperative. One will generally refrain from the more complicated forms of psychotherapy.

The handling of cases of mental deficiency is a problem in itself. I refer those interested to the book by Pierce Clark. One should keep in mind that an organism with a defect from the point of view of efficiency is still an organism and therefore a whole. The mentally deficient individual has to deal with the same basic problems as the individual with full intelligence. He will naturally have greater difficulties in handling these problems. The emotional outbursts and the erotic conflicts are likely to be particularly severe. I have seen this in a mentally deficient girl who was deeply in love with her companion, towards whom she even made homosexual approaches, which were tactfully kept in proper limits by the companion, who understood the situation. The girl went into a state of extreme agitation when the companion had to leave. For fourteen days she shouted continually, did not sleep, and did not eat. The symptoms disappeared immediately when the parents recalled the companion. Emotional conflicts in defectives very often crystallize in a set pattern. One of the boys observed by Walter Bromberg waved a handkerchief for hours, standing at the window and saying, "I surrender." This was the substitute for a masturbation phantasy and an expression of masochism. Such patients often do well with properly conducted treatment. They will gain an insight appropriate to their intellectual level. The emotional adaptation of the defective is a problem of great practical importance which can be solved on the basis of the general principles evolved in this book.

Manic-depressive Psychosis

The biological factor in the genesis of the severe manic-depressive psychosis is obvious. There are such distinct hereditary relations that we have the right to consider the manic-depressive psychosis as an organic constitutional disease. There are probably also nonconstitutional organic factors at play. We know very little about it. How much these biological factors will come into appearance depends on the degree of the organic change and also on the total psychic situation. At any rate, things being as they are, we have to approach the problem with modesty. I have mentioned that in many cases it will be advisable to put the patient under the routine of the modern psychiatric hospital. This is of course imperative in those cases which become dangerous to themselves and to others. The hospital has the primary duty of putting the patient into a simpler situation and a simpler reality. He should be released from tasks which are too difficult for him. This principle is true for the manic as well as for the depressive picture. The suicidal danger of depressive pictures should be considered. I think that at any rate the physician has a duty to discuss the present situation as openly as possible with the patient. He may feel that it is not wise to put any tasks before the patient, and he must, of course, carefully avoid any problems that might be upsetting for the patient. In many cases it will be advantageous to lead the patient into a deeper insight of his situation and the structure of his psychic life.

I agree with the general psychoanalytic interpretation that one finds in these cases an enormous aggressiveness, often in connection with oral and cannibalistic tendencies. Anal problems may be obvious, and also in the anality the aggressiveness may be paramount. Besides the aggressiveness against other persons, there is an aggressiveness against one's own self. The aggressiveness may originate from an identification with aggressive objects on the outside. Freud has stressed that the aggressiveness against oneself is an aggressiveness against the love object introjected into one's ego. There obviously is also a tendency to self-punishment for aggressive instincts which originates in one's own ego. There is also obviously a feeling of guilt and a tendency to self-punishment and even to self-annihilation in the depressive state. Rado has emphasized that the depressive case depreciates himself so that he can later again have the love of his mother and father and their images in the superego. The symptomatology of depressive pictures is variable.

The psychological theory, in spite of considerable work done in this respect, is still incomplete. It is difficult to judge the result of psychoanalysis, although Freud reports that psychoanalysis has prevented the return of attacks. The problem can be definitely solved only by statistical methods. I myself have observations at my disposal which seem to indicate that some depressions react favorably to psychoanalysis. In group psychotherapy I have seen only two cases, both severe. There was no result in either of these cases. One patient committed suicide, owing to a lapse in supervision by the family. There is no definite indication for an attempt at deep psychotherapy in depressive cases. We are not yet reasonably sure which cases will react and which will not. However, the depressive case needs psychic help, which sooner or later must lead to an enlargement of his psychic horizon. Whenever one is in doubt whether one deals with a true depression or a psychogenic depression, intensive psychotherapy should be tried. Even chronic psychogenic depressions react favorably to psychoanalysis. I have no definite opinion about the efficiency of psychological treatment in the interval in order to prevent further attacks. I have the definite impression that many of the patients suffering from manic-depressive psychosis show more or less severe difficulties also in the interval. It is obvious that these difficulties should be accessible to psychotherapy, and I think persons who have gone through depressive attacks should have a psychological treatment for whatever character difficulties they may have. Whether that can prevent further manic-depressive attacks is an undecided question. The psychotherapeutic routine concerning depressive cases should be as follows:

Simplification of the life situation, psychic help, and the revealing of problems as far as this would not too much complicate the situation of the patient. Deeper treatment during the depressive attack is at the present time not definitely indicated but is permissible if the patient responds. This usually can be decided in the first two or three weeks of the treatment. An appreciation of the total personality after the depression is over should be tried. Deep psychotherapy may prove to be indicated. In psychogenic depressions, or in doubtful cases, or in cases which appear to be so light that psychogenesis cannot be excluded, psychotherapy should be done, appropriate to the depth of the problem. The manic states are, according to present opinion, an attempt to overcome the same problems which are present in a depressive state. If they are more severe, they are not accessible for a direct psychotherapeutic approach. In light cases one may try such an approach but should not extend it for too long a time, if unsuccessful. The state of transference should be especially watched in this trial period. From a theoretical point of view, it is interesting that the manifest sex functions are very often not impaired in the psychosis. But the opposite has also been observed.

Suicide

Suicide is obviously merely a symptom and not a clinical entity. Suicidal preoccupations occur in the normal. The idea that death is an escape from insupportable difficulties plays an important part. One may also expect a greater amount of love when one is dead. One punishes, by death, the person who denied love. Death is peace, reunion with a love object. Death is also aggression directed towards oneself. It may be a self-punishment for aggression previously directed against others, especially love objects. According to Freud, the depressive case identifies himself with his love object and directs reproaches and aggression against the introjected love object. In the suicidal act he kills the introjected person.

It is of importance in which setting suicide ideas or threats occur. One may expect that the suicidal danger is the greater, the greater the aggression. Accordingly, depressions are indeed particularly endangered. In statistics by Jamieson of 100 cases which were observed in a mental hospital and committed suicide either in the hospital (24 per cent) or after discharge (76 per cent), 46 belonged to the manic-depressive group and 19 were involutional melancholias. The remainder belonged to the other groups of neuroses and psychoses. Most of the suicides in adults have a very long history, and in a careful psychotherapy it should be possible to evaluate the degree of aggressiveness and the danger of suicide. In many cases it is possible to analyze the various factors which let death appear desirable to the patient. If one can give the patient an insight into the structure of his death ideology he can be liberated from his suicidal urge.

Schizophrenia

The psychological treatment in schizophrenia has been discussed by Hinsie. I am convinced that schizophrenia is an organic disease in the same sense as the manic-depressive psychosis. Full success, therefore, should not be expected as a rule. That there are cases in which the patient seems to have been cured by psychotherapy cannot be denied. The definite scientific proof can lie only in statistics, since our knowledge concerning this disease is so limited that the reliability of the diagnosis is not great, even when the physician has long experience. If there is any doubt concerning the diagnosis, whether one deals with a neurosis or with a beginning schizophrenia, a therapy fit for a severe neurosis should be inaugurated. One has stated that a therapy which brings forward the hidden complexes might damage the patient. His ego (in the psychoanalytic sense) is too weak to handle the libidinous forces liberated. On the basis of a rather extensive experience, I cannot consider that this so-called danger exists. If one handles a psychotherapeutic situation wrongly, one can do harm to any patient. The dangers of harming the schizophrenic are no greater than those of harming the nonschizophrenic. In every psychotherapy we have to be careful not to bring forward material which the patient either does not understand or cannot handle. One also can drive the neurotic into helplessness and shock by exposing him to interpretations and orders which either are not correct or not correct in relation to the therapeutic situation.

A few theoretical remarks are necessary. There is no doubt that in schizophrenia the patient goes back to a more primitive mode of existence. One generally defines this regression by saying that the patient goes back to the state of primary narcissism and gives attention merely to his body. On the way back to this very primitive stage of existence, other primitive attitudes are revived, so that one finds all the prior stages of psychosexual development. One may, for instance, see the return of the Oedipus complex, of anal and homosexual trends, and, finally, a reorganization concerning the body image and magic thinking may appear. During this regressive process, the superego, as representative of social adaptations, undergoes changes, too. It glides down to a lower level. Since the schizophrenic is not contented with his primitive stage of adaptation (narcissism), he tries again and again to come to new adaptations, and we find not only regressive phenomena but one might also say progressive tendencies by which the patient tries to get into closer contact with the world again. In cases which lead to recovery, this progressive tendency gets the upper hand.

I still consider this description as correct, but I do not think that the current formulation that narcissism is an increased interest in one's body and a lack of interest in the world is a correct description. The primitive stage of development is far from being objectless, but the relation between subject and object is changing and in a continuous state of construction. I have repeatedly pointed out that the knowledge of one's own body is dependent upon one's knowledge of the world. They develop parallel to each other. One has pointed to the particular strength of the superego in schizophrenics and has doubted the greater primitivity of the superego in schizophrenics, but such an objection overlooks the fact that it is one of the signs of primitivity in psychic life that patterns prematurely developed crystallize and may develop a great strength. The organization of the superego is on a lower level in schizophrenia, and this is the most important point. There is no state in which relation to love objects is completely absent. There is always transference, only this transference is unreliable and difficult to handle. This description puts the emphasis on the primitivity in the libidinous structure, and the primitivity of the superego parallel to it.

Some psychoanalysts, for instance Alexander, are of the opinion that the structure of the ego in the psychoanalytic sense is impaired by these conflicts. I often have emphasized that one should not make too schematic a differentiation between ego, superego, and id. There is no question that every conflict is a conflict of the person and, therefore, has to influence the structure of the ego also in the psychoanalytic sense. It is also obvious that the disturbance in the structure of the ego will be the greater, the more severe and the more primitive the libidinous conflict. A further great difficulty lies in the indefiniteness of the psychoanalytic connotation of the ego. Freud defines it as the apparatus which serves perception and motility and in some degree also self-observation and is connected with awareness. On the other hand, he ascribes to it a synthetic function; it is called an organization which has to correlate the demands of reality, id, and superego. The first function mentioned, perception-action, has of course much more obvious relations to physiologic functions. The so-called synthetic function of the ego has no obvious physiological correlations. It is more or less characteristic of the psychic function in general and to ascribe it to any one part of psychic life is obviously an arbitrary decision.

We have, of course, reason to believe that the synthetic function is a good indicator of the general state of psychic development. The child's attitude is certainly less unified than the attitude of the adult. It is obvious, therefore, that the ego function in the psychoanalytic sense has to show a disturbance in proportion to the severity of the regression, and one may speak in this sense about the impairment of the ego function in schizophrenia; but such a statement is merely a repetitious formulation of the fact that one deals with a far-reaching disturbance in the psychosexual structure. I prefer to emphasize that in schizophrenia the basic functions pertaining to perception, action, and judgment are chiefly perturbed by the conflicts and the regressions. This is fundamentally different from the psychic disturbances one finds in organic processes affecting the brain tissue. I prefer to call the psychological disturbances observed in these cases, disturbances in the ego function. However, the terminology is not important, but one should keep in mind that the schizophrenic is an individual overwhelmed by primitive libidinous material.

Our knowledge of the psychogenesis of these cases is limited. The disease very often originates from the psychological conflicts inherent in the biological cycles of life—puberty, childbirth, and also, though much less frequently, involution. We know little about the conflicts in the early development in these cases. Very often we find overwhelming homosexual and anal fixations in relation to the Oedipus situation but reaching to still earlier phases of development. We do not know what is their etiologic significance. At any rate they have a great influence on the symptomatology. I have more and more come to the conclusion that the schizophrenic in his earliest childhood felt confronted with terrific dangers. One of my patients was, at the age of three, extremely afraid of shadows and sacrificed to them buttons and pieces of sugar. Details of the analysis, which I cannot repeat here, make it probable that these shadows were magic fathers. In his later psychosis, homosexual fears played a very great part and he finally ended in a picture of extreme anxiety in which he feared that he might be attacked by everybody and that he might be poisoned by food. I would venture the preliminary hypothesis that the schizophrenic is an individual who experiences an extreme threat in the early stages of development. When this threat is revived in later life, he answers it by reconstructing the world by hallucinations and delusions so that he can face it better; he may also react to this threat by withdrawing into apathy and finally stupor. Another way of escaping the dangerous situation is in catatonic negativism, a defense against any change in the outward world, and the automatic giving in to any order given which is the psychological equivalent of catalepsy. The sterner forms of schizophrenic outbursts with aggressiveness correspond to attempts to maintain their relation to the world by primitive and often sadistic actions. Staercke has justly pointed to the importance of the castration complex. But I may here interpret the castration complex as a general danger symbol.

In the stormier cases of schizophrenia one will, therefore, have to eliminate the threat from the outside situation as much as possible. One may put the patient into a world which is simple; routine is very important in this respect. One will bring the patient to believe that there is no hostility against him, and one will show him love and consideration when he is ready to accept them and not to consider them as an attack. In a more active type of psychotherapy one will analyze situation after situation, find out its meaning with the patient, and give him the possibility of seeing that this situation has less danger than he anticipated. In cases in which the patient has retained closer relations to the outside world, psychotherapy of a more searching type can be tried. One very often has debated whether the techniques in these cases should be the same as in neurosis, or whether another type of technique should be used. Every technique has to be adapted to the particular problem, and since the psychotic and the neurotic are different, I do not see how one can avoid adapting one's technique to the problem in question. Of course, we always follow the basic principle of bringing forward material which has to be interpreted according to the patient's possibilities for insight.

We have, furthermore, to take care of the transference situation. Also, in the treatment of neurosis we have to make the patient understand that his positive transference and his negative transference are different from the emotions displayed in life, that they cannot be transformed into actual life situations. The demands of the schizophrenic patient concerning satisfaction in the positive transference very often will be much more outspoken. If he or she demands intercourse, one has to explain that this is impracticable. He may then feel that this is a hostile act, and an attempt to hurt the physician physically may follow. It is obvious that the patient has to learn, early, the limitations of possible gratifications. In addition, he must be assured of our interest and sympathy. We may do favors for him and so retain the valuable transference of the patient, connected with the insight that the whole world is not hostile towards him, and he may, on the basis of this, get a better insight concerning earlier situations. On the whole, there will very often arise the necessity of convincing the patient of one's good intentions towards him. One may consider this activity in the countertransference as a deviation from the usual psychoanalytic technique. One should keep in mind that even in the most passive psychoanalysis of neurotics, the patient must be sure of having a sympathetic and attentive listener. If in some corner of his mind he is not sure that the analyst has sympathy and good will towards him, he will leave the analyst.

Ferenczi has advocated stronger expressions of countertransference by the physician. We may draw the general conclusion that the expression of countertransference has to change according to the psychotherapeutic situation. We have, anyhow, declined the point of view that the psychotherapist can be passive in any phase of psychotherapy. Schizophrenia merely makes it clear that the problem of countertransference is continually present in psychotherapy and the handling of the countertransference is not less important than the handling of the transference. We have to show our positive countertransference more openly to the schizophrenic.

How far one should go in the analysis of early infantile material of schizophrenics is not always easy to decide. Malamud, Kempf, and Sullivan, to name only a few, report good results although the elucidation of the past in their cases was not very complete. Zilboorg reports a good result in one analyzed case. I see no reason why one should not try to be as complete as possible. In the majority of cases, a complete analysis will be impossible, anyhow. Since the schizophrenic very often retains his distrust and fear concerning the outward world and is, therefore, hindered in his object relations, especially on the heterosexual level, he very often will need continued help from the analyst. The breaking of the transference in the last stage of treatment will, therefore, often be either impossible or not advisable. At any rate, one should not ask too much from the schizophrenic, who suffers so much from the dangers of the world. The analysis of paranoid and paranoiac cases, even if it were possible, might prove a heavy burden or a danger to the physician, who frequently will be an object of a too strong positive and subsequent negative transference, for which the patient cannot get insight. He will become a part of the paranoiac system. Such developments may even take place in cases in which the paranoid signs played a secondary part in the symptomatology. I saw a patient who, after several years of analysis (finally without payment), tried to force the analyst, by threatening letters, to continue the analysis till the cure was complete.[5]

I am, so far, very much gratified with the results achieved in the limited number of cases I have treated in group psychotherapy. In one case who had complained about sensations in the anus (as if after anal intercourse), lack of concentration, and stomach trouble, and had refused to do anything, a complete disappearance of the symptoms was observed; the patient has remained healthy and active now for about two years. Homosexual experiences in early childhood played an important part. His difficulties centered, however, around the very active and energetic mother, who had crushed him from earliest childhood. She was also responsible for the outbreak of the psychosis by forcing him into overwork of a type which he detested. In about eight months, the treatment elucidated a great part of his early experiences.

In another case which could be treated for only a comparatively short time, in which indifference and lack of emotional contact prevailed, a preliminary adaptation was reached. Of great interest is the case of S., a twenty-three-year-old clerk, who, after having had intercourse with prostitutes, entered a love relation which culminated in an intercourse. He was perturbed because this intercourse was not different from the intercourse with prostitutes and developed a severe picture of depersonalization. The analysis showed that he had resented in early childhood that his mother proved unreliable. He had, at the age of six, attempted intercourse with his sister. The mother found out about it and told the grandmother. He felt betrayed. There were also early homosexual experiences with a boy cousin, and at three his eye was hurt by a stone thrown at him. He still has a corneal scar which makes this eye almost useless. After a passing improvement, the patient did not bring any more material. He stopped working completely and stayed at home, but he remained amenable and, according to the report of the mother, did some housework, which he had never done before. He continued, however, to come to the group treatment, mostly complaining there about the analyst, and refusing to bring any material. Once he reported a

[5] A good deal more work has been done in psychotherapy and psychoanalysis of schizophrenia since this was written. See Paul Federn, Frieda Fromm-Reichmann, John Rosen, Mann, Menzer and Standish. See also Melanie Klein for psychotherapy of schizophrenic children. [L.B., Ed.]

dream that he had been kept by the analyst on another planet with a boy cousin with whom he had had sexual relations at five and they had escaped. He did not participate in the group, for the most part. Occasionally he made scathing remarks about the analyst, which provoked the defense of the other patients. The patient has been seen now for more than a year and a half. The other patients consider him supercilious and bossy, and occasionally express the wish to punch him in the nose, but they consider him an equal. He is carefully and neatly dressed. I do not know whether further improvement will take place. The result of the treatment is far from being satisfactory, but I have the impression that the relation of the patient to the analyst and the group has protected him against more dangerous manifestations of his difficulties.

As stated, I consider schizophrenia an organic process. One should not be too optimistic concerning the chances of psychotherapy. There are a great many cases in which the psychotherapeutic approach is without effect, and an equally great number in which it is insufficient in its results; in a small number of cases, results are achieved. The doubt remains whether in some cases one does not deal merely with the spontaneous course and whether in some other cases the results will be only temporary. One may hesitate, of course, under such circumstances to use methods which take so much of the time and energy of the physician as psychoanalysis, and will be inclined to rely upon the enlightened routine of the modern hospital or on work therapy in the sense of H. Simon. It is, at any rate, alarming from the point of view of psychotherapy that the number of schizophrenics in state hospitals does not decrease, even in states like New York and Massachusetts, where the psychological approach to the schizophrenia problem is prevalent. Psychotherapy of schizophrenia has been, at least so far, sociologically ineffective.

Considerations very similar to those for schizophrenia in the narrower sense are valid for paranoiac cases. When one attempts to treat such patients, one often will have to start with an effort to have the patient gain an insight without doubting the reality of his delusions and persecutions. When insight progresses, one may attempt to explain to the patient the psychological mechanisms upon which his delusions and persecutions are based; this should not be omitted in any treatment which is complete. (Cf. Waelder.) It is obvious that this is also true about the schizophrenia in the narrower sense, and it is obviously true that the schizophrenic as well as the paranoiac should be put into a situation where he can choose a world and an occupation which are satisfactory to him. It would not be worth while to discuss schizophrenia and paranoia in such detail if such a discussion would not focus more clearly general principles of treatment which are of importance also for the treatment of neurosis.

The leading American institutions which believe in the psychogenesis of schizophrenia have never published statistics which prove their contention that psychotherapeutic methods are of decisive value in the treatment.[6] We do not doubt the value of psychotherapeutic procedures in psychosis. However, the number of cases in which the long-lasting psychotherapeutic cures are effective is limited. Obviously a specific constellation is necessary so that the psychological influence on the organic process of schizophrenia becomes decisive. The number of such cures in diagnostically clear cases is so small that it is almost impossible to find any statistical proof for the efficiency of psychotherapy in procuring cures in schizophrenia. The New York State hospital system can be credited with a far-going understanding of the psychological problems involved in the psychotherapy of schizophrenics. Nevertheless the number of schizophrenics in state hospitals has not changed in an appreciable way. Psychotherapy doubtless helps almost every schizophrenic patient in his adaptation to circumstances. However, in the majority of cases this help is more or less symptomatic and does not lead to an adaptation to reality, which makes an independent life possible. The basic psychological conflict of the schizophrenic is obviously in connection with the organic character of the disease and is only rarely accessible for the psychological methods which are at hand. It might be that psychological methods become more efficient when there is some preparation of the organic sphere to receive the psychological influence.

3. THE PSYCHOLOGICAL STUDIES OF THE ORGANIC TREATMENT OF SCHIZOPHRENIA

The question arises: To which organic layers can the psychological treatment of schizophrenia progress? Another problem deals with

[6] Reprinted from Leo Orenstein and Paul Schilder, "Psychological Implications of Insulin Treatment in Schizophrenia," *Journal of Nervous & Mental Disease* 88:397–413, 644–60, 1938. [L.B., Ed.]

the psychological changes and their meaning produced by the organic treatment. Such questions are not merely theoretical. They may sooner or later lead to changes and innovations in technique.

Since the state of psychotherapy in schizophrenia is unsatisfactory, on the whole, it is not to be wondered at that many attempts have been made to treat schizophrenia by organic methods. These have been ineffective in the majority of cases. The treatment with hormones is still in the stage of experimentation. I mention three treatments in this connection, in which psychological factors are of importance. In fever treatment, especially by malaria inoculation, the patient becomes helpless and dependent, gets a closer relation to the persons around him, and may be benefited by gaining a closer contact with reality. According to my own experience this is rare, and I am rather doubtful about this effect, which mostly disappears as soon as the fever and the helplessness are over.

Klaesi has inaugurated the so-called sleep treatment of schizophrenics. The patient receives hyoscin, in the beginning. Later on, he receives barbital derivatives in large doses which keep him asleep from ten to fourteen days. Somnifen has been used at first; later on one has used luminal, dial, and others. One has to be careful about the bladder function and temperature. The treatment is not without dangers. Pneumonia may occur. One can use any other type of sleeping medicine, as, for instance, paraldehyde. Favorable results have been reported not only in schizophrenics, but also in manic-depressive states, especially in the manic phase. (M. Cloetta and H. W. Maier.) I have occasionally seen good results but found the method unreliable. The possibility that there is an organic factor working cannot be denied. Klaesi himself stresses the psychological dependence which the patient develops during the treatment and emphasizes how completely he takes care of the patient when he becomes helpless. A part of the reorganization of the patient, if it takes place, may be due to such psychological factors.

Insulin treatment has been used by Sakel. He exposes the patient to a series of hypoglycemic shocks. We are here not interested in the details of the technique, which have been described by Sakel himself, by Dussik and Sakel, and by Glueck. We are merely interested in the psychological implications of the problem. The results reported so far are decidedly favorable, and it looks as if there would be a specific organic curative factor in this treatment. For, as Benedek and

Glueck state, the patients regress deeply during the stupor, and out of this regression a new adaptation may originate. The relation of the patient to the physician, during the stupor and during the disappearance of the stupor, is therefore of very great importance. We may deal here with an independent psychological factor or with the reflection of biological factors in the psychological sphere, or with the combination of both. It is at any rate probable that psychological factors have to be utilized carefully, even if, as we hope, the treatment has a deep biologic effect on the organic processes of the schizophrenia.

The large series of cases collected by Max Mueller (Muensinger) and the Viennese Clinic, where the method originated (Dussik), gave unmistakable proof for the efficiency of the method. The European cases have been observed (1937) now for several years and relapses are seemingly infrequent. The experiences of Bellevue Hospital, about which Karl Bowman, Joseph Wortis, and Leo Orenstein have reported (1937–1938), are favorable. It seems that there is an efficient method for the treatment of schizophrenia for the first time at hand, and it seems that the metrazol treatment of schizophrenia introduced by Meduna is another pharmacological approach in the treatment of schizophrenia which is successful.[7]

The psychological problem which offers itself at first is the problem of what is going on in the insulin shock. Dussik reviewed his own cases and the experiences of others by saying that, at first, slight somatic and vasomotor symptoms, tremors, and sweating appear. With the increase of the somatic signs, the patients come into a state of apathy which becomes more and more similar to normal sleep. Sometimes the psychotic manifestations become outspoken in this phase. Sometimes the psychotic manifestations disappear. Later on, excitement may prevail or sleep may occur until a deep coma appears. Sometimes epileptic attacks take place. Epileptoid twitchings are common. In the phase of awakening after the ingestion of sugar, specific symptoms like aphasia or more general symptoms like perseveration may occur. Such symptoms may also be present during the coma. Immediately after the awakening, states of excitement may

[7] For the most recent comprehensive review of the use and value of the shock treatments, see Selinski, Kalinowsky and Hoch, Sargent and Slater, and Granville L. Jones. Paul Schilder had not written about electric shock treatment or the lobotomies. For the psychoanalytic scrutiny of lobotomy, see Jan Frank, *Psychiatry* 13:25–42, 1950. [L.B., Ed.]

occur which are connected with violent restlessness, tossing, and, according to Dussik, with choreoathetotic movements.

Benedek carefully studied the influence of the insulin shock on perception. He observed disturbances in the perception of movements similar to those observed by Redlich and Poetzl, and Goldstein and Gelb in occipital lobe lesions. One of his first cases complained that the movement of other people had become machine-like, as if interrupted. Instead of an uninterrupted movement he saw the object first in one and then in another place. Quick movements were particularly disagreeable. After awakening, he perceived the world as very beautiful. Another of his patients saw everything turning around; the persons seemed to turn ten to fifteen times in the air. A third patient saw the room increase in length; the persons were at a great distance away and seemed small. One person seemed to turn around and incline; another looked like a mirror image; another patient saw the nurses and visitors smaller, sometimes thinner, and sometimes fatter. Still another patient reported about megalopsia. Primitive optic hallucinations were observed. Colors were sometimes perceived as less impressive during the shock but appeared more saturated after the shock was over. He observed further that during the insulin shock the caloric reactions were changed. He also reported about dysarthrias and paresis in the bulbar innervated muscles. Angyll studied the motor phenomena during the insulin shock and observed tonic phenomena, which he refers to the frontal lobe. Pisk observed a patient who experienced an acceleration in the flow of time.

A psychological theory concerning the mode of action in insulin therapy has to take careful consideration of what is going on during and immediately after the shock. Bychowski and Glueck reported patients wakening from the insulin shock showing great dependence on the persons about them. We want to emphasize that the question of the psychological theory of insulin treatment has nothing at all to do with the problem whether the insulin acts as a physiological or psychological agent. Nevertheless the psychological problem as such remains. Our own investigation concerns cases from Bellevue Hospital (Bowman, Wortis and Orenstein). Patients were observed carefully during the insulin shock and were examined concerning their speech faculty, their tonic and clonic phenomena, as far as the general plan of the treatment allowed. Furthermore the patients were urged to copy the visual motor gestalt figures (Lauretta Bender).

In nineteen cases it was observed that there were difficulties in perception and naming of objects both during the stupor and after awakening. There was a general retardation in all reactions but especially in naming objects. Perseveration was outstanding. Cataleptic phenomena were observed.

The problem arises, what does the insulin shock mean from the point of view of psychology, and furthermore, does the psychology of the insulin shock give any hint of the mechanisms of the recovery process in schizophrenia under insulin therapy?

The insulin hypoglycemia obviously influences deeply the whole central nervous system. It seems that its beginning is not so very different from sleep and has therefore an influence on the subcortical sleep center. It is obvious that when the dosage is increased, sleep is replaced by coma, and it is probable that all of the centers of consciousness down to the medulla oblongata are more or less involved. In the motility there is a slight evidence of impairment of the pyramidal system (positive Babinski sign). However, the bulk of the symptoms point to lesions in the apparatuses of the extrapyramidal motility. The rigidities have generally not the character of the pyramidal tract rigidities. They obviously are of the type that one sees in lesions of the prefrontal area and the subcortical tracts. However, there is not only a release of subcortical tonicity but there are twitchings of epileptiform character and other epileptiform phenomena. We generally have the opinion that these are irritation phenomena originating from the motor area involving also extrapyramidal-subcortical apparatus. Our investigations do not give any proof for the theory proposed that the dominant hemisphere is affected first and stays so longest. We have observed the course of paresis of pyramidal tract character. As the coma progresses, the reflexes finally disappear. It seems almost hopeless to come to an exact classification of these phenomena.

In addition to neurological phenomena in the narrower sense, very often motor phenomena occur which seem to be partially voluntary. The patients toss around, make all kinds of threatening gestures, try to jump out of bed, turn around, groan, grunt, purse their lips, move their tongues, salivate, howl, grimace, clutch, tear pillows apart, and show all kinds of more or less violent mannerisms. In some cases patients express anxiety in connection with this state of manneristic excitement. However, this is not always so. Not all patients show such states. They may occur before, during, or even after the interruption of the coma. Sometimes it appears as if they could be stopped voluntarily. In patients who become quiet in the coma, catalepsy may be present.

The manneristic syndromes occur in cases which do not show any trace of it without the insulin coma. The conclusion might be drawn that in schizophrenia at least this might have an organic background. This conclusion is the more probable since some of us (S. Parker, B. Wortis, and P. Schilder) have observed a similar syndrome in severely alcoholic Negroes. We came to the conclusion that in these patients this syndrome is an attenuated form of alcoholic encephalopathy and postulated that its pathology is to be sought especially in the subcortical extrapyramidal motility. However, it is worth while mentioning that the disturbance in the consciousness and in the visual motor gestalt function is much more outspoken in the insulin shock than in the alcoholics. This manneristic syndrome in schizophrenia is generally not connected with disturbances in consciousness. As one sees it, it is almost impossible to differentiate between the so-called organic and the so-called psychological disturbances.

If there would be any doubt that cortical apparatuses are also involved in the insulin shock one could point to the aphasic symptoms that occur so often in the shock and after awakening. The aphasia is, of course, colored by the presence of the disturbance in consciousness. However, there is a decided difficulty in naming objects. Some tendency to perseveration which shows the typical features is outstanding. It is astonishing how quickly this aphasia can clear up. The patients uniformly remember that they could not find words. One patient could only find the Hungarian word for *nose*. Others substituted for *thumb* the more general *finger* or *digit*. In some cases complex material colors the paraphasic reaction. The aphasia is never isolated. It is connected with a deep disturbance in the gestalt function.

The disturbances in the visual motor gestalt function included perseveration, substitution of loops for points, curves for angles, lines for series of dots, right angles for diagonal crossings, and rotations of various types. There were other forms of exaggeration of more primitive gestalt principles which all of these disturbances suggest.

These gestalt function disturbances appear as a combination of the disturbances observed by L. Bender in cases with toxic infections and organic confusions and in cases of sensory aphasia. On the whole, the gestalt disturbances add another argument for a lesion of the temporal, parietal, and occipital lobes. We therefore come to the conclusion that also the functions of large parts of the cortex are disturbed by the insulin shock.

It is difficult to come to an understanding of the time-sense disturbances in these cases. Some experience the duration of the shock in an appropriate way, and to some the shock seems to last a long time, while to others it seems to last only a short time. The same variations have been found in purely psychogenic gaps in memory.

Some patients experience towards the end of the shock and at the beginning of awakening either an acceleration or a retardation in the flow of time. These phenomena remind us of those observed in intoxication with mescal and hashish. They have obviously an organic genesis which cannot be brought into connection with specific apparatuses at the present time. Pisk, however, has come to the conclusion of an occipital lesion in his case of time-sense disturbance in the insulin shock, and refers to observations of Hoff and Poetzl in local lesions of the brain. It is true that Benedek's observations speak also for such an occipital lesion since he noticed disturbances in the visual perception of movement, a phenomenon which, according to Redlich and Poetzl, has to be referred to the occipital lobe. The metamorphosis observed also by Benedek belongs to the same category. It is remarkable that derealization is also observed in some of these cases. This speaks for the correctness of my assumption (1914) that the occipital lobe lesions and depersonalization symptomatology have something in common.

After the insulin shock, most of the patients feel obviously relaxed, freer from anxieties, and ready to have a greater confidence in the persons around them. Hypomanic attitudes are not uncommon. Many patients during the insulin shock feel danger and uncertainty and the experience of a struggle against the unconsciousness which means death.

These are the data, and it is obvious that the psychology of the insulin shock is the psychology of an individual with a severe organic disturbance of the central nervous system. Material relative to the individual life history can obviously be obtained only at the beginning and towards the end of the shock. The shock appears to the patient in two aspects. It is a complete escape and a complete withdrawal. It is also a threat of death and complete annihilation. It is obviously the second part which has the greatest importance. The individual struggles against this danger and rejoices when it is over. The psychology of the shock is in this respect rather similar to the psychology of the epileptic fit. It seems that the danger of the shock in its organic massiveness supersedes all the other dangers in connection with schizophrenia. The way seems to be cleared, after the shock is over, for an attitude of confidence in the person who is near by, the physician or the nurse. "Overcoming the danger of organic destruction" would be in some way the motto of the insulin shock. The psychological formulations of this type are clumsy in so far as they give comparatively little help in differentiating this organic danger from any other organic danger.

One would come to the conclusion that the greater depth in the disturbance of consciousness and an involvement in cortical and subcortical structure are of importance for the therapeutic results on the schizophrenic process. The formulation is independent from the question whether the insulin shock acts immediately on the central nervous system or by the metabolic intermediaries. In the final analysis the central nervous system has to be influenced in order to change a disturbance which appears in the psychological field. The severity of the disturbance in the cerebral function, as well as its distribution, has to express itself in the psychology of the shock. The postulate seems to be reasonable that a physiological agent with a specific effect on the mental disturbance should express itself in a specific psychological picture. However, this is not true; the effect of fever therapy upon a paralytic process cannot be anticipated by the study of the general paresis case under the influence of fever. Physiological curative agents can therefore express themselves in psychological terms but do not necessarily do so.

This discussion of the psychopathology of the patient during the insulin shock may help us to a deeper understanding of the attitude to his psychosis after he recovers as a result of this therapy. The attitude of the schizophrenic when his psychosis has passed without organic therapy has been described by Mayer Gross and Bertschinger. Schizophrenics may experience their psychosis as a great revelation and an important part of their lives. They may try to push it aside as something which is uncanny. They may try to forget it completely, or they may see it as a symbol of life which has to be realized. When we treat the schizophrenic psychologically, we try to give him an increased insight into his own problems and into the situation which he has to face. One may characterize this procedure by saying that it gives him a deeper understanding of his emotional problems and their relation to his symptoms, so he can use his psychic energies, pent up in his symptoms, for the purpose of everyday life. It is obvious that the insight into the psychodynamics of a symptom, or the psychic cause of a symptom in connection with the inner-life history, does not always help the schizophrenic patient. The schizophrenic often has a spontaneous insight into many psychodynamic problems. It helps him only when this spontaneous insight is directed by another person, and even then, results are not often obtained. When a patient is cured by psychotherapy he knows that his delusions and hallucinations were such and that he was mentally sick (objective insight). In addition he has some knowledge of his inner-life history and its connection with the symptoms (psychodynamic insight). When one has suffered from a cancer and been successfully operated on and cured, one may have a complete objective insight into what has happened. A psychodynamic insight is obviously neither necessary nor desired even if there should be strong psychological components in the genesis of the cancer which is at least highly improbable.

In the cancer case and in the organic case in general even objective insight is not indispensable. Although it is desirable that the patient should know about his having been sick, there is no absolute necessity that he should know that he had cancer. In psychosis, of course, objective insight, as well as the capacity to act according to one's insight, is at least one of the criteria of recovery, and if there should be others, it is at least the most important one. We would not expect more in general paresis. The patient knows that he has had ideas of grandeur, defects of memory and in judgment. He has, therefore, objective insight when he is cured with malaria-fever treatment. Psychodynamic insight is not possible concerning the majority of his symptoms and superfluous concerning the symptoms in which it would be possible. Indeed, the attitude of the general paresis case concerning the general paresis which has been cured is objective. He considers it an organic disease which does not concern the vital problems of his personality. He has not only objective insight but also an objective attitude. It is in connection with this attitude that the patient is not very much interested in the details of his psychosis and intends not to care about it or to forget it.

One can venture the general statement that the schizophrenic patient does not gain psychodynamic insight by insulin therapy but merely objective insight. His resistance against understanding his symptoms is in no way lessened by the insulin therapy. In one case the resistance against an understanding was even particularly strong and the antipathy against the physician who had tried to give this insight into his psychosis was lasting. We may summarize by saying that the schizophrenic patient has objective but not dynamic insight into his psychosis when recovered under insulin. Furthermore he does not show any particular interest in the psychosis. It is not a great event in his life, does not reveal anything to him; it is merely an organic disease, something like a catastrophe coming merely from the outside. The experiences of the psychosis become pale and unimportant. Furthermore the patient does not change his general attitude towards life. He does not come out enriched by new insight. Sometimes one even gets the impression of a particular emotional flatness. At least the one or the other of the patients adapts well after the treatment is finished.

One is justified to say that the insulin treatment helps the individual to go back to his previous prepsychotic self. In psychoanalytical terminology, we might say it detracts libido from the symptom and uses this libido to cement the forces of the ego. The dynamic forces which perform this come obviously from a layer which is not merely what one usually terms psychological. It is obviously a physiological change. The protocols show clearly the transference phenomena which played some part in the process of fortifying the ego against the id. However, as far as one can judge the quantity of such phenomena, it is far from overwhelming and is obviously merely the reflection of deeper physiological processes, the appreciation of which transgresses the psychological limits. The psychological experiences speak therefore decidedly in favor of the theory that the insulin shock acts chiefly as a physiological agent. One should beware of generalizations. A suggestive treatment of any kind or a treatment which cures merely a transference also detracts libido from the symptoms and lets them appear pale although one deals with a process which we call psychological with our present nomenclature.

This psychological description contains everything which we can say at the present time about the theory of insulin shock therapy. We may suspect that the threat of danger for the patient experienced during shock provokes restitutive psychological processes. The regeneration put into motion in this way brings with it regeneration also in those spheres of the personality which seem to be less organically fixated. In other words, the shock acts on organic structures which are generally more crystallized and more rigid (psychologically, in the periphery of the ego). The shock involves a regeneration of the "organic sphere." The process in these deeper-lying organic layers brings with it a revaluation of emotional problems which belong to a sphere nearer to the center of the personality which is more plastic than the structuralized sphere which constitutes the periphery of the personality. These contents are purely psychological and merely draw conclusions concerning the processes going on from a physiological point of view. Sakel has evolved the theory that the insulin therapy destroys the new faulty associations. This is actually not very different from the remarks I have made.

The question remains as to what psychological treatment and how much psychological treatment the patients need in insulin therapy. The problem has come into the foreground in the investigation of Glueck. The problem cannot be as to whether there is psychotherapy or no psychotherapy, since psychological factors are always present in the way we handle the patient. Reassurance and friendliness are psychotherapeutic too, and there is no question that patients coming out of the shock need such reassurance. The question remains however of how much understanding of his psychosis we should try to give the patient. Shall we use psychoanalytic technique? It is understandable that at the height of the stress, deep-going psychotherapeutic measures will probably not be of any particular advantage and may even hinder the physiological consolidation. However, the patients who show improvement are frequently free from symptoms in the afternoon. And the possibility exists to discuss their psychosis with them. Sakel advises against such active procedure. Glueck seems to be generally more in favor of it, although he shows a high degree of cautiousness. The experiences at hand are not sufficient for a definite decision whether and in which degree and when active psychotherapy should be done with the patient. Sufficient evidence is present that active psychotherapy is not necessary in order to obtain the state of remission. Whether psychotherapy can prevent relapses is not known. Since the insulin therapy alone does not increase the insight of the patient, one feels that psychotherapeutic attempts which would better adapt the patient to the tasks of his life seem to be advisable. During the metrazol treatment the patient feels threatened at first by the injection as such but during the aura a much more fundamental threat is experienced.[8] It is the threat of annihilation and death and indeed during the epileptic fit and the following coma the patient comes very near to death. He experiences after the fit a slow revival of his interest in the world and an enormous feeling of relief in which he grasps for any contact offered him. The confusional state after the epileptic attack is filled with perseverations and expresses the organic inability to come in close contact with the world, which the individual desires after his revival from psychological death. Schilder, Clark and others have shown previously that the epileptic experiences death and rebirth. Hypomanic elation which follows so often the epileptic attack is the joy of rebirth. The epileptic fit provoked by metrazol is in this respect not different from the epileptic fit due to other causes. In comparison with these experiences other experiences lose their importance. The individual's psychic energy is free once more again. The previous fixations of libido have lost their importance and there is renewed interest in the persons next to the patient. The victory over the death threat, expressed in the epileptic fit and lingering on in the perceptual and aphasic difficulty, enables the individual to start life and relations to human beings all over again. The previous fixations of libido lying in a more personal layer of experience are washed away by the recovery from a cataclysmic catastrophe in the depth of the organism.

This is the same explanation which Jelliffe has given for the curative effect of the insulin shock. "There are innumerable death threats from without that entail increased object libido investments and many threats from within. The hypoglycemic death threat however is unique. Genetically considered it may be thought of as a very primordial, primitive and massive type of threat which strikes at the very initial stages of life's unfolding." Indeed, the psychological phenomena following the insulin shock are very similar to the phe-

[8] Reprinted from Paul Schilder, "Notes on the Psychology of Metrazol Treatment of Schizophrenia," *Journal of Nervous and Mental Diseases* 89: 133–44, 1939. [L.B., Ed.]

nomena observed after the metrazol injection. It seems that perseverations are in the insulin picture more outspoken than in the metrazol case. There is a greater variability of psychotic pictures in and after the hypoglycemic shock. The phase of excitement between deep coma and consciousness is more elaborate and more grotesque. These are however minor differences. There are the same aphasic and gestalt disturbances in insulin and metrazol treatment. Orenstein and myself didn't find any proof that insulin affects the dominant hemisphere first, or more. To be sure the anatomic phenomena point to the left hemisphere but the right hemisphere even when affected remains silent. Insulin as well as metrazol affects psychic structures which are fundamentally different from the psychic structures involved in the regressive process of schizophrenia. Both therapies provoke objective but not psychodynamic insight.

The patients do not know the psychic conflicts which are reflected in their symptoms and their fundamental attitude towards life problems remains unchanged. We do not know yet whether the remissions observed after metrazol treatment (and after insulin treatment) will last without the help of psychotherapy. However, we also do not know whether they will last with psychotherapy. Both approaches should be tried. We may expect that similarly as in the insulin therapy, permanent remissions may come also without psychotherapy. However, even if that would be so there is no reason why we should not treat the psychological maladaptation of the organically treated schizophrenic case as we treat any other psychological adaptation difficulty.

It is not permissible to bring the therapeutic success of shock therapy in connection with the fact that amnesias occur. The amnesias after metrazol clear up completely. The psychosis and the psychotic symptoms are not forgotten but the individual has changed his emotional attitude.

This is a psychological interpretation. The fact that we can understand the results of the treatment with the help of the tools of modern psychology does not say that the metrazol treatment acts as a psychological agent in the ordinary sense. Its effects are deeper than the effects of what we call psychic influence. The treatment is an organic treatment reflected in psychological attitudes. Quite in the same way as in insulin treatment it looks as if the organic processes of regeneration which are put in action by metrazol bring with themselves a reconstruction which serves also the more labile organic structures which serve emotions and which are damaged by the process of schizophrenia. The forces liberated by the metrazol and insulin treatment come from layers which are generally not accessible to the organic processes which we usually call psyche.

We have come to a unified attitude to schizophrenic psychology.[9] The schizophrenic threatened in early childhood withdraws into positions more secure. He tries to heighten the importance or the strength of his own personality. Furthermore he uses primitive methods of defense either by giving in to immobility and catalepsy or by negativism. He may also use the technique of violent attack. He does not dare to retain higher forms of object relations. Primitive types of libidinous development occur. In addition to that we find primitive stages of ego-ideal development. The primitive attitude comes also into appearance in the formation of language and thought processes. Symbolism, projection, renewed identifications, belong in this sphere. The primitive threat is revived by the dangerous situations of everyday life. The threat of being destroyed leads to outbursts of aggressiveness which appear particularly clearly in the schizophrenia of children. Many of these manifestations of primitive motor faculties are disturbed in a sphere which is not the same as in gross lesions of the brain.

During and after metrazol and insulin shock, aphasic and confusional states occur of clear-cut organic type. They may be studied with the help of gestalt tests and the Goodenough test. These phenomena belong to another order than the phenomena in schizophrenia. After the insulin shock and after the metrazol fit, the individual has an increased capacity for transference. It is as if the individual would feel that he is safe now from a psychological point of view and would form now a better relation to the world and would consider a psychotic experience as of no importance. One may talk with Jelliffe of "a death threat overcome" if one keeps in mind that this death threat comes from the depth of the organism and is a reflection of organic occurrences. At any rate the individual reorganizes his attitudes in connection with the physiological reorganization within the organism.

The amnesia does not play an important part in the psychophysiological reorganization. The individual regains by the treatment an

[9] Reprinted from Paul Schilder, "The Psychology of Schizophrenia," *Psychoanalytic Review* 26:380–98, 1939. [L.B., Ed.]

objective but no psychodynamic insight into the occurrences of the psychosis. He may need at any rate psychological help although we do not know if it can prevent relapses. At any rate psychological help does not seem to be essential for the immediate curative effect.

Schizophrenia can be understood at least in some degree. From a psychological point of view, we may say that the organic process of schizophrenia is modifiable in some degree by psychological methods. The organic methods of treatment are even at the present time more effective, and it is to be hoped that their psychological analysis will help us to deeper understanding of schizophrenia and will improve our psychotherapeutic and organic approach.

BIBLIOGRAPHY

ABELES, MILTON, AND SCHILDER, PAUL: "Psychogenic Loss of Personal Identity," *Arch. Neurol. & Psychiat.* 34:587–604 (Sept. 3, 1935).

Abraham, Karl: *Selected Papers on Psychoanalysis* (London, Internat. Psychoanalytic Press and Hogarth Press, 1927).

Adler, Alexandra: "Unfallhaeufung und ihre persoenliche Bedingtheit," *Zentralblatt f. Neurol. u. Psychiat.* 60:141 (1931).

———: *Guiding Human Misfits, Practical Application of Individual Psychology,* 2nd. ed. (New York, Philosophical Library, Inc., 1948).

Adler, Alfred: *The Neurotic Constitution: Outlines of a Comparative Individualist* (New York, Moffat, Yard and Co., 1917).

———: *A Study of Organ Inferiority and Its Psychical Compensations,* translated by Smith Ely Jelliffe (New York, Nerv. & Ment. Dis. Publishing Co., 1917).

———: *What Life Should Mean to You* (Boston, Little, Brown & Co., 1931).

———: *Social Interests: A Challenge to Mankind* (New York, Putnam, 1939).

Adrian, E. D.: "Electrical Activity of the Nervous System," *Arch. Neurol. & Psychiat.* 32:1125–1136 (Dec., 1934).

Adrian, E. D., and Matthews, B. H. C.: "The Berger Rhythm: Potential Changes from the Occipital Lobes in Man," *Brain* 57:355 (1934).

Alcoholics Anonymous: *The Story of How One Hundred Men Have Recovered from Alcoholism* (New York, Works Publishing Co., 1937).

Alexander, Franz: "Schizophrenic Psychosis. Critical Consideration of Psychoanalytic Treatment," *Arch. Neurol. & Psychiat.* 26:815–838 (1931).

———: *Fundamentals of Psychoanalysis* (New York, W. W. Norton & Co., 1948).

Alexander, Franz, and French, Thomas M.: *Psychoanalytic Therapy* (New York, Ronald Press, 1946).

———: *Studies in Psychosomatic Medicine* (New York, Ronald Press, 1948).

Alexander, Franz, and Healy, William: *Roots of Crime, Psychoanalytic Studies* (New York, Alfred A. Knopf, 1935).

Angyll, L. von: "Ueber die motorischen und tonischen Erscheinungen des Insulin Schocks," *Ztschr. Neurol.* 35:157 (1937).

Association for Research in Nerv. & Ment. Dis.: *Schizophrenia (Dementia Praecox) Investigation* (New York, Paul Hoeber, Inc., 1928).

Babinski, S.: *Oeuvre scientifique Part IX Hysteria et pithiatisme* (Paris, Masson, 1934), pp. 457 ff.

Beerd, George M.: *A Practical Treatise on Nervous Exhaustion; Neurasthenia, Its Symptoms, Nature, Sequences and Treatment* (New York, W. Wood & Co., 1880).

Bell, Marjorie: *Bulwarks against Crime* (New York, National Probation and Parole Assoc., 1940).

Bellak, Leopold: *Dementia Praecox, the Past Ten Years' Work* (New York, Grune & Stratton, 1948).

Bender, Lauretta: "Psychoses Associated with Somatic Diseases That Distort the Body Structure," *Arch. Neurol. & Psychiat.* 32:1000–1029 (1934).

———: *A Visual Motor Gestalt Test and Its Clinical Use,* Research Mono. No. 3 (New York, Amer. Orthopsychiat. Assoc., 1938).

———: "Treatment of Aggression," *Amer. J. Orthopsychiat.* 13:392–399 (1943).

———: "Organic Brain Conditions Producing Behavior Disturbances," in *Modern Trends in Child Psychiatry,* edited by N. D. C. Lewis and B. Pacella (New York, Grune & Stratton, 1945), pp. 155–193.

———: "Psychopathic Behavior Disorders in Children," *Handbook of Correctional Psychology,* edited by R. M. Lindner and R. V. Seliger (New York, Psychological Library, 1947), pp. 360–377.

———: "Genesis of Hostility in Children," *Amer. J. Psychiat.* 105:241–245 (1948).

———: "Psychological Problems in Children with Organic Brain Disease," *Amer. J. Orthopsychiat.* 19:404–415 (1949).

———: "Anxiety in Disturbed Children," *Anxiety,* edited by P. Hoch (New York, Grune & Stratton, 1950).

———: *Child Psychiatric Techniques: A Diagnostic and Therapeutic*

Approach to Normal and Abnormal Development Through Patterned Expressive and Group Behavior (Springfield, Illinois, Charles C. Thomas, 1950).

Bender, Lauretta, and Blau, Abram: "The Reaction of Children to Sexual Relations with Adults," *Amer. J. Orthopsychiat.* 7:500–518 (1937).

Bender, Lauretta, and Cottington, Frances: "The Use of Amphetamine Sulphate (Benzedrine) in Child Psychiatry," *Amer. J. Psychiat.* 99:116–121 (1942).

Bender, Lauretta, Keiser, S., and Schilder, P.: "Studies in Aggressiveness," *Genetic Psychol. Mono.*, Vol. 18, Nos. 5 and 6 (1936), pp. 357–564.

Bender, Lauretta, and Schilder, P.: "Impulsions, a Specific Disorder in the Behavior of Children," *Arch. Neurol. & Psychiat.* 44:990–1008 (1940).

Bender, Lauretta, and Woltmann, A. G.: "The Use of Puppet Shows as a Psychotherapeutic Method for Behavior Problems in Children," *Amer. J. Orthopsychiat.* 6:341–354 (1936).

Bender, Lauretta, and Yarrell, Zuleika: "Psychoses among Followers of Father Divine," *J. Nerv. & Ment. Dis.* 27:418–449 (1938).

Benedek, L.: *Insulinschockwirkung auf die Wahrnehmung* (Berlin, S. Karger, 1935).

Benedek, Therese: *Insight and Personality Adjustment, a Study of the Psychological Effects of War* (New York, Ronald Press, 1946).

———: "Climacterium a Developmental Phase," *Psychoanalyt. Quart.* 19:1–27 (1950).

Benedek, Therese, and Rubenstein, B.: "The Sexual Cycle in Women, the Relation between Ovarian Function and Psychodynamic Processes," *Psychosomatic Monog.* III, Nos. 1 and 2 (1942).

Bennett, A. E.: "Convulsive Shock Therapy in Depressive Psychoses," *Amer. J. Med. Science* 196:420 (1938).

Benussi, V. H.: "Die Atmungssymptome der Luege," *Arch. f. d. ges. Psychol.* 31:244–273 (1914).

Bergler, Edmund: "Psychoanalysis of a Case of Agoraphobia," *Psychoanalyt. Rev.* 22 (1935).

———: "Obsession Neurosis in Its Last Stage. Four Mechanisms in the Narcissistic Pleasure in the Compulsion," *Internat. Ztschr. f. Psychoanal.* 22:238–248 (1936).

———: *The Basic Neurosis; Oral Aggression and Psychic Masochism* (New York, Grune & Stratton, 1949).

Bergler, Edmund, and Eidelberg, L.: "Der Mechanismus der Depersonalization," *Internat. Ztschr. f. Psychoanal.* 21:258 (1935).

Bierer, Joshua (ed.): *Therapeutic Social Clubs* (Adlerian Group Therapy) (London, H. K. Lewis & Co., 1948).

Billings, E. G.: *A Handbook of Elementary Psychobiology and Psychiatry* (New York, The Macmillan Co., 1943).

Binswanger, Ludwig: *Wandlungen in der Auffassung u. Deutung des Traumes von den Griechen bis zur Gegenwart* (Berlin, Springer, 1928).

Blanton, Smiley, and Blanton, Margaret: *For Stutterers* (New York, D. Appleton-Century Co., 1936).

Bleuler, E.: *Dementia Praecox,* translation by Joseph Zinkin (New York, International Universities Press, 1950).

Bowlby, John: *Forty-four Juvenile Thieves: Their Character and Home-life* (London, Baillière, Tindall & Cox, 1946).

Bowman, Karl M.: "Psychoses with Pernicious Anemia," *Amer. J. Psychiat.* 92:371–396 (1935).

Braun, Ludwig: *Herz und Angst* (Leipzig-Vienna, Franz Deuticke, 1932).

Brenman, M., and Gill, M. M.: *Hypnotherapy. A survey of the literature,* publication of Josiah Macy, Jr.; Foundation Review Series, Vol. II, No. 3 (New York, International Universities Press, Inc., 1944).

Brentano, Franz: *Psychologie vom empirischen Standpunkt* (Leipzig, Meiner, 1924).

Breuer, A., and Freud, S.: *Studien ueber Hysterie* (Vienna, Springer, 1895).

Brill, A. A.: "Psychic Suicide," *J. Nerv. & Ment. Dis.* 80:63–64 (1934).

Bromberg, Walter: *Report of the Psychiatric Clinic, Court of General Sessions* (New York City, 1936, 1937, 1938).

———: *Crime and the Mind, an Outline of Psychiatric Criminology* (Philadelphia, J. B. Lippincott Co., 1948).

Bromberg, Walter, and Schilder, Paul: "Psychologic Considerations in Alcoholic Hallucinosis-Castration and Dismembering Motives," *Int. J. Psychoanal.* 14:206 (1933).

———: "Death and Dying," *Psychoanalyt. Rev.* 20:133 (1933).

Brunswick, Ruth Mack: "A Follow-up on Freud's Story of an Infantile Neurosis," *Int. J. Psychoanal.* 9:439–476 (1928).

Burrow, Trigant: *The Neuroses of Man, an Introduction to the Science of Human Behavior* (London, Routledge, & K. Paul, 1949).

CHADWICK, MARY: *The Psychological Effects of Menstruation* (New York, Nerv. & Ment. Dis. Publishing Co., 1932).

———: *Women's Periodicity* (London, Noel Douglas, 1933).

Clark, L. Pierce: "What Is the Psychology of Organic Epilepsy?" *Psychoanalyt. Rev.* 20:79–85 (1933).

———: *The Nature and Treatment of Amentia* (London, Baillière, Tindall & Cox, 1933).

Cleckley, H.: *The Mask of Sanity* (St. Louis, C. V. Mosby Co., 1941).

Cloetta, M., and Maier, H. W.: "Concerning an Improvement of the Psychiatric Prolonged Sleep Treatment," *Amer. J. Psychiat.* 91:1409–1412 (1935).

Conrad, Agnes: "The Psychiatric Study of Hyperthyroid Patients," *J. Nerv. & Ment. Dis.* 79:505, 656 (1934).

Coriat, Isador H.: *Stammering, a Psychoanalytic Interpretation* (New York, Nerv. & Ment. Dis. Publishing Co., 1928).

Coué, E.: *How to Practice Suggestion and Autosuggestion* (New York, Amer. Library Institute, 1933).

Cowdry, E. V. (ed.): *Problems of Aging; Biological and Medical Aspects* (Baltimore, The Williams & Wilkins Co., 1939).

Curran, Frank J.: "Personality Studies in Alcoholic Women," *J. Nerv. & Ment. Dis.* 86:645–667 (1937).

———: "Psychotherapeutic Problems of Puberty," *Amer. J. Orthopsychiat.* 10:510–521 (1940).

———: "The Adolescent and His Emotional Problems," *Dis. of the Nerv. System* 1:144–147 (1940).

Curran, Frank, and Schilder, Paul: "A Constructive Approach to the Problems of Childhood and Adolescence," *J. Clin. Psychopath.* 2:125–142, Pt. I (1940); 2:305–320, Pt. II (1941).

DAVIS, HALLOWELL, AND DAVIS, PAULINE A.: "Action Potentials of the Brain in Normal States of Cerebral Activity," *Arch. Neurol. & Psychiat.* 36:1214–1224 (1936).

Despert, Louise, *et al:* "Psychosomatic Studies of Fifty Stuttering Children," *Amer. J. Orthopsychiat.* 16:100–133 (1946).

Deutsch, Felix: "Biologie u. Psychologie der Krankheitsgenese," *Int. Ztschr. f. Psychoanal.* 19:130–146 (1933).

———: *Applied Psychoanalysis, Selected Objectives of Psychotherapy* (New York, Grune & Stratton, 1949).

Deutsch, Helene: *The Psychology of Women,* Vols. I and II (New York, Grune & Stratton, 1944, 1945).

Diethelm, Oskar: *Treatment in Psychiatry,* 2nd ed. (Springfield, Ill., Charles C. Thomas, 1950).

Draper, G.: *Human Constitution: Its Significance in Medicine* (Baltimore, The Williams & Wilkins Co., 1928).

Dreikurs, Rudolf: *An Introduction to Individual Psychology,* Introduction by Alfred Adler (London, Kegan Paul, Trench & Trubner & Co., Ltd., 1935).

Dubois, P.: *The Psychic Treatment of Nervous Disorders,* 6th. ed. (New York, Funk & Wagnalls, 1909).

Dunbar, Flanders: *Psychosomatic Diagnosis* (New York, Paul B. Hoeber, Inc., 1945).

———: *Emotions and Bodily Changes. A Survey of Literature on Psychosomatic Interrelationship,* 1910–1945 (New York, Columbia University Press, 1945).

Dussik, K. T.: "Three and a Half Years of Hypoglycemic Therapy of Schizophrenia; Results and Problems," *Amer. J. Psychiat.* 94:296 (1938).

Eissler, Kurt R. (ed.): *Searchlights on Delinquency—New Psychoanalytic Studies* (New York, International Universities Press, 1948).

English, O. Spurgeon: "Role of Emotion in Disorders of the Skin," *Arch. Dermatol. and Syphil.* 60:1063–1076 (1949).

Erickson, Milton E.: "A Clinical Note on a Word Association Test," *J. Nerv. & Ment. Dis.* 84:5 (1936).

Federn, Paul: "Some Variation in Ego Finding," *Internat. J. Psychoanal.* 7:434 (1926).

———: "Narcissism in the Structure of the Ego," *Internat. J. Psychoanal.* 9:401 (1928).

———: "The Severe Laws of Compulsion," *Internat. J. Psychoanal.* 19:616–620 (1933).

———: "Principles of Psychotherapy in Latent Schizophrenia," *Amer. J. Psychother.* 1:29 (1947).

———: "Mental Hygiene of the Psychotic Ego," *Amer. J. Psychother.* 3:356–371 (1949).

Fenichel, Otto: *Perversionen, Psychosen, Charakterstoerungen* (Vienna, Internat. Psychoanalytic Verlag, 1931).

———: *Outline of Clinical Psychoanalysis* (New York, W. W. Norton & Co., 1934).

Fenichel, Otto: *The Psychoanalytic Theory of Neurosis* (New York, W. W. Norton & Co., 1945).
Ferenczi, S.: *Contributions to Psychoanalysis* (Boston, Richard G. Badger, 1916).
———: *Theory and Technique of Psychoanalysis* (London, Hogarth Press, 1926).
Ferenczi, S., and Hollos, S.: "Psychoanalysis and the Psychic Disorder of General Paresis," *Nervous and Mental Disease Monograph* (1925).
Forel, August H.: *Hypnotism or Suggestion and Psychotherapy,* translated from the 5th German ed. (New York, Retman, 1906).
Foulkes, S. H.: *Introduction to Group-Analytic Psychotherapy Studies in Social Integration of Individuals and Groups* (New York, Grune & Stratton, 1949).
Foxe, Arthur N.: *Studies in Criminology* (New York, Nerv. & Ment. Dis. Publishing Co., 1950).
Frank, Jan: "Lobotomy under Psychoanalytic Scrutiny," *Psychiatry* 13:35–42 (1950).
Frank, L.: *Die psychokathartische Behandlung nervoeser Stoerungen* (Leipzig, G. Thieme, 1927).
Freud, Anna: *Introduction to the Technic of Child Analysis* (New York, Nerv. & Ment. Dis. Publishing Co., 1928).
———: *The Ego and the Mechanisms of Defense* (London, Hogarth Press, 1937).
Freud, Sigmund: *The Interpretation of Dreams* (New York, The Macmillan Co., 1922).
———: *Beyond the Pleasure Principle* (London, Internat. Psychoanalytic Press, 1922).
———: *Collected Papers,* Vols. I–IV (London, Internat. Psychoanalytic Press & Hogarth Press, 1924–1925), Vol. V (1950).
———: *Introductory Lectures on Psycho-Analysis* (London, G. Allen & Unwin, 1929).
———: *Civilization and Its Discontents* (New York, Jonathan Cape & Harrison Smith, 1930).
———: *New Introductory Lectures on Psychoanalysis* (New York, W. W. Norton & Co., 1933).
———: *Inhibitions, Symptoms, and Anxiety* (London, Hogarth Press, 1936).
———: *The Basic Writings of Sigmund Freud,* with an introduction by

A. A. Brill; Modern Library ed. (New York, Random House, Inc., 1938).

———: *Group Psychology and the Analysis of the Ego* (London, Hogarth Press, 1940).

———: *General Introduction to Psychoanalysis* (Garden City Publishing Co., 1943).

———: *An Outline of Psychoanalysis* (New York, W. W. Norton & Co., 1949).

Friedjung, Josef K.: "Acute Psychoneurosen in Kindheit," *Ztschr. f. Kinderheilkunde* 40:126–132 (1925).

Fromm, Erich: *Escape from Freedom* (New York, Farrar and Rinehart, Inc., 1941).

———: *Man against Himself* (New York, Rinehart & Co., 1947).

Fromm-Reichmann, Frieda: "Recent Advances in Psychoanalytic Therapy" and "Remarks on Philosophy of Mental Disorder," in *A Study in Inter-Personal Relations,* edited by Patrick Mullahy (New York, Hermitage Press, Inc., 1949).

Fry, Clements C.: *Mental Health in Colleges* (New York, New York Commonwealth Fund, 1942).

Galdston, Iago: "On the Etiology of Depersonalization," *J. Nerv. & Ment. Dis.* 105:25–39 (1947).

Gesell, Arnold, and Amatruda, C. S.: *Developmental Diagnosis, Normal and Abnormal Child Development* (New York, Paul B. Hoeber, Inc., 1947).

Ginsberg, Raphael: "Psychology in Everyday Geriatrics," *Geriatrics* 5:36–43 (1950).

Glover, Edward: "Psychological Groundwork in Group Psychology," *Internat. J. Psychoanal.* 10:1929.

———: "Etiology of Drug Addiction," *Internat. J. Psychoanal.* 13:298–328 (1932).

———: "A Psychoanalytic Approach to the Classification of Mental Disorders," *J. Ment. Science* 87:819–842 (1932).

Glueck, Bernard: "Criteria for Estimating the Value of Psychiatric Services in the Field of Criminology," *Amer. J. Psychiat.* 91:693–702 (1934).

———: "Induced Hypoglycemic State in the Treatment of Psychoses," *New York State J. Med.* 36:1473–1484 (1936).

———: "Clinical Experience with the Hypoglycemic Treatment of the Psychoses," *J. Nerv. & Ment. Dis.* 85:564 (1937).

Glueck, Eleanor T.: "Mental Retardation and Juvenile Delinquency," *Mental Hygiene* 19:549–569 (1935).

Glueck, Sheldon, and Glueck, Eleanor T.: *500 Criminal Careers* (New York, Alfred A. Knopf, 1930).

———: *500 Delinquent Women* (New York, Alfred A. Knopf, 1934).

Goldfarb, William: "The Effects of Early Institutional Care on Adolescent Personality," *J. Exper. Educat.* 12:106–120 (1943).

Goldman, George S.: "A Care of Compulsive Hand Washing," *Psychoanalyt. Quart.* 7:96–121 (1938).

Greenacre, Phyllis: "The Predisposition to Anxiety," *Psychoanalyt. Quart.* 10:66–95, 610–639 (1941).

Greene, James S.: "Treatment of the Stutter-type Person in the Medicosocial Clinic," *J. Nerv. & Ment. Dis.* 81:313–317 (1935).

Grinker, Roy R., and Spiegel, John P.: *Men under Stress* (Philadelphia, Blakiston, 1945).

Groddeck, G.: *The Book of the Id* (New York, Nerv. & Ment. Dis. Publishing Co., 1927).

Gutheil, Emil: *The Language of the Dream* (New York, The Macmillan Co., 1939).

Guttmann, E., and Maclay, W. S.: "Mescalin and Depersonalization," *J. Neurol. and Psychopath.* 16:103 (1935–1936).

Hartmann, H.: "Cocainismus und Homosexualitaet," *Ztschr. f. d. ges. Neurol. u. Psychiat.* 95:79–94 (1925).

Hartmann, Heinz, and Kris, Ernst: "The Genetic Approach in Psychoanalysis," *The Psychoanalytic Study of the Child I* (New York, International Universities Press, Inc., 1945).

Hassin, G. B., Schaub, C. F., and Voris, H. C.: "Spasmodic Torticollis," *Arch. Neurol. & Psychiat.* 26:1043 (1931).

Haug, K.: *Die Stoerungen des Persoenlichkeitsbewusstseins* (Stuttgart, Enke, 1936).

Hausner, E., and Hoff, H.: "Zur Pathogenese des Angstgefuehls in Angina Pectoris," *Anfall. Ztschr. f. Klin. Med.* (1933), pp. 493–507.

Healy, Wm. H., Bronner, August F., and Bowers, Anna M.: *The Structure and Meaning of Psychoanalysis* (New York, Alfred A. Knopf, 1930).

Heilig, Robert, and Hoff, Hans: "Psychische Beeinflussung von Organfunktionen," *Allg. aerzt. Ztschr. f. Psychotherapie* 1:268–280 (1928).

Hendrick, Ives: *Facts and Theories of Psychoanalysis,* 2nd ed. (New York, Alfred A. Knopf, 1941).

Heyer, G. R.: *Der Organismus der Seele* (Munich, J. F. Lehmann, 1932).

———: *Praktische Seelenheilkunde* (Munich, J. F. Lehmann, 1935).

Hinsie, Leland: *Treatment of Schizophrenia* (Baltimore, The Williams & Wilkins Co., 1930).

———: *Concepts and Problems of Psychotherapy* (New York, Columbia University Press, 1937).

———: *The Person in the Body* (New York, W. W. Norton & Co., 1945).

Hoch, Paul H.: "The Present Status of Narco-Diagnosis and Therapy," *J. Nerv. & Ment. Dis.* 103:248–258 (1946).

———: *Failures in Psychiatric Treatment* (New York, Grune & Stratton, 1948).

Hoff, H.: "Die Psychische Beeinflussung der Organfunktion," *Vienna med. Wochenschrift* 79:932 (1929).

Horney, Karen: "The Problem of Feminine Masochism," *Psychiat. Rev.* 22:241–257 (1935).

———: "Conception and Misconception of the Analytical Method," *J. Nerv. & Ment. Dis.* 81:399–411 (1935).

———: *The Neurotic Personality of Our Time* (New York, W. W. Norton & Co., 1937).

———: *New Ways in Psychoanalysis* (New York, W. W. Norton & Co., 1939).

———: *Our Inner Conflicts* (New York, W. W. Norton & Co., 1945).

Horsley, J. S.: *Narco-analysis* (London, Oxford Medical Publication, 1943).

Huddelson, J. H.: *Accidents, Neurosis, and Compensation* (Baltimore, The Williams & Wilkins Co., 1932).

Hurst, Arthur: "Some Disorders of the Esophagus," *J. Amer. Med. Assoc.* 102:582–587 (1936).

Hyman, H. T.: "Value of Psychoanalysis as a Therapeutic Procedure," *J. Amer. Med. Assoc.* 107:326–329 (1936).

Institute for Psychoanalysis, Chicago: *Proceedings of the Second Brief, Psychotherapy Council, 1944.*
I. War Psychiatry
II. Psychosomatic Medicine
III. Psychotherapy for Children
IV. Group Psychotherapy
Proceedings of the Third Brief, Psychotherapy Council, 1946.

Jacobi, Jolan: *The Psychology of Jung,* translated by K. Bash (New Haven, Yale University Press, 1943).

Jacobson, E.: *Progressive Relaxation* (Chicago, University of Chicago Press, 1929).

Jaensch, E. R.: "Ueber den Farbenkontrast und die sogenannte Beruecksichtigung der farbigen Beleuchtung," *Ztschr. f. Sinnesphysiol.* 52: 165–180 (1917).

Jameison, G. R.: "Suicide and Mental Disease," *Arch. Neurol. & Psychiat.* 36:1–11 (1936).

Janet, Pierre: *Psychological Healing* (New York, The Macmillan Co., 1925).

Jelgersma, H. C.: "Psychoanalyse der Dementia Senilis," *Ztschr. f. d. ges. Neurol. u. Psychiat.* 135:657–670 (1931).

Jelliffe, Smith Ely: *Psychopathology of Forced Movements in Oculogyric Crises* (New York, Nerv. Ment. Dis. Publishing Co., 1932).

———: "Discussion on Insulin Treatment," *J. Nerv. & Ment. Dis.* 85:575–578 (1937).

———: *Sketches in Psychosomatic Medicine* (New York, Nerv. & Ment. Dis. Publishing Co., 1939).

Jellinek, E. M.: *Alcohol Addiction and Chronic Alcoholism* (New Haven, Yale University Press, 1942).

Jones, Ernest: *What Is Psychoanalysis?* (New York, International Universities Press, Inc., 1950).

Jones, Granville L.: *Psychiatric Shock Treatment, Current Views and Practices,* sponsored by the Manfred Sakel Foundation (New York, The National Com. for Mental Hygiene, 1949).

Jong, H. de: "Die Hauptgesetze . . . koerperlicher Erscheinungen beim psychischen Geschehen," *Ztschr. f. d. ges. Neurol. u. Psychiat.* 69:61 (1921).

Jung, Carl G.: *Studies in Word Association* (London, William Heinemann, 1918).

———: *Psychological Types in the Psychology of Individuation,* translated by H. Goodwin Baynes (New York, Harcourt, Brace & Co., 1926).

———: *The Psychology of the Unconscious,* translated by Beatrice M. Hinkle (New York, Dodd, Mead & Co., 1927).

———: *Two Essays on Psychoanalytical Psychology,* translated by H. G. and C. F. Baynes (New York, Dodd, Mead & Co., 1928).

———: "Problems in Modern Psychotherapy," *Schweiz med. Woch.* 12:810 (1931).

———: *Modern Man in Search of a Soul,* translated by W. S. Dill and H. G. Baynes (New York, Harcourt, Brace & Co., 1933).

———: *Psychology of Dementia Praecox,* translated by A. A. Brill (New York, Nerv. & Ment. Dis. Publishing Co., 1936).

———: *Psychology and Religion* (New Haven, Yale University Press, 1938).

———: *The Integration of the Personality,* translated by S. M. Dell (New York, Farrar and Rinehart, Inc., 1939).

Kahn, Eugene: *Psychopathic Personalities* (New Haven, Yale University Press, 1931).

Kalinowsky, Lothar B.: "Present Status of Electric Shock Therapy," *Bull. N.Y. Acad. Med.* 25:541–553 (1949).

Kalinowsky, Lothar B., and Hoch, Paul H.: *Shock Treatments and Other Somatic Procedures in Psychiatry* (New York, Grune & Stratton, 1946).

Kanner, Leo: *Child Psychiatry,* 2nd ed. (Springfield, Ill., Charles C. Thomas & Co., 1948).

Kaplan, O. J.: *Mental Disorders of Later Life* (Stanford University Press, 1945).

Kardiner, Abram: "The Bio-analysis of Epileptic Reaction," *Psychoanalyt. Quart.* 1:375 (1932).

———: *The Individual and His Society* (New York, Columbia University Press, 1939).

———: *The Traumatic Neuroses of the War* (New York, Paul B. Hoeber, Inc., 1947).

Kardiner, Abram, and Spiegel, H.: *War Stress and Neurotic Illness* (New York, Paul B. Hoeber, Inc., 1947).

Karpman, B.: *The Individual Criminal* (New York, Nerv. & Ment. Dis. Publishing Co., 1935).

———: "The Mental Roots of Crime," *J. Nerv. & Ment. Dis.* 9:89–142 (1939).

——— (chairman): "The Psychopathic Delinquent Child," *J. Amer. Orthopsychiat.* 20:223–265 (1950).

Kauders, Otto, and Schilder, Paul: *Hypnosis* (New York, Nerv. & Ment. Dis. Publishing Co., 1927).

Kempf, E. L.: "Bisexual Factors in Curable Schizophrenia," *J. Abnorm. & Soc. Psychol.* 44:414–419 (1949).

Kennard, Margaret A.: "The Value of the Electroencephalogram as an Index of Generalized Cortical Activity," *Confinia Neurologica* 9:193–205 (1949).

Kessel, L., and Hyman, H. T.: "Value of Psychoanalysis as a Therapeutic Procedure," *J. Amer. Med. Assoc.* 101:1612–1615 (1933).

Kinsey, Alfred C., Pomeroy, W. B., and Martin, C. E.: *Sexual Behavior in the Human Male* (Philadelphia, W. B. Saunders, 1948).

Klaesi, J.: "Einiges ueber Schizophreniebehandlung," *Ztschr. f. d. ges. Neurol. u. Psych.* 78:606–620 (1922).

———: "Ueber die therapeutische Anwendung des 'Dauernarkose' Mittels Somnifens bei Schizophrenie," *Ztschr. f. d. ges. Neurol. u. Psych.* 74:557–592 (1922).

Klauder, T. V.: "Psychogenic Aspects of Diseases of the Skin," *Arch. Neurol. & Psych.* 33:221–223 (1935).

Klein, Melanie: *Psychoanalysis of Children* (New York, W. W. Norton & Co., 1932).

———: *Contribution to Psychoanalysis, 1921–1945* (London, Hogarth Press, 1948).

———: "A Contribution to the Theory of Anxiety and Guilt," *Internat. J. Psychoanal.* 29:114–123 (1948).

Klein, Viola: *The Feminine Character* (New York, Internat. Universities Press, 1950).

Kleist, Karl: "Schreckpsychosen," *Allg. Ztschr. f. Psychiatrie* 74:432–510 (1918).

Kluever, H.: "Studies on the Eidetic Type and on Eidetic Imagery," *Psychol. Bull.* 25:69 (1928).

———: "Eidetic Imagery," in *A Handbook of Child Psychology,* ed. by Murchison (Worcester, Mass., Clark University Press, 2nd. ed., 1933), pp. 699–722.

Koenig-Fachsenfeld, E.: *Wandlungen des Traumproblems* (Stuttgart, Enke, 1935).

Lennox, W. G.: "Psychiatry, Psychology and Seizures," *Amer. J. Orthopsychiat.* 19:432–446 (1949).

Levine, Maurice: *Psychotherapy in Medical Practice* (New York, The Macmillan Co., 1942).

Levy, David M.: "Use of the Play Technic as Experimental Procedure," *Amer. J. Orthopsychiat.* 3:266 (1933).

———: "Hostility Patterns in Sibling Rivalry Experiments," *Amer. J. Orthopsychiat.* 6:183–258 (1936).

Lewin, Bertram D.: *The Psychoanalysis of Elation* (New York, W. W. Norton & Co., 1950).

Lewin, Kurt: *A Dynamic Theory of Personality* (New York, McGraw-Hill Book Co., 1935).

Lindemann, E., and Malamud, W.: "The Neurophysiological Effects of Intoxicating Drugs," *Amer. J. Psychiat.* 13:853–879, 1007–1037 (1934).

Lief, Alfred (ed.): *The Commonsense Psychiatry of Dr. Adolf Meyer, Fifty-two Selected Papers Edited with Biographical Narrative* (New York, McGraw-Hill Book Co., 1948).

Lipton, Edgar L.: "The Amytal Interview, a Review," *Amer. Practitioner and Digest of Treatment,* Vol. I, No. 2 (1950).

Lorand, Sandor: *The Technique of Psychoanalytic Therapy* (New York, Internat. Universities Press, Inc., 1946).

Maeder, Alphonse: "Sexualitaet und epilepsie," *Jahrbuch f. Psychoanal. Forsch.* (1909).

Malamud, W.: "Psychogenic Motor Disturbances, an Analysis of Their Etiology and Manner of Development," *Arch. Neurol. & Psych.* 32:1173–1186 (1934).

Malamud, W., and Miller, W. R.: "Psychotherapy in Schizophrenics," *Amer. J. Psychiat.* 11:457–480 (1931).

Mann, James, Menzer, Doris, and Standish, C.: "Psychotherapy of Psychosis," *Psychiatry* 13:17–23 (1950).

———: "Some Observations on Individual Psychotherapy with Psychotics," *Psychiat. Quart.* 24:144–152 (1950).

Mayer-Gross, W.: "On Depersonalization," *Brit. J. M. Psychol.* 15:103 (1935).

Meduna, L. von: "Common Factors in Shock Therapies," *Dis. Nerv. System* 6:283–285 (1945).

———: *Die Konvulsiontherapie der Schizophrenie* (Halle, Carl Marbold, 1937).

Meduna, L. von, and Friedmann, E.: "The Convulsive-irritative Therapy of the Psychoses," *J. Amer. Med. Assoc.* 112:6 (1939).

———: "New Method of Medical Treatment of Schizophrenia," *Arch. Neurol. & Psych.* 35:361 (1936).

Meige, H., and Feindel, E.: *Tics and Their Treatment* (New York, William Wood & Co., 1907).

Menninger, Wm. C.: *Psychiatry in a Troubled World* (New York, The Macmillan Co., 1948).

Miller, Emmanuel (ed.): *The Neuroses of War* (New York, The Macmillan Co., 1940).

Moorhead, J.: *Traumatherapy* (Philadelphia, W. B. Saunders Co., 1931).

Moreno, J. L.: *Psychodrama* (New York, Beacon House, 1946).

Mueller, M.: "Insulin und Cardiazolschockbehandlung der Schizophrenie," *Fort. d. Neurol. u. Psych.* 9:131 (1937).

Mullahy, Patrick: *Oedipus—Myth and Complex* (New York, Hermitage Press, Inc., 1948).

Muncie, Wendell: *Psychobiology and Psychiatry; a Textbook of Normal and Abnormal Human Behavior,* Foreword by Adolf Meyer (St. Louis, The C. V. Mosby Co., 1939).

Nunberg, H.: "Ueber Depersonalizationszustaende im Lichte der Libidotheorie," *Internat. Ztschr. f. Psychoanal.* 10:17 (1924).

Oberndorf, C. P.: "Depersonalization in Relation to Erotization of Thought," *Internat. J. Psychoanal.* 15:271 (1934).

Oberndorf, C. P., Greenacre, P., and Kubie, L.: "Symposium on the Evaluation of Therapeutic Results," *Internat. J. Psychoanal.* 29:1–27 (1948).

Orenstein, L. L., and Schilder, P.: "Psychological Considerations of the Insulin Treatment in Schizophrenia," *J. Nerv. & Ment. Dis.* 88:397–644 (1938).

Orenstein, L. L., Rosenbaum, I. J., and Schilder, P.: "Application of Convulsive Therapy in Schizophrenia," *New York State J. Med.* 38:1506 (1938).

Pap, Z. von: "Erfahrungen mit der Insulinschocktherapie bei Schizophrenie," *Monatsch. f. Psychiat. u. Neurol.* 94:318 (1937).

Pavlov, Ivan Petrovich: *Conditioned Reflexes* (London, Oxford University Press, 1927).

———: *Lectures on Conditioned Reflexes* (London, Oxford University Press, 1941).

———: *Lectures on Conditioned Reflexes,* translated by W. H. Gantt (New York, Internat. Publish., 1941).

Peoples, S. A., and Guttmann, E.: *Hypertension Produced with Benzedrine Lancet* 16:1107 (1936).

Pisk, Gerhard: "Ueber die Aenderung der hysterischen Symptome in den letzen Jahren," *Wiener Kl. Woch.* 2:938–939 (1936).

———: "Ueber ein 'Zeitraffer' Phaenomen nach Insulinkoma," *Ztschr. Neurol.* 156:777 (1936).

Poetzl, Otto: "Ueber einige Wechselwirkungen hysterischer und organischer cerebraler Stoerungsmechanismen," *Jahrbuch f. Psychiat.* 37:269–373 (1917).

Poetzl, Otto, and Economo, C. von: "Der Schlaf," *Jahreskurse f. Aerztliche Fortbildung* 5:1–65 (1920).

Prinzmetal, M., and Bloomberg, W.: "The Use of Benzedrine in Narcolepsy," *J. Amer. Med. Assoc.* 105:2057 (1935).

Rado, S.: "Das Problem der Melancholie," *Ztschr. f. Psychoanal.* 13:439–455 (1927).

———: "The Psychoanalysis of Pharmacothymia" (drug addiction), *Psychoanal. Quart.* 2:1 (1933).

Rank, Otto: *The Myth and the Birth of the Hero* (New York, Nerv. & Ment. Dis. Publishing Co., 1914).

———: *The Trauma of Birth* (New York, Harcourt, Brace & Co., 1929).

———: *Will Therapy and Truth and Reality* (New York, Alfred A. Knopf, 1947).

Rank, Otto, and Ferenczi, Sandor: *The Development of Psychoanalysis* (New York, Nerv. & Ment. Dis. Publishing Co., 1925).

Rapaport, David: *Organization and Pathology of Thought* (New York, Columbia University Press, 1950).

Reich, Wilhelm: *Der triebhafte Character* (Wien, Internationaler Psychoanalytischer Verlag, 1925).

———: *The Function of the Orgasm* (New York, Orgone Institute Press, 1942).

———: *The Sexual Revolution* (New York, Orgone Institute Press, 1945).

———: *Character Analysis,* 3rd ed. (New York, Orgone Institute Press, 1949).

Reik, Theodor: *Strafbeduerfnis u. Gestaendniszwang* (Leipzig, Int. Psychoanal. Verlag, 1925).

———: *Wie man Psychologe wird* (Leipzig, Int. Psychoanal. Verlag, 1927).

———: *Ritual* (New York, Farrar, Strauss, 1946).

———: *Listening with the Third Ear* (New York, Farrar, Strauss, 1948).

Reiwald, Paul: *Society and Its Criminal* (New York, International Universities Press, Inc., 1950).

Remington, R. E.: "The Social Origin of Dietary Habits," *Scientific Monthly* 43:193–205 (1936).

Rennie, Thomas A.: *Mental Health in Modern Society* (New York, Commonwealth Fund, 1948).

Rickman, John: "A Survey: The Development of the Psychoanalytical Theory of the Psychoses, 1894–1926," *Brit. Med. Psychol.* 6:270–294; 7:94–124, 321–374 (1926).

Riese, W.: *Traumatic Neuroses as a Problem of Contemporary Medicine* (Stuttgart, Hippocrates Publishing Co., 1929).

Rosen, John N.: "Treatment of Schizophrenic Psychosis by Direct Analytic Therapy," *Psychiat. Quart.* 21:3–37 (1947).

———: "Methods of Resolving Acute Catatonic Excitement," *Psychiat. Quart.* 20:83–198 (1946).

Rosenthal, Pauline: "Death of the Leader in Group Psychotherapy," *Amer. J. Orthopsychiat.* 17:266–277 (1947).

Ross, T. A.: *An Inquiry into Prognosis in the Neuroses* (Cambridge, Eng., University Press, 1936).

———: *The Common Neuroses, Their Treatment by Psychotherapy,* 2nd. ed. (Baltimore, Md., The Williams & Wilkins Co., 1937).

Rubin, Sidney, and Bowman, Karl M.: "Electroencephalographic and Personality Correlates in Peptic Ulcer," *Psychosom. Med.* 4:309–318 (1942).

Sadger, D. J.: "Neue Studien sur Kastration," *Fortsch. der Med.* 37:1 (1920).

Sadger, I.: "Ueber Depersonalization," *Internat. Ztschr. f. Psychoanal.* 14:315 (1928).

Sakel, Manfred: "Schizophreniebehandlung mittels Insulin Hypoglykaemie sowie hypoglykaemischer Schock," *Wien. Med. Woch.* 84:11 (Nov. 3, 1934, to Feb. 9, 1935).

———: *Pharmacological Shock Therapy of Schizophrenia* (New York, Nerv. & Ment. Dis. Publishing Co., 1938).

Sargent, W., and Slater, E.: *Somatic Methods of Treatment in Psychiatry* (Baltimore, The Williams & Wilkins Co., 1946).

Saul, Leon J.: *Emotional Maturity, Development and Dynamics of Personality* (Philadelphia, J. B. Lippincott Co., 1947).

Scheid, K. F.: "Die Psychologie des erworbenen Schwachsinns," *Zentralbe. f. d. ges. Neurol. u. Psychiat.* 67:1 (1933).

Scherner, Karl Albert: *Das Leben des Traumes* (Berlin, Verlag von Heinrich Schwindler, 1861).

Schilder, Paul: *Selbstbewusstsein und Persoenlichkeitsbewusstsein* (Berlin, Springer, 1919).

———: *Introduction to Psychoanalytic Psychiatry* (New York, Nerv. & Ment. Dis. Publishing Co., 1928).

———: "The Somatic Basis of the Neuroses," *J. Nerv. & Ment. Dis.* 70:502–519 (1929).

———: "Problems in the Technique of Psychoanalysis," *Psychoanalyt. Rev.* 17:1–19 (1930).

———: *Studien zur Psychologie u. Symptomatologie der progressiven Paralyse* (Berlin, S. Karger, 1930).

———: *Brain and Personality* (New York, Nerv. & Ment. Dis. Publishing Co., 1931).

———: "Principles of Psychotherapy in Psychosis," *Psychiat. Quart.* 5:423–431 (1931).

———: *Meaning of Neurosis and Psychosis, in Psychoanalysis Today,* ed. by S. Lorand (New York, International Universities Press, 1944).

———: *The Image and Appearance of the Human Body* (London, Psych. Mono. No. 4, Kegan Paul, Trench & Trubner & Co., 1935).

———: "Psychic Disturbances after Head Injuries," *Amer. J. Psychiat.* 91:155–188 (1935).

———: "Psychophysiology of the Skin," *Arch. Neurol. & Psychiat.* 33:223–224 (1935).

———: "Psychoanalysis of Space," *Internat. J. Psychoanal.* 16:274 (1935).

———: "Psychotherapeutic Approach to Medicine," *Psychoanalyt. Rev.* 24:264–276 (1937).

———: "Health as a Psychic Experience," *Arch. Neurol. & Psychiat.* 37:1322–1337 (1937).

———: "The Psychological Implications of Motor Development in Children," *Proceedings of Fourth Institute on the Exceptional Child of the Child Research Clinic of The Woods School, Langhorne, Pa.* (Oct. 1937), pp. 38–59.

———: "The Child and the Symbol," *Scientia* (July, 1938), pp. 21–26.

———: "Psychoanalytic Remarks on 'Alice in Wonderland' and Lewis Carroll," *J. Nerv. & Ment. Dis.* 87:159–168 (1938).

———: "The Social Neurosis," *Psychoanalyt. Rev.* 25:1–19 (1938).

———: "The Psychological Effects of Benzedrine Sulphate," *J. Nerv. & Ment. Dis.* 87:384–387 (1938).

———: "The Organic Background of the Obsessions and the Compulsions," *Amer. J. Psychiat.* 94:1397–1413 (1938).

———: "Notes on the Psychology of Metrazol Treatment of Schizophrenia," *J. Nerv. & Ment. Dis.* 89:132–144 (1939).

Schilder, Paul: "The Psychology of Schizophrenia," *Psychoanalyt. Rev.* 26:380–398 (1939).

———: "The Treatment of Depersonalization," *Bull. New York Acad. Med.* 15:258–266 (1939).

———: "The Concept of Hysteria," *Amer. J. Psychiat.* 95:1389–1409 (1939).

———: "Mental Hygiene of the Medical Student," *Medical Bulletin of the Student Association of the New York University College of Medicine* 4:68–70 (1939).

———: "Neurosis Following Head and Brain Injuries," Chapter 12, in *Injuries of the Skull, Brain and Spinal Cord,* ed. by Samuel Brock (Baltimore, The Williams & Wilkins Co., 1940).

———: "Influence of Psychoanalysis on Psychiatry," *Psychoanalyt. Quart.* 9:216–228 (1940).

———: "The Structure of Obsession and Compulsion," *Psychiatry* 3:549–560 (1940).

———: "Introductory Remarks on the Group," *J. Social Psychol.* 12:83–100 (1940).

———: "The Cure of the Criminal and the Prevention of Crime," *J. Clin. Psychopath.* 2:146–161 (1940).

———: "Psychiatric Aspects of Old Age and Aging," *Amer. J. Orthopsychiat.* 10:62–69 (1940).

———: "Types of Anxiety Neuroses," *Internat. J. Psychoanal.* 22:193–208 (1941).

———: "The Psychogenesis of Alcoholism," *Quart. J. Alcohol* 2:277–293 (1941).

———: "Success and Failure," *Psychoanalyt. Rev.* 29:353–372 (1942).

———: "The Body Image in Dreams," *Psychoanalyt. Rev.* 29:113–126 (1942).

———: "*Goals and Desires of Man, a Psychological Survey of Life* (New York, Columbia University Press, 1942).

———: *Mind: Perception and Thought in Their Constructive Aspects* (New York, Columbia University Press, 1942).

Schilder, Paul, and Kauders, Otto: *Hypnosis* (New York, Nerv. & Ment. Dis. Publishing Co., 1927).

Schilder, Paul, and Wechsler, David: "The Attitudes of Children toward Death," *J. Genetic Psychol.* 45:406–451 (1934).

———: "What Do Children Know of the Interior of Their Bodies?" *Internat. J. Psychoanal.* 16:355 (1935).

Schmideberg, Melitta: "The Treatment of Criminals," *Psychoanalyt. Rev.* 36:403–410 (1949).

Schnyder, P.: "Commotio cerebri post-concussion Neurosis und Stoerung der Sexualfunktion," *Schweiz. Med. Woch.* 17:242 (1936).

Schwarz, Oswald: "Das psycho-physische Problem in d. Sexualpathol.," *Wien. Klin. Woch.* 11 (1922).

———: *Psychogenese u. Psychotherapie koerperlicher Symptome* (Vienna, Springer, 1925).

———: *Ueber Homosexualitaet* (Leipzig, Thieme, 1931).

Seguin, C. Alberto: *Introduction to Psychosomatic Medicine* (New York, Internat. Universities Press, 1950).

Selinski, Herman: "The Selective Use of Electro-shock Therapy as an Adjuvant to Psychotherapy," *Bull. New York Acad. Med.* 19:245–252 (1943).

Sharpe, Freeman Ella: *Dream Analysis* (London, Internat. Psychoanal. Publishing Co., 1937).

Sherif, M., and Cantril, H.: *The Psychology of Ego-Involvements* (New York, Wiley, 1947).

Simon, H.: "Arbeitstherapie in der Irrenanstalt und ihre moderne Ausgestaltung," *Allg. Ztschr. f. Psychiat.* 86:466 (1927).

———: "Psychotherapie in der Irrenanstalt," *Bericht ueber den 2 Allg. Aerztl. Kongr. f. Psychotherapie* (Leipzig, S. Hirzel, 1927).

Slavson, S. R.: *Introduction to Group Therapy* (New York, Commonwealth Fund, 1943).

——— (ed.): *The Practice of Group Therapy* (New York, Internat. Universities Press, Inc., 1947).

Staercke, Johan: "Neuere Traumexperimente im Zusammenhang mit spaeteren und neueren Traumtheorien," *Jahr. f. Psychoanal. u. Psychopath. Forsch.* 5:233–307 (1913).

Stekel, W.: *Conditions of Nervous Anxiety and Their Treatment* (New York, Dodd, Mead & Co., 1923).

———: *Techniques of Analytic Psychotherapy* (New York, W. W. Norton & Co., 1940).

Stengel, Erwin: "On the Disturbances of the Instincts and the Defense Reactions of the Ego in Brain Disease," *Internat. Ztschr. f. Psychoanal.* 21:544–560 (1935).

Stephen, Karen: *Psychoanalysis and Medicine* (New York, The Macmillan Co., 1933).

Stern, Robert: "Ueber die Aufhellung der Amnesien bei pathologischen

Rauschzustaenden," *Ztschr. f. d. ges. Neurol. & Psychiat.* 108:4, 601–624 (1927).

Stierlin: "Psychische Stoerungen nach der Katastrophe von Courrieres," *Deutsche Med. Woch.* (1911).

Storch, Alfred: *The Primitive Archaic Forms of Inner Experiences and Thoughts in Schizophrenia* (Washington and New York, Nerv. & Ment. Dis. Publishing Co., 1924).

Strauss, Hans: "Clinical and Electroencephalogram Studies," *Amer. J. Psychiat.* 101:42–50 (1944).

Strauss, I., and Savitzky, N.: "The Sequelae of Head Injuries," *New York State J. Med.* 37:13 (1937).

Strecker, E. A., Appel, K. E., Palmer, H. D., and Braceland, F. J.: "Psychiatric Studies in Medical Education," *Amer. J. Psychiat.* 92:937–957 (1936); 93:1197–1229 (1937).

Sullivan, Harry S.: "Modified Psychoanalytic Treatment of Schizophrenia," *Amer. J. Psychiat.* 10:977–991 (1930–1931).

———: *Conceptions of Modern Psychiatry* (Washington, William A. White Psychiatric Foundation, 1947).

Szondi, L.: "Der Neurotiker im Lichte der psychoanalytischen, Neuroendokrinen und erbpathologischen Forschungen," *Schweizer Arch. f. Neurol. u. Psychiat.* 155:758–783 (1936).

Tanner, H.: "Physiological and Psychological Factors in Electric Shock Treatment as Criteria in Therapy," *J. Nerv. & Ment. Dis.* 111:232–238 (1950).

Teicher, Joseph D.: "The Preliminary Survey of Motility in Children," *J. Nerv. & Ment. Dis.* 94:277–304 (1941).

Thomas, Giles W.: "Group Psychotherapy; a Review of the Recent Literature," *Psychosom. Med.* 5:166 (1943).

Thompson, Clara: *Psychoanalysis, Evolution and Development* (New York, Hermitage House, Inc., 1950).

Tulchin, S. H.: *Intelligence in Crime* (Chicago, University of Chicago Press, 1939).

Waelder, R.: "Schizophrenia and Creative Thinking," *Internat. J. Psychoanal.* 7:366–376 (1926).

Weber, Ernst: *Der Einfluss psychischer Vorgaenge auf den Koerper, insbesondere auf die Blutverteilung* (Berlin, Springer, 1910).

Wechsler, David: *The Range of Human Capacities* (Baltimore, The Williams and Wilkins Co., 1935).

Weiss, Edward, and English, O. Spurgeon: *Psychosomatic Medicine, the*

Clinical Application of Psychopathology to General Medical Problems (Philadelphia and London, W. B. Saunders, 1943).

Wender, Louis: "The Dynamics of Group Psychotherapy and Its Application," *J. Nerv. & Ment. Dis.* 84:1 (1936).

Wertham, Frederic: "Progress in Psychiatry," *Arch. Neurol. & Psychiat.* 24:150–160 (1930).

Wetterstrand, Otto Georg: *Hypnotism and Its Application to Practical Medicine* (New York, Putnam, 1897).

———: "Ueber den kuenstlich verlaengerten Schlaf besonders bei der Behandlung der Hysterie," *Ztschr. f. Hypnotismus* (1892).

Wilder, J.: "Aenderung in den Manifestationen der Hysterie in Deutschland und Oesterreich in den letzen Jahren," *G. di Clinica Medica* 7:239–248 (1930).

Wilson, S. A. Kinnier: *Neurology* (ed. by Bruce A. Ninian), Vol. I (Baltimore, William & Wilkins Co., 1940).

Wilson, S. A. Kinnier, and Cottrell, Samuel Smith: "The Affective Symptomatology of Disseminated Sclerosis," *J. Neurol. Psychopath.* 7:1–30 (1926).

Wilson, G. W.: "Report of a Case of Acute Laryngitis Occurring as a Conversion Symptom during Analysis," *Psychoanalyt. Rev.* 21:408–414 (1934).

———: "The Analysis of a Transitory Conversion Symptom Stimulating Pertussis," *Internat. J. Psychoanal.* 16:474–480 (1935).

Wiss, M. H.: "Vegetative Reactionen bei psychischen Vorgaengen," *Schweiz. Arch. f. Neurol. u. Psychia.* 19:3–41 (1926).

Witt, G. F., and Cheavens, T. J.: "Prolonged Barbital Narcosis in the Treatment of the Acute Psychosis," *South. Med. J.* 29:574 (1936).

Wittels, Fritz: *Freud and His Time* (New York, Liveright, 1931).

Wolberg, Lewis R.: *Medical Hypnosis* (New York, Grune & Stratton, 1948).

Wolf, Alexander: "The Psychoanalysis of Groups," *Amer. J. Psychother.* 3:525–558 (1949); 4:16–50 (1950).

Wortis, Joseph: "On the Response of Schizophrenic Subjects to Hypoglycemic Shock," *J. Nerv. & Ment. Dis.* 84:497 (1936).

———: "Sakel's Hypoglycemic Insulin Treatment of Psychosis, History and Present Status," *J. Nerv. & Ment. Dis.* 85:581 (1937).

———: "Experiences at Bellevue Hospital with Hypoglycemic Treatment of Schizophrenia," *J. Nerv. & Ment. Dis.* 85:561 (1937).

Wortis, Joseph, Bowman, Karl M., and Orenstein, Leo I.: "Further Experiences at Bellevue Hospital with Hypoglycemic Treatment of Schizophrenia," *Amer. J. Psychiat.* 94:153–158 (1937).

Wulff, M.: "Ueber den hysterischen Anfall," *Internat. Ztschr. f. Psychoanal.* 19:584–612 (1933).

Wundt, Wilhelm: *Grundzuege der physiologischin Psychologie,* 3 vols. (Leipzig, W. Englemann, 1902–8).

Zilboorg, G.: "Affective Reintegration in Schizophrenias," *Arch. Neurol. & Psychiat.* 24:335–347 (1930).

———: "Deeper Layers of Schizophrenic Psychoses," *Amer. J. Psychiat.* 11:493–511 (1931).

INDEX